Concise Clinical Oncology

Dedicated to
Rhonwen, Carys, Mum, Dad and Derek

For Elsevier

Senior Commissioning Editor: Heidi Harrison
Development Editor: Catherine Jackson
Project Manager: Joannah Duncan
Designer: George Ajayi
Illustration Manager: Bruce Hogarth

Concise Clinical Oncology

Clive Peedell BM MRCP FRCR

Consultant in Clinical Oncology,
James Cook University Hospital, Middlesbrough

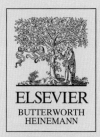

ELSEVIER
BUTTERWORTH
HEINEMANN

EDINBURGH LONDON NEW YORK OXFORD PHILADELPHIA ST LOUIS
SYDNEY TORONTO 2005

ELSEVIER
BUTTERWORTH
HEINEMANN

First published 2005

ISBN 0 7506 8836 X

British Library Cataloguing in Publication Data
A catalogue record for this book is available from the British Library

Library of Congress Cataloging in Publication Data
A catalog record for this book is available from the Library of Congress

your source for books,
journals and multimedia
in the health sciences

www.elsevierhealth.com

The
Publisher's
policy is to use
**paper manufactured
from sustainable forests**

Printed in China

Contents

Contributors

Andrew John Ashcroft MA MB BChir MRCP MRCPath
Research Fellow, Academic Unit of Haematology and Oncology, University of Leeds, Leeds, UK

Lisa J. Barker MB ChB BSc
Specialist Registrar in Histopathology, Department of Histopathology, Leeds General Infirmary, Leeds, UK

Rhidian Bramley BSc(Hons) MBChB MRCP FRCR
Consultant Radiologist, Department of Radiology, Christie Hospital NHS Trust, Withington, Manchester, UK

Suzanne Kite MA MRCP
Consultant in Palliative Medicine, Leeds General Infirmary and Cookridge Hospitals, Leeds Teaching Hospitals Trust, Leeds, UK

Richard Milton MB ChB FRCSEd
Specialist Registrar, Department of Cardiothoracic Surgery, Leeds General Infirmary, Leeds, UK

D.P.H. Stark MB BChir MRCP PhD
Senior Lecturer in Cancer Medicine at the University of Leeds, and Honorary Consultant in Medical Oncology at Bradford Teaching Hospital and Leeds Teaching Hospital NHS Trusts, Leeds, UK

Preface

Cancer will affect one in two of the population by the year 2015 and large amounts of money are currently being invested in improving and reorganising UK cancer services. Most healthcare professionals will at some point be involved in the management of cancer patients. In spite of this, oncology has traditionally had a low profile when it comes to medical education.

During my training as a clinical oncologist, I found it a time-consuming and often frustrating exercise trying to extract useful information relevant to UK oncological practice from the huge body of cancer literature. This made me realise how difficult it would be for medical students, junior doctors, nurses and other busy healthcare professionals to grasp a full understanding of the principles and practice of modern oncology. I therefore decided to write a concise textbook on clinical oncology with the aim of condensing a large amount of cancer information into an easily accessible and readable form that was relevant to everyday UK practice.

The book is divided into three main parts:

The first part is concerned with general principles of oncology and covers the basic biology and pathology of cancer, as well as the main investigation and treatment modalities, and principles of palliative and supportive care. The roles of screening and clinical trials are also discussed.

The second part deals with the individual types of cancer, and for the sake of quick and easy reference, these are listed in alphabetical order. The background information section of each chapter covers epidemiology, aetiology, pathology and overall prognosis. Other sections then cover diagnosis, staging, clinical presentation, management and future perspectives. The final section of each chapter describes the typical problems encountered in advanced disease and offers practical advice on managing these problems.

The third part is concerned with complications of cancer and oncological emergencies. Background information, diagnosis, management and prognosis are discussed.

The appendix provides information about radiation tolerances of normal tissues, chemotherapy drugs, useful websites and definitions of performance status.

In order to keep the book as concise as possible, I have only included figures and photographs where I felt they would make a significant contribution to the understanding of the text. The style of writing aims to pack as much information in as possible whilst still being very readable. The chapters on the more common cancers are purposely longer and more detailed than the less common cancers. I have very much concentrated on UK oncology practice and included the up-to-date National Institute for Clinical Excellence (NICE) recommendations for the relevant cancer sites. In addition, information on cancer incidence and mortality is from UK sources such as Cancer Research UK and the Office for National Statistics.

The book is mainly aimed at medical students, junior doctors in both medical and surgical specialties, palliative care doctors, GPs, oncology trainees in their first few years of training, nursing staff, radiographers and other healthcare professionals involved in managing cancer patients. It will also be useful for oncology consultants who need a very brief refresher course in the cancer sites they no longer specialise in.

I hope this book will be very educational, informative and fun to read. Most importantly I hope it gives the reader an accurate overview of the modern management of cancer in the UK without needing to spend hours in the library!

Clive Peedell, 2005

Acknowledgements

I would first of all like to thank all of the contributors to the book, as well as the staff at Elsevier for their helpful advice in the preparation of the manuscript.

I would also like to acknowledge the help of the following consultant oncologists who offered invaluable expert advice, suggestions and feedback:

Dr David Bottomley, Dr John Chester, Dr Mehmet Zen, Dr Jane Orton, Dr Adrian Crellin, Dr David Sebag-Montefiore, Dr Georg Gerrard, Mr Ian Rothwell, Mr J. A. C Thorpe, Dr Mike Snee, Dr David Dodwell, Dr Geoff Hall, Professor Gareth Morgan, Dr Sri Kumar, Dr Fiona Roberts, Dr Di Gilson, Dr Dan Ash, Dr Roger Taylor, Dr Anne Kiltie, Dr Alan Anthony and Dr Catherine Coyle.

I am grateful to many work colleagues and medical students for useful feedback information to make the book more readable and informative. In particular, thanks to Jane Garrud for help and ideas with the medical illustrations.

Special thanks to Dr Peter Kaye, who inspired me to write the book and to Dr L. W. Blazewicz who inspired me to study medicine.

Most of all, I would like to thank three people. Firstly, my wonderful wife who put up with me constantly writing and updating the book over the last five years. Her help and support have been immeasurable and I hope she can cope with the second edition! Secondly, Dr Rhidian Bramley for his continued support, advice, information technology expertise and suggestions throughout this project, as well as his chapter on Principles of Radiology. Finally, I would like to thank my mum for her dogged persistence in making sure that I received a good education, despite never having the same educational opportunities of her own.

Abbreviations

AA	Anaplastic astrocytoma
AFP	Alpha-fetoprotein
ALL	Acute lymphoblastic leukaemia
AML	Acute myeloblastic leukaemia
APC	Adenomatous polyposis coli
ARDS	Adult respiratory distress syndrome
ASCT	Autologous stem cell transplant
ATRA	All-*trans*-retinoic-acid
BCC	Basal cell carcinoma
BCG	Bacille Calmette – Guérin
BMT	Bone marrow transplant
BSA	Body surface area
CD	Cluster designation
CEA	Carcinoembryonic antigen
CHART	Continuous hyper-fractionated accelerated radiotherapy
CIS	Carcinoma in situ
CLL	Chronic lymphocytic leukaemia
CML	Chronic myeloid leukaemia
CNS	Central nervous system
CRM	Circumferential resection margin
CRP	C-reactive protein
CRT	Conformal radiotherapy
CSF	Cerebrospinal fluid
CT	Computed tomography
CTV	Clinical target volume
CUP	Cancer unknown primary site
CXR	Chest X-ray
DCC	Deleted in colorectal cancer
DIC	Disseminated intravascular coagulation
DRE	Digital rectal examination

EBRT	External beam radiotherapy
EPP	Extrapleural pneumonectomy
ERCP	Endoscopic retrograde cholangiopancreatography
ESR	Erythrocyte sedimentation rate
EUA	Examination under anaesthesia
EUS	Endoscopic ultrasound
FAB	French-American-British
FAP	Familial adenomatous polyposis
FBC	Full blood count
FFP	Fresh frozen plasma
FIGO	International Federation of Gynecology and Obstetrics
FNA(C)	Fine needle aspiration (cytology)
FOB	Faecal occult blood
5FU	5-Fluorouracil
GBM	Glioblastoma multiforme
GCT	Germ cell tumour
GTV	Gross tumour volume
HAI	Hepatic arterial infusion
HBV	Hepatitis B virus
HCC	Hepatocellular carcinoma
β-HCG	Human chorionic gonadotrophin
HCV	Hepatitis C virus
HNPCC	Hereditary non-polyposis colorectal cancer
HPOA	Hypertrophic pulmonary osteoarthropathy
HPV	Human papilloma virus
HRCT	High resolution computed tomography
HRPC	Hormone relapsed prostate cancer

HRT	Hormone replacement therapy	NSCLC	Non-small cell lung cancer
HSA	Human serum albumin	NGT	Nasogastric tube
ICP	Intracranial pressure	OCP	Oral contraceptive pill
IFN	Interferon	OLT	Orthotopic liver transplantation
IHC	Immunohistochemistry		
IL-2	Interleukin 2	PBSCT	Peripheral blood stem cell transplant
ILT	Intraluminal therapy	PCP	*Pneumocystis carinii* pneumonia
IMRT	Intensity modulated radiotherapy		
IORT	Intraoperative radiotherapy	PCR	Polymerase chain reaction
		PEG	Percutaneous endoscopic gastrostomy
ITGCN	Intratubular germ cell neoplasia		
		PEI	Percutaneous ethanol injection
kV	Kilovolts	PEL	Primary effusion lymphoma
		PET	Positron emission tomography
LDH	Lactate dehydrogenase		
LHRH	Luteinising hormone releasing hormone	PNET	Primitive neuroectodermal tumour
		PNS	Peripheral nervous system
MDR	Multidrug resistance	PS	Performance status
MDS	Myelodysplastic syndrome	PSA	Prostate specific antigen
MEN	Multiple endocrine neoplasia	PSC	Primary sclerosing cholangitis
MeV	Mega electronvolt	PTC	Percutaneous transhepatic cholangiography
MFH	Malignant fibrous histiocytoma		
		PTH	Parathyroid hormone
MGUS	Monoclonal gammopathy of uncertain significance	PTHrP	Parathyroid hormone related protein
MIBG	Meta-iodobenzylguanidine	PTV	Planning target volume
MLC	Multileaf collimator		
MM	Multiple myeloma	RAI	Radioactive iodine
MRC	Medical Research Council	Rb	Retinoblastoma
MRCP	Magnetic resonance cholangiopancreatography	RFA	Radiofrequency ablation
		RT	Radiotherapy
MRI	Magnetic resonance imaging		
		SCLC	Small cell lung cancer
MV	Megavolt	SCC	Squamous cell carcinoma
		SIADH	Syndrome of inappropriate antidiuretic hormone
NAP	Neutrophil alkaline phosphatase		
		SOL	Space-occupying lesion
NET	Neuroendocrine tumour	SRS	Somatostatin receptor scintigraphy
NHL	Non-Hodgkin's lymphoma		
NSAID	Non-steroidal anti-inflammatory drug		
NSGCT	Non-seminomatous germ cell tumour	TENS	Transcutaneous electrical nerve stimulation

TSET	Total skin electron therapy
TNF	Tumour necrosis factor
TURBT	Transurethral resection of bladder tumour
TVUS	Transvaginal ultrasound
VAIN	Vaginal intraepithelial neoplasia
VATS	Video-assisted thoracoscopic surgery
VEGF	Vascular endothelial growth factor
WBRT	Whole brain radiotherapy

Dosage abbreviations

b.d.	twice a day
IM	intramuscular(ly)
IV	intravenous(ly)
o.d.	once a day
p.o.	by mouth
PR	per rectum
p.r.n.	as required
q.d.s.	four times a day
s.c.	subcutaneous(ly)
t.d.s.	three times a day

SECTION ONE

Principles of oncology

CHAPTER 1

Introduction – the cancer problem

INTRODUCTION

Cancer is a major public health problem with significant associated morbidity and mortality. In 2000, there were over 270 000 newly diagnosed cancers (excluding non-melanoma skin cancer) registered in the UK (Table 1.1). The lifetime risk of developing cancer is now more than one in three and by 2015 this is expected to rise to one in two. There are over 200 different types of

TABLE 1.1 UK cancer incidence 2000: cancers that contribute 1% or more to the total cancer burden	
Type	Number (%)
Breast	40 710 (15)
Lung	38 410 (14)
Large bowel	35 300 (13)
Prostate	27 150 (10)
Bladder	11 080 (4)
Stomach	9 660 (4)
NHL	9 190 (3)
Head and neck	7 950 (3)
Oesophagus	7 360 (3)
Pancreas	7 090 (3)
Malignant melanoma	6 970 (3)
Leukaemia	6 800 (3)
Ovary	6 730 (2)
Kidney	6 200 (2)
Uterus	5 620 (2)
CNS	4 660 (2)
Myeloma	3 730 (1)
Cervix	2 990 (1)
Liver	2 620 (1)
Testicular	2 010 (1)
Others	28 200 (10)
Total (excludes non-melanoma skin cancer)	270 430 (100)

cancer, but four cancers account for more than half of all cases. These are lung cancer, breast cancer, prostate cancer and large bowel cancer. The disease predominantly affects the elderly population with approximately 65% of cancers diagnosed in patients over the age of 65 years. The ageing population only partially explains why the overall incidence of cancer is rising.

In 2002, there were 155 180 deaths from cancer, representing over a quarter of all deaths in the UK (Table 1.2). Over one-fifth (22%) of cancer deaths were from lung cancer, with a further quarter (24%) from cancers of the bowel, breast and prostate. A third of all cancer deaths are linked to cigarette smoking. It is estimated that a quarter of the UK population smoke.

The modern practice of oncology requires a multidisciplinary integrated approach involving the specialties of general practice, radiology, medicine, surgery/surgical oncology, medical oncology, radiotherapy, palliative care, nursing care, pain management teams, public health, and social and psychological/psychiatric services. New advances in the science of oncology and cancer research are increasing our understanding of cancer. This has enabled the development of new anti-cancer agents as well as improvements in diagnostic methods, screening programmes, radiotherapy delivery systems, surgical techniques, and supportive/palliative care. These advances are now leading to improved outcomes for many cancer patients and overall

TABLE 1.2 UK cancer mortality 2002: cancers that contribute 1% or more to total cancer mortality

Type	Number (%)
Lung	33 600 (22)
Large bowel	16 220 (10)
Breast	12 930 (8)
Prostate	9 940 (6)
Oesophagus	7 250 (5)
Pancreas	6 360 (4)
Stomach	6 450 (4)
Bladder	4 910 (3)
NHL	4 750 (3)
Ovary	4 690 (3)
Leukaemia	4 310 (3)
CNS	3 370 (2)
Kidney	3 360 (2)
Head and neck	3 000 (2)
Myeloma	2 600 (2)
Liver	2 510 (2)
Mesothelioma	1 760 (1)
Melanoma	1 640 (1)
Cervix	1 120 (1)
Uterus	1 070 (1)
Others	22 910 (15)
Total	155 180 (100%)

mortality rates are falling. However, despite these advances, prevention rather than cure of cancer is currently the most likely way to reduce the cancer burden. Therefore, the importance of public health programmes aimed at reducing smoking and obesity levels, reducing viral infection transmission rates (e.g. HPV, HBV, EBV, HIV), screening of cancer, and improving public education on other risk factors for cancer cannot be overestimated. In addition, people from lower socioeconomic groups are more likely to get certain cancer types (e.g. lung cancer) and are more likely to die from cancer once they develop it. Therefore, tackling socioeconomic inequality is also an important way to reduce the cancer burden.

Cancer survival rates in the UK have been poor in comparison to other European countries mainly due to chronic underinvestment in NHS infrastructure. Fortunately, cancer has now become a government priority and this has led to the development and publication of the Calman Hine report in 1995 and the NHS cancer plan in September 2000. These documents form the cornerstones of the national service framework (NSF) for cancer.

THE CALMAN HINE REPORT

An Expert Advisory Group on Cancer (EAGC) was established by the Chief Medical Officers for England and Wales. Amongst its priorities was to prepare a policy framework for commissioning cancer services, which was published in April 1995 – the 'Calman Hine report'. The general aim of this framework is to create a network of care in England and Wales that will enable a patient wherever he or she lives to be sure that treatment and care is of a uniformly high standard.

Three levels of care are proposed:

1. Primary care   This is seen as the focus of care. Detailed discussions between Primary Care Teams, Cancer Units and Cancer Centres will be necessary to clarify local guidelines for the identification and management of malignancies, what constitutes best care, the establishment of local referral patterns, effective communication and discharge information.

2. Designated Cancer Units   These should be created in many district general hospitals to manage the more common cancers, such as breast, lung and colorectal malignancies. Involvement of the multidisciplinary team in the care of cancer patients is important and nursing care for patients must be planned and led by specialist oncology nurses. Nursing expertise must also be available for cytotoxic chemotherapy administration, site-specific expertise e.g. breast care, and also for counselling and symptom control. Each Cancer Unit has to appoint a lead clinician who organises and coordinates the whole range of cancer services provided. Cancer Units are identified as playing an important role in education and research.

3. Designated Cancer Centres These should provide expertise in the management of all cancers, including common cancers within their immediate geographical locality and less common cancers by referral from Cancer Units. They will provide specialist diagnostic and therapeutic techniques including a full range of radiotherapy services, medical oncology including intensive chemotherapy, bone marrow transplantation and peripheral blood stem cell support, paediatric and adolescent cancer services and specialist surgical services including plastic and reconstructive surgery.

The Cancer Centres would work in close collaboration with the Cancer Units. Cancer Centres are also identified as being centres that will be involved in education and research, playing a focal role for coordinating clinical trials.

Furthermore, all cancers must now be seen in outpatients within 2 weeks of referral. Another important aspect is the involvement of palliative care early in the course of the patient's disease. Palliative care should not be associated exclusively with terminal care.

NHS CANCER PLAN

The four main aims of the NHS cancer plan are:

1. To save more lives
2. To ensure patients receive the right professional support and care as well as the best treatments
3. To tackle health inequalities between different social groups
4. To build for the future with increased investment in the cancer workforce, research, and facilities.

The government hopes to achieve these aims in the following ways:

1. Reducing cancer risk by reducing smoking and improving diet.
2. Detecting cancer earlier by raising public awareness, extending cancer screening programmes for breast and cervical cancer. The roles of screening in colorectal, prostate cancer and ovarian cancer are being researched.
3. Improving community care.
4. Faster access to treatment by introducing targets to reduce waiting time at all stages of the pathway of care.
5. Investment in staff and equipment and redesigning services.
6. Ending the 'postcode lottery'. The National Institute for Clinical Excellence (NICE) will publish guidance on the use of new cancer treatments and the organisation of services. Standards will be assessed by the Commission for Health Improvement (CHIMP).
7. Investment in support services, hospices and palliative care.
8. Investment in research and the development of the new National Cancer Research Institute (NCRI).

The challenge faced by the NHS is formidable, but with increased organisation of cancer services due to the national service framework (NSF) for cancer, progress is already being made. With technological advances and the unravelling of the molecular mechanisms of cancer, the next few decades will be interesting and exciting for oncology and will hopefully result in improved quality of life and survival for patients with cancer.

FURTHER READING

The Calman Hine report and the NHS cancer plan can be downloaded from the Department of Health websites: www.doh.gov.uk/pub/docs/doh/cancerfr.pdf and www.doh.gov.uk/cancer respectively.

CHAPTER 2

Basic cancer biology

Clive Peedell and D.P.H. Stark

WHAT IS CANCER?

Cancer includes many related diseases that are characterised by the uncontrolled growth and spread of abnormal cells.

THE MOLECULAR GENETIC BASIS OF CANCER

Recent advances in molecular biology and genetics have greatly increased the understanding of the malignant process.

Cancer results from mutations affecting genes that regulate cell growth and division and is therefore a 'genetic' disease. However, these mutations are predominantly acquired and only rarely inherited. Out of the 30 000 or so genes within the human genome, there are only a small number that are particularly important in the development of cancer. Mutations of these important genes lead to uncontrolled cell growth and proliferation, with further mutations leading to invasive properties and spread. Many of these genes have been identified. They may result in a cancer by excessive function, malfunction or non-function and can be classified into three broad categories:

- oncogenes
- tumour suppressor genes
- DNA repair genes.

To understand these genes it is necessary to review normal cell growth and its control.

NORMAL CELL GROWTH AND THE CELL CYCLE

For tissues to grow, renew, repair and function normally, a careful balance between proliferation of cells, differentiation of cells and cell loss is needed. Control of the cell cycle is pivotal to achieving this balance and dysregulation of this key process is a fundamental feature of cancer.

All dividing cells pass through the cell cycle (Fig. 2.1), which is divided into distinct phases:

G1-phase – gap phase. Enzymes necessary for DNA synthesis are produced.
S-phase – synthesis of DNA leads to doubling of the total amount (DNA is replicated).
G2-phase – second gap period. Specialised proteins and RNA are synthesised.
M-phase – mitosis stage, when cell division occurs. The four main stages are prophase, metaphase, anaphase and telophase.
G0-phase – resting phase. The cell is not committed to division, but certain stimuli such as local growth factors can stimulate the cell into the cell cycle.

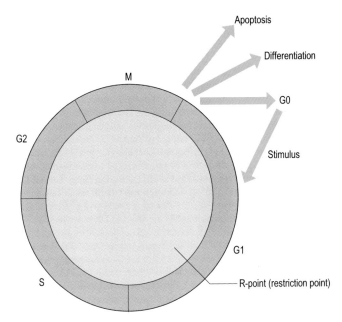

FIGURE 2.1 The cell cycle.

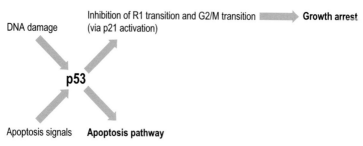

FIGURE 2.2 Role of p53 in cell cycle arrest and apoptosis.

Progression through each of the four distinct phases (G1, S, G2 and M) is carefully regulated by multiple components, which control transition between the stages at various checkpoints through the cycle (e.g. the restriction point (Fig. 2.1)). Regulation allows DNA replication and cell division to be coordinated, and cells to protect against DNA damage. The presence of DNA damage will normally prevent passage through the main checkpoints of the cell cycle, leading to 'cell cycle arrest'. Arrest of the cell cycle allows minor DNA damage to be repaired prior to replication, or if damage is more severe, cells die a programmed death, called apoptosis. Thus, DNA damage/mutations are prevented from being passed on to daughter cells (Fig. 2.2).

Control of the cell cycle and apoptosis are central to the development of cancer. The mechanisms and pathways controlling these processes are increasingly understood to be complex, but several principal pathways have been defined. One important group of proteins involved in these pathways are the cyclins. They regulate the transition from one stage of the cell cycle to the next at the checkpoints. They bring about control by regulating cyclin-dependent kinases (CDKs). One important checkpoint controls the transition from the G1-phase to S-phase, which commits the cell to divide. It is controlled by a complex between a nuclear transcription factor E2F, and the retinoblastoma protein (pRb). When E2F is bound to pRb it is inactive. When a CDK-cyclin phosphorylates the pRb–E2F complex, active E2F is released, which then activates expression of genes involved in DNA replication. This process can be inhibited by proteins such as p53 and CDK inhibitors or enhanced by mitogenic signals such as growth factors (Fig. 2.3). The other main checkpoint is between the G2- and M-phases. Failure of the checkpoints to control the cell cycle leads to excessive cell proliferation. Genomic instability also increases as damaged DNA is replicated in daughter cells.

The genes involved in regulating these crucial processes, which have been identified as integral to the development of cancer, are called oncogenes, tumour suppressor genes and DNA repair genes and are discussed below.

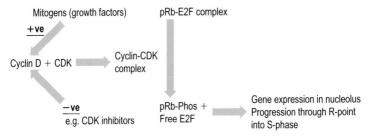

FIGURE 2.3 Transition through the R-point.

ONCOGENES

Oncogenes are hyperfunctional forms of normal genes called proto-oncogenes. The protein products of proto-oncogenes normally help to regulate cellular functions such as proliferation, differentiation and apoptosis. They include growth factors, growth factor receptors, intracellular cell signalling proteins, anti-apoptosis proteins and nuclear transcription proteins. When a proto-oncogene becomes abnormal to form an oncogene, overproduction leads to dysregulation of normal cell growth, increased proliferation, loss of apoptosis and potential transformation to a malignant state. Over one hundred oncogenes are now recognised (see Table 2.1 for some examples).

Several mechanisms have been identified whereby proto-oncogenes may become oncogenes:

1. Point mutations. A single DNA base pair mutation may result in the production of a hyperfunctioning protein (e.g. *Ras* G protein).
2. Chromosomal rearrangements. A chromosomal 'translocation' may result in a proto-oncogene being relocated to a part of the genome controlled by an active promoter nearby, causing excessive expression. Translocation may also result in the production of fusion genes with fusion protein products that are hyperfunctional. For example, in chronic myeloid leukaemia (CML), the t(9;22) translocation produces the Philadelphia chromosome, resulting in the bcr-abl fusion gene/protein that functions as an overactive cell signalling tyrosine kinase, stimulating cell division.
3. Gene amplifications. Multiple copies of a proto-oncogene lead to excessive production of the protein product. For example, in small cell lung cancer *L-myc* and *C-myc* are amplified, leading to excessive activation of genes involved in cell proliferation.
4. Viral insertional mutagenesis. Insertion of viral genes may cause activation of proto-oncogenes.

TABLE 2.1 Oncogenes and their products

Oncogenes and oncogene products	Function
Growth factors: platelet derived growth factor (PDGF) (v-sis) epidermal growth factor (EGF)	Stimulate cell division after binding to growth factor receptor
Growth factor receptors: e.g. epidermal growth factor receptor family, e.g. c-erb-B2	Persistent activation of growth factor receptors leads to continuous mitogenic signalling. Trastuzumab (Herceptin) is a monoclonal antibody drug that blocks the c-erb-B2 receptor
G proteins: H-ras, K-ras, N-ras oncogenes	Membrane associated proteins that stimulate intracellular signalling cascade leading to gene activation. Overexpression leads to increased cell proliferation
Cytoplasmic tyrosine kinase family: includes bcr-abl oncogene product that is found in chronic myeloid leukaemia (c.f. Philadelphia chromosome)	This large group of proteins is involved in intracellular cell signalling cascades
Cell cycle regulator proteins: e.g. cyclin D, cyclin-dependent kinases	Key proteins involved in the control of the cell cycle
Nuclear transcription proteins: e.g. C-myc, N-myc oncogenes	Bind to DNA to activate genes involved in cell proliferation
Anti-apoptosis proteins: e.g. bcl-2	Overexpression of bcl-2 disrupts normal apoptosis (programmed cell death) process

TUMOUR SUPPRESSOR GENES

The normal function of tumour suppressor genes (TSGs) is to prevent abnormal cellular proliferation and genetic instability. The protein products of TSGs are thus involved in a variety of cellular functions such as cell cycle control, checkpoint control, cell signalling, promotion of apoptosis and DNA repair (see Table 2.2 for some examples). Inactivation or loss of these genes by mutation or deletion will lead to loss of function, reducing restrictions on cell growth and division, causing genetic instability and loss of apoptosis, thereby increasing the likelihood of malignant behaviour.

These genes normally act recessively, i.e. both copies of the gene (alleles) must be mutated to produce loss of function. Patients who inherit a germline mutation in one of the copies of a TSG often have a syndrome with a predisposition to cancer. For example, Li–Fraumeni syndrome results from a germline mutation of the p53 gene. This greatly increases the lifetime risk of cancer (usually breast, brain, lung, sarcomas and leukaemia), with many developing multiple cancers. There is a case report of a patient with Li–Fraumeni syndrome developing 17 different malignancies!

TABLE 2.2 Examples of tumour suppressor genes (TSGs) and their products

Tumour suppressor gene	Function of TSG product	Clinical example
p53	Involved in arrest of the cell cycle, apoptosis, and DNA repair pathways	Seen in most human cancers and the most commonly mutated gene in human cancer. Li–Fraumeni syndrome is due to an inherited defect in p53
Retinoblastoma	Regulator of the cell cycle at the restriction checkpoint	Retinoblastoma, lung cancer
BRCA I and 2	Transcription factors, DNA repair	Familial breast and ovarian cancer
APC	Inhibitors of cell signal transduction	Familial adenomatous polyposis coli, colon, stomach, pancreas cancer
WT-I	Nuclear transcription	Wilms' tumour
p16INK 4	Inhibitor of CDKs, checkpoint cell cycle arrest	Pancreatic, oesophageal cancers, melanoma

The retinoblastoma (Rb) gene was the first TSG to be identified, following studies of families with a predisposition to developing retinoblastoma, a rare childhood tumour of the retina. This cancer is familial in ~40% of cases and sporadic in the rest. In the familial form the propensity to tumours is inherited in a Mendelian autosomal dominant pattern, i.e. children have a 50% chance of developing disease if a parent is affected. Patients often develop multiple and bilateral tumours much earlier in life than in sporadic cases. Familial patients are also more likely to develop other types of cancer later in life. The familial form is caused by a germline mutation of one copy of the Rb gene, so that only one further 'hit' is required for loss of function of the gene. The sporadic form requires both alleles to be hit, which is a very rare chance event. The Rb protein is central to the control of the restriction checkpoint (R-point) of the cell cycle (see above). Loss of this protein removes checks from the cell cycle, resulting in cellular proliferation. Although our understanding of the Rb gene began with the study of retinoblastoma, many common human tumours have also been found to contain mutant Rb genes.

The p53 tumour suppressor gene is the most commonly mutated gene in human cancers. As well as a role in cell cycle arrest and control of some DNA repair genes, importantly p53 is also involved in apoptosis following recognition of DNA damage (Fig. 2.2). Following chemotherapy- or radiotherapy-induced DNA damage, cells may undergo p53-mediated apoptosis. However, loss of the function of p53 results in survival of cells damaged by treatment. Therefore, p53-deficient cells are more resistant to chemotherapy and radiotherapy.

TSGs may be inactivated by:

1. Point mutations or small deletions/insertions of genetic material
2. Chromosomal abnormalities, e.g. translocations or insertions
3. Epigenetic changes, e.g. DNA methylation.

DNA REPAIR GENES

DNA repair genes have the 'caretaker' function of preserving genomic stability. These genes encode proteins involved in repairing DNA damage. Loss of DNA repair results in persistent DNA damage with consequent further mutations and genomic instability. This may lead to loss of TSGs and conversion of proto-oncogenes to oncogenes, resulting in an increased susceptibility to cancer. Examples of DNA repair genes include the human mismatch repair genes. A germline mutation in these genes is observed in patients with hereditary non-polyposis colorectal cancer (HNPCC). Xeroderma pigmentosum is another example of a disease due to defective DNA repair and patients with this condition develop multiple skin cancers.

TUMOUR PROGRESSION AND METASTASES

Cancers may evolve from a single abnormal cell that has acquired several critical gene mutations following a long process of competition and natural selection from other host cells, often over a period of many years. This process is known as multistage carcinogenesis. One of the best understood examples of this process is the adenoma–carcinoma sequence in the development of colorectal cancer (Fig. 2.4). After initial DNA damage, further mutations lead to the development of tumour heterogeneity. As the tumour grows, heterogeneity increases, increasing the likelihood of developing invasive or metastatic potential.

When tumours reach a few millimetres in size, simple diffusion of oxygen and nutrients is no longer enough to sustain tumour growth. Tumours overcome this problem by developing new blood vessels by a complex process known as angiogenesis, which is regulated by various angiogenic (e.g. vascular endothelial growth factor – VEGF) and anti-angiogenic (e.g. angiostatin) factors. Tumour angiogenesis is currently a promising target for new cancer treatments.

Tumours become invasive when cells lose adhesion to adjoining cells and breach the basement membrane. This is made possible by further specific gene mutations leading to the loss of the normal cellular anchorage mechanisms (e.g. loss of E-cadherin) and production of enzymes that destroy the extracellular matrix and basement membrane (e.g. matrix

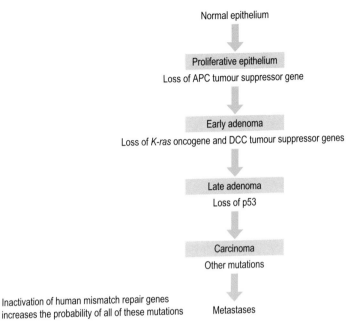

Normal epithelium

Proliferative epithelium
Loss of APC tumour suppressor gene

Early adenoma
Loss of *K-ras* oncogene and DCC tumour suppressor genes

Late adenoma
Loss of p53

Carcinoma
Other mutations

Inactivation of human mismatch repair genes
increases the probability of all of these mutations

Metastases

FIGURE 2.4 Multistage carcinogenesis.

metalloproteinases). Migration into the lymphovascular channels allows the cells to metastasise.

In order to survive the cancer cells must also be able to avoid the immune system and find a suitable tissue microenvironment to grow in. Escape from immune surveillance can be achieved in a number of ways including:

1. Reduced expression of tumour antigens
2. Reduced major histocompatibility complex (MHC) expression
3. Production of anti-T-cell factors (e.g. TGF-β)
4. 'Hiding' from immune response in sanctuary sites, e.g. testes and the central nervous system (CNS).

Immunotherapies, such as interferon and interleukin-2, may act by modifying tumour immunogenicity.

Finally, cancer cells' inherent genetic instability promotes further mutagenesis. Treatments may then bring about a natural selection process favouring cancer cells with multidrug resistance genes and radiation resistance genes. This has obvious implications for resistance mechanisms to further treatments.

WHAT ARE THE CAUSES OF CANCER?

Genetic abnormalities form the basis of cancer. These abnormalities can be inherited, but are more frequently acquired probably in response to environmental mutagens. As mentioned above, the chain of events leading to the development of cancer is known as carcinogenesis and there are three main classes of carcinogens that cause the mutations responsible for this process:

- chemicals
- radiation
- biological factors.

CHEMICALS AND CHEMICAL CARCINOGENESIS

Chemical carcinogenesis can be considered as having three main steps – initiation, promotion and progression.

The initiation step is caused by chemicals that cause permanent non-lethal DNA damage to the cell. The list of sources of exposure to these carcinogens is very large and includes industrial chemicals, medical drugs, and tobacco smoke (see below). Specific chemicals implicated include alkylating agents, aromatic amines, polycyclic aromatic hydrocarbons, asbestos, and nickel and chromium compounds.

Promotion is a partially reversible process whereby, after initiation, cells proliferate under the influence of chemicals that stimulate cell division. This is thought to lead to the development of benign lesions such as polyps, hyperplasia or adenomas etc. These chemicals do not usually cause DNA damage themselves. Some examples include hormones (e.g. oestrogens, androgens), growth factors, and vitamins A and D.

Progression is the process whereby cells become malignant as further mutations lead to tumour growth, invasive properties and the capacity to metastasise. This may occur many years or decades after the initiation process.

TOBACCO

Smoking is a cause of a third of all cancers and a major public health problem. Cigarette smoking is a major cause of cancers of the lung, head and neck, and oesophagus and is a contributing cause in the development of cancers of the bladder, pancreas, uterine cervix, kidney, stomach, and some leukaemias. About 4000 chemicals have been identified in tobacco smoke of which over 40 are carcinogens. Smokers who quit before age 50 have half the risk of dying in the next 15 years compared with those who continue to smoke. Those who quit by age 35 avoid 90% of the risk attributable to tobacco.

RADIATION CARCINOGENESIS

Both ionising radiation and ultraviolet light may be carcinogenic. Ionising radiation may be electromagnetic (e.g. X-rays and gamma rays) and particulate (e.g. electrons, protons, neutrons, alpha particles etc.). Exposure to ionising radiation may result from manmade (e.g. therapy and imaging, nuclear industry) or natural sources. Radiation from natural sources is termed background radiation, and results from cosmic rays, radon, terrestrial radioisotopes (soil and rocks) and internal sources within the body (e.g. carbon-14 and potassium-40).

Ionising radiation causes DNA damage and is therefore mutagenic and potentially carcinogenic to any tissue in the body. Radiation damage may particularly lead to loss of DNA repair genes, and tumour suppressor genes. Further mutations, over a period of many years, may result in malignant transformation.

A single exposure to ionising radiation may be sufficient to induce cancer. The odds of cancer induction depend on the dose and type of tissue irradiated. Myeloid cells are particularly sensitive to ionising radiation, and breast, thyroid and lung are also vulnerable tissues. The 'latency' period between exposure and cancer induction also varies. For leukaemia, the average period is 7 years, whereas for solid malignancies it is usually at least 10 years.

UV radiation exposure increases the risk of both non-melanoma skin cancers (NMSC) and melanoma. NMSCs may be induced by multiple exposures to UV (mainly UVB) light. The mechanism involves damage to the p53 gene and DNA repair processes. Patients with xeroderma pigmentosum are less able to repair UV-induced DNA damage due to inherited defective DNA repair mechanisms and have a particularly high risk of multiple skin cancers after UV light exposure. Melanomas have been associated with a history of acute sunburn episodes rather than chronic exposure to sunlight, but no direct causal link is proven at present.

BIOLOGICAL FACTORS

Age

The incidence of cancer increases dramatically with increasing age. This is consistent with the multi-hit model of cancer, which suggests that several gene mutations that occur over a period of many years are required to cause cancer. The ageing process itself also increases the likelihood of sporadic somatic mutations.

Diet, obesity and alcohol

After smoking, diet is the next biggest contributor to cancer deaths. Obesity is a particularly strong risk factor. There is good evidence that eating more than five portions of fruit or vegetables per day reduces cancer risk, especially colon and stomach cancers. A good diet should also aim to decrease the intake of red meats, salt, sugar and fat. Physical exercise reduces cancer risk (especially colon cancer) and is helpful for reducing obesity.

Excessive alcohol intake is associated with cancers of the oral cavity, pharynx and oesophagus. The risk of these cancers dramatically increases in drinkers who also smoke. Primary liver cancer is also more common in heavy drinkers.

VIRUSES AND INFECTIONS

Many RNA retroviruses, DNA viruses and some bacteria are known to be causative agents in human cancers (Table 2.3). It is estimated that viruses cause 15% of all tumours worldwide. This figure is much lower in the UK as rates of hepatitis B and HIV infection are much lower than in the developing world. Most individuals infected with viruses do not develop cancer.

The viruses that cause human cancers normally establish chronic infections and latency periods are many years. Viruses are also rarely complete carcinogens so additional changes are usually required for cancer to develop. There are numerous mechanisms involved in viral carcinogenesis. These include:

1. Viral oncogene integration into host DNA; e.g. Epstein–Barr virus (EBV) encodes a transforming oncoprotein that acts as a cell surface growth factor receptor (direct acting virus).
2. Chromosomal translocations; e.g. EBV increases the probability of chromosomal translocation (direct acting virus).

TABLE 2.3 Examples of carcinogenic biological agents

Agent	Human cancer
Viruses	
Human papilloma virus (HPV)	Squamous carcinomas of the cervix, anus, vulva, penis
Hepatitis B and C viruses (HBV, HCV)	Hepatocellular carcinoma
Epstein–Barr virus (EBV) – (herpes family)	Burkitt's lymphoma, Hodgkin's disease lymphomas in the immunosuppressed, nasopharyngeal cancer
Human immunodeficiency virus (HIV/AIDS)	Kaposi's sarcoma, non-Hodgkin's lymphoma, cervical squamous carcinoma
Kaposi's sarcoma associated herpes virus (KSHV)	Kaposi's sarcoma
Human T-cell leukaemia virus (HTLV-1)	Adult T-cell leukaemia
Bacteria	
Helicobacter pylori	Gastric B-cell lymphomas Gastric carcinoma

3. Inactivation of host tumour suppressor gene protein products by viral oncoproteins; e.g. the HPV virus produces the E6 and E7 proteins that bind to and inactivate the p53 and pRb proteins respectively (direct acting virus).
4. Activation of host proto-oncogenes by insertion of promoter sequences – 'insertional mutagenesis' (indirect acting virus).
5. Chronic cellular injury due to immune response to virus, e.g. HBV causes chronic injury and cirrhosis of the liver, which may eventually lead to hepatocellular carcinoma (indirect acting virus).
6. Immunosuppression predisposes to certain cancers, e.g. HIV and Kaposi's sarcoma (indirect acting virus).

HEREDITARY/FAMILIAL CANCER AND CANCER PREDISPOSITION

Hereditary cancer is an uncommon subset of cancer in which an inherited germline mutation confers an increased genetic predisposition towards developing cancer. Only 5–10% of the common cancers have a hereditary basis, with sporadic cancers accounting for the vast majority of cases.

The main characteristics of hereditary cancers include:

1. Germline mutations, which mainly affect TSGs, but can also affect oncogenes and DNA repair genes.
2. Earlier onset of cancer.
3. The development of multifocal cancers or bilateral cancers in paired sites (e.g. retinoblastoma).
4. The development of multiple primary tumours (e.g. Li–Fraumeni syndrome).
5. A strong family history of cancer, usually of the same type.
6. An association with congenital abnormalities.

A germline mutation results in every cell in the body containing that mutation. However, there are two copies of every gene and in the case of a TSG, both copies of the gene need to be inactivated to cause a cancer. The probability of this occurring is extremely high if one copy is already affected in each cell, as is the case with a germline mutation. In those without a germline mutation, two separate 'hits' on both sister genes (alleles) in the same cell are required and this is an extremely rare event in comparison. This is the basis of Knudsen's 'two hit hypothesis' and explains why patients with germline mutations are at much higher risk of cancer development.

Examples of some familial cancer syndromes and the genes involved are given in Table 2.4.

TABLE 2.4 Examples of some familial cancer syndromes

Syndrome	Cancer	Genes affected
Familial breast/ovarian cancer	Breast, ovary, prostate, colon	BRCA 1
	Breast, ovary, prostate, pancreas, others	BRCA 2
Hereditary non-polyposis colorectal cancer (HNPCC)	Colon, uterus, GI tract, bladder, head and neck, melanoma	Human mismatch repair genes
Hereditary prostate cancer	Prostate	HPC 1 and 2
Familial melanoma	Melanoma	p16, p15, CDK4
Papillary renal cancer	Papillary renal cancer	MET
Li–Fraumeni	Breast, sarcoma, brain, leukaemia, others	p53
Retinoblastoma	Retinoblastoma, osteosarcoma	Rb
Familial polyposis coli	Colon, upper gastrointestinal tract, desmoids	APC
Neurofibromatosis types 1 and 2	Optic glioma, neurofibrosarcomas (type 1)	NF1
	Acoustic neuroma, brain/spinal tumours	NF2
Von Hippel–Lindau	Haemangioblastomas, renal cancer, phaeochromocytoma	VHL
Ataxia telangiectasia	Leukaemias and lymphomas	ATM
Familial medullary thyroid cancer	Medullary thyroid cancer	RET

FURTHER READING

Kruh G D, Tew K D 2000 Basic science of cancer. Current Medicine, Philadelphia
McKinell R G, Parchment R E, Perantoni A O, Pierce G B 1998 The biological basis of cancer. Cambridge, Cambridge University Press

CHAPTER 3

Principles of cancer pathology

Lisa J. Barker

INTRODUCTION – IMPORTANCE OF PATHOLOGICAL DIAGNOSIS

Cancer has profound emotional and physical consequences for a patient including significant morbidity and possible mortality from treatment. The diagnosis of cancer must therefore be as certain and as accurate as possible to ensure the most appropriate treatment decisions are made. There are very few circumstances in which a pathological tissue diagnosis is not required in a patient with suspected cancer.

The pathological diagnosis gives vital information regarding prognosis, response to treatment, and genetic implications. It also provides epidemiological data essential for our future understanding of the disease.

PATHOLOGICAL TERMS AND THE BASIC FEATURES OF MALIGNANCY

The hallmark of malignancy is the ability to invade and metastasise. Although benign tumours lack this ability, they may still prove fatal due to local effects.

BASIC NOMENCLATURE

Tumour simply means 'swelling'.

Neoplasia means 'new growth'.
Cancer is a term for a malignant neoplasm/tumour.

TABLE 3.1 Basic nomenclature of some benign and malignant tumours

Tissue of origin	Benign	Malignant
Epithelium	Adenoma Papilloma Squamous cell papilloma Liver cell adenoma Renal tubular adenoma	Adenocarcinoma Papillary adenocarcinoma Squamous cell carcinoma Hepatocellular carcinoma Renal cell carcinoma
Mesenchymal tissue (connective tissue)	Fibroma Lipoma Chondroma Osteoma Haemangioma Rhabdomyoma Leiomyoma	Fibrosarcoma Liposarcoma Chondrosarcoma Osteosarcoma Angiosarcoma Rhabdomyosarcoma Leiomyosarcoma
Totipotential cells in gonads or embryonal tissue	Mature teratoma, dermoid cyst	Immature teratoma

Tumours are named according to their anatomical site, tissue or cell type of origin and their biological behaviour (i.e. benign or malignant). (See Table 3.1 for examples.)

EARLIEST STAGES OF CANCER DEVELOPMENT

The first microscopically evident abnormality of cell maturation is termed 'dysplasia'. The finding of dysplasia in an epithelial tissue is acknowledged to be a premalignant change. Defective maturation results in architectural disorder, nuclear irregularity, increased and abnormal mitoses, and an increase in apoptotic cells (i.e. cells undergoing programmed death). When severe, these changes are termed carcinoma in situ. The abnormalities by definition are limited by the epithelial basement membrane. Without penetration of the membrane, there is no opportunity for lymphatic permeation and therefore carcinoma in situ is unable to metastasise.

Intramucosal carcinoma implies that this process has extended into the connective tissue of the mucosa but is still confined by the muscularis mucosae layer and is therefore an early stage of cancer.

GROWTH, INVASION AND METASTASIS

The rate of tumour growth is due to an imbalance between cell division and cell loss, and varies greatly between tumours. Angiogenesis – the production of new blood vessels to supply oxygen and nutrients – is critical for growth. It is promoted by tumour-associated angiogenic factors such as vascular endothelial growth factor (VEGF).

Tumour spread into adjacent tissue is facilitated by decreasing adhesion between tumour cells (by loss of E-cadherin and catenin expression). Tumour cells attach to the extracellular matrix (by binding factors such as laminin receptors and integrins), degrade the matrix (by metalloproteinases) and migrate outward. The tumour may grow in an infiltrating or expansile manner. In the latter case it may develop a fibrous capsule by compression of surrounding connective tissue. The pattern of invasion is important as it has implications for the ease of surgical excision. Invasion is often more extensive than it appears clinically or at operation.

Tumours may spread by:

- direct local invasion
- lymphatic spread (usually following the natural lymphatic drainage route)
- vascular spread
- transcoelomic (peritoneal, pleural) spread, e.g. ovarian cancer, mesothelioma
- cerebrospinal fluid (CSF) spread, e.g. medulloblastoma, ependymoma.

Metastases result from tumour spread to a site distant from the original tumour and may become apparent before, at the same time as, or many years after the appearance of the primary tumour. Histologically, metastases usually resemble the primary tumour, although not always, and this may pose a particular diagnostic problem if the site of the primary tumour is unknown.

For any tumour, the possibility of a metastasis from an unrecognised primary must be considered, as this will significantly affect treatment. This is especially the case for tumours arising in the lung, liver and brain.

Sometimes metastases that were not apparent clinically are diagnosed histologically, e.g. microscopic deposits in axillary lymph nodes removed in the treatment of breast cancer.

The prognostic significance of micrometastases detected by immunohistochemistry remains uncertain and these are not routinely sought.

USES OF PATHOLOGICAL DIAGNOSIS

TYPING, CLASSIFYING AND GRADING TUMOURS

Certain tumours are associated with particular sites and presentations, but the unexpected often happens in medicine. An unusual tumour may occur, which requires special treatment. This is why a tissue diagnosis is usually essential before planning treatment.

Grading is a measure of the degree of differentiation of the tumour, i.e. how closely it resembles the tissue of origin. Poorly differentiated (or anaplastic) tumours tend to behave more aggressively than well-differentiated tumours. Poorly differentiated tumours have lost most of the features that characterise the tissue of origin, such that poorly differentiated lymphoma, carcinoma and sarcoma may all look very similar. This poses difficulties in pathological diagnosis, but is usually resolved by immunohistochemical investigation (see later).

STAGING

Staging is a measure of spread, i.e. the local and distant extent of the tumour. Precise staging is essential to determine optimum treatment, as a baseline for response to treatment, and as a guide to the prognosis. Ideally, clinical, biochemical, haematological, radiological and isotope assessments are combined with pathological staging.

The TNM staging system is widely recognised and accepted. The tumour is given a pT stage (usually related to size or tissue layers penetrated, with 'Tis' representing in situ disease). The lymph nodes are given a pN stage (which may be related to the number of nodes involved, or the position of these nodes, including the involvement of the node furthest from the tumour) and, if this information is available, distant metastases are given a pM stage. In general, the number '0' denotes no disease, and 'X' denotes unknown extent. A prefix 'r' rather than 'p' denotes a recurrent tumour.

ASSOCIATED FEATURES

Particular histological features may give a guide to the characteristics of the disease; e.g. a lymphocytic reaction can be associated with microsatellite instability in colorectal carcinoma (which may suggest a hereditary non-polyposis colonic carcinoma syndrome). Perineural spread is an adverse prognostic factor for head and neck cancer and prostate cancer, and lymphovascular invasion is an adverse prognostic factor for many tumour types.

TREATMENT-RELATED FACTORS

The expression of tumour markers and receptors may characterise the tumour origin, predict prognosis, and predict response to treatment. A good example is the oestrogen receptor in breast cancer, which, if present, predicts a better prognosis and high response rates to hormonal therapy.

ASSESSMENT OF COMPLETENESS OF EXCISION

Another most important part of the pathological examination is to determine the completeness of excision. Tumour involvement of surgical margins is a high risk factor for local recurrence, and is usually an indication for further surgery or other local treatment such as radiotherapy.

BASIC PROCESSES IN PATHOLOGICAL DIAGNOSIS

SAMPLING

In general the least invasive procedure is used. The options available are cytology, needle biopsy (e.g. Trucut), an incisional biopsy (with no attempt at complete removal), or an excisional biopsy or resection.

Cytology

Cytology is the study of cells separated from the tissue structure. Samples may be taken for cytology from fluids (e.g. ascites, pleural effusion, CSF) or by removing cells by scraping (e.g. bronchial brushing, cervical cytology) or by fine needle aspiration – FNA (e.g. thyroid, breast, lymph nodes).

The specimen processing for cytology differs from that for histology, which means a more rapid result can be given. The cells do not require overnight fixing and are either smeared directly on a slide or in the case of fluids, centrifuged to produce a more concentrated specimen, before putting on a slide and staining. However, by the nature of cytology, little or no tissue structure remains and the diagnosis rests on the features of the individual cells. Information that depends upon the relationship to surrounding tissue, e.g. invasion, cannot be given.

LABORATORY PROCEDURE

When tissue is sent for histopathological evaluation it is given a unique code, which remains with it throughout its processing and examination. Fresh tissue may occasionally be taken for freezing or to be put into tissue culture medium for cytogenetic analysis, or glutaraldehyde for electron microscopy. Otherwise tissue is fixed as an intact specimen. This means that it is immersed for approximately 24–48 hours in formalin, which halts cellular metabolism and autolysis, and preserves the tissue structure.

Macroscopic examination

Once fixed, the tissue is examined and described by the pathologist. The specimen may vary from a whole organ, e.g. lung (pneumonectomy), to a collection of tissues (e.g. lymph nodes from a neck dissection), to a tiny single fragment of biopsy tissue (e.g. in an endoscopic biopsy).

Clinical details such as the site and operative procedure are essential for correct orientation of the specimen. Photographs are used to record the appearance of large specimens. Marker sutures positioned during surgical excision are very useful at this point – otherwise the specimen may not be accurately mapped to its position in the body.

Selected small samples of tissue ('blocks') are taken to build up a picture of the tumour and its relationship to the tissue in which it has arisen. The margins of excision are often painted with ink in order to check for margin involvement or measure the distance between the tumour and this margin.

If the specimen is a small biopsy the whole piece is taken for microscopic examination.

Microscopic examination

The blocks of tissue taken for microscopy are approximately 2 cm × 2.5 cm. They are further fixed in formalin, then embedded in paraffin wax to aid the cutting of fine slices ('sections'), which are laid on slides and stained (usually with haematoxylin and eosin). This whole process may take several days, which explains why there is an inevitable delay in the reporting of larger histopathological specimens.

Every slide is examined for both abnormal and uninvolved tissues, and their relation to each other.

Frozen section

Where a very rapid result is absolutely essential, freezing can replace the fixation stage. The tissue is frozen solid rapidly and sections cut and stained. However, the resulting slides are more difficult to interpret and this method is therefore not suitable for routine use.

This procedure should only be used where intraoperative diagnosis is vital to determine the progress of the operation. In oesophageal cancer surgery, for example, frozen section examination of coeliac and para-aortic nodes at operation may prevent unnecessary oesophageal resection by establishing the presence of distant spread to these sites.

EXTRA TESTS

Special stains

Special stains are used to give further information about the tumour. For example, stains exist for detecting characteristics of cells such as the mucin of secretory cells, the pigment of melanocytes, or neuroendocrine granules.

Stains can also help identify the way the tumour has spread by highlighting whether tumour is limited by the basement membrane of an epithelium, or the elastic lamina of an anatomical plane, or demonstrating vessels permeated by tumour.

They may also be used to identify 'foreign' substances, e.g. asbestos bodies, iron granules or amyloid.

Immunohistochemistry

Immunohistochemistry is used to identify the proteins expressed by cells. This is achieved by attaching an antibody to the protein, amplifying this signal, and then using an enzyme reaction to produce a coloured pigment at the site of attachment.

The use of immunohistochemistry has increased substantially over recent years, and this technique is now very prominent in tumour diagnosis. It can now be performed on formalin-fixed tissue. Immunohistochemistry can be performed on cytological samples by preparation of a cell block (cells which have been concentrated and then embedded in gel and treated like a tissue sample).

Immunohistochemistry can be used to identify characteristics such as cytokeratins, which vary in molecular weight between types of epithelia, or proliferation markers such as Ki67, which only occur in cells during the process of mitosis. A group of markers used to distinguish immune cells is called the cluster designation (CD) system.

The use of immunohistochemistry is constantly being explored and refined (Table 3.2). It should be noted that no marker can be said to be truly specific for only one cell type, and the interpretation of immunohistochemical results must be done in the light of other features.

Genetics

Molecular diagnosis is carried out on various types of tissue – fresh tissue is usually preferable, but techniques are increasingly being developed to obtain results from fixed tissue when there is no access to fresh material.

TABLE 3.2 Examples of immunohistochemical stains and their uses

Immunohistochemical stain	Examples of tissue identified
S100/chromogranin/synaptophysin	Neural origin
CD56	Neuroendocrine including small cell lung carcinoma
CK7	Epithelia of gynaecological, urinary and upper gastrointestinal tract
CK20	Epithelia of lower gastrointestinal tract
CK14	Squamous epithelia
CD34/31	Blood vessels
HMB45	Immature melanocytes
ER/PR	Hormone receptors (oestrogen and progesterone)
CD68	Macrophages
Calretinin/thrombomodulin/CK5/6	Mesothelial
TTF1	Lung and thyroid epithelium
CA125	Ovarian epithelium
c-kit(CD117)	Gastrointestinal stromal tumour
CD45	Leucocytes
Desmin	Muscle
Actin/myosin	Smooth muscle or myoepithelium
Vimentin	Mesenchymal
MNF116/CAM 5.2/BerEP4	General epithelial markers
RCC	Renal cell carcinoma
CD99	Ewing's/PNET
CD3/4/8	T-lymphocytes
CD20	B-lymphocytes

TABLE 3.3 Some tumours and their associated genetic abnormalities

Tumour	Genetic abnormality looked for
Synovial sarcoma	Translocation X;18
Ewing's/PNET	Translocation 11;22
Alveolar rhabdomyosarcoma	Translocation 2;13 or 1;13
Breast carcinoma	Her 2 amplification
Wilms' tumour	11p13 (WT1) mutation or deletion
Neuroblastoma	1p deletion
Embryonal rhabdomyosarcoma	11p deletion
Burkitt's lymphoma	Translocation 8;14
Retinoblastoma	13q14 mutation or deletion

Techniques include flow cytometry, fluorescent in-situ hybridisation (FISH) and the polymerase chain reaction (PCR).

Aneuploidy, gene mutations, translocations, deletions and amplifications can be detected, and some give a very accurate guide to the diagnosis, e.g. a chromosome 11 to 22 translocation in PNET/Ewing's sarcoma. (See Table 3.3 for more examples.)

However, as with immunohistochemistry, many results are non-specific. A negative finding cannot exclude the diagnosis and therefore results need to be interpreted with care.

Molecular diagnositc studies should be requested:

- to narrow down the differential diagnosis of certain difficult tumours
- to confirm the suspected identity of a tumour with a closely associated genetic defect
- after the diagnosis of a syndrome-associated tumour, or one which may be inherited, when it is necessary to screen family members.

COMMUNICATION

CLINICIAN TO PATHOLOGIST – THE REQUEST FORM

In order to give the maximum useful information, the pathologist needs to know the context of the case. The following details are essential to interpreting the pathology and should be included on the request form:

1. The patient's history, particularly any history of malignancy or premalignant lesions
2. The presentation and extent of the lesion
3. Whether preoperative radiotherapy or chemotherapy was used.

Any specific questions that the clinician would like answered should also be included.

PATHOLOGIST TO CLINICIAN – THE PATHOLOGY REPORT

The report issued by a pathologist will contain as much relevant information as can be obtained about the case, and in dealing with many tumours there is a minimum of information that in good practice must be provided – the minimum dataset.

The following information should be expected: size; appearance; tissue of origin; benign/malignant; primary/secondary; differentiation; local invasion (blood vessels, lymphatics, nerves, organ capsule, lymph nodes); host immune response; completeness of excision.

The pathologist will try to answer the clinical questions, but it must be remembered that looking at a tissue in isolation cannot always predict the situation in the patient, and that appearances and special techniques have to be interpreted with care.

The use of terms such as 'in keeping with' or 'suggestive of' is an attempt to give a guide as to the likelihood of a lesion being part of an overall clinical picture.

THE MULTIDISCIPLINARY MEETING

In this forum, a discussion can take place between representatives of all the oncology specialties, i.e. pathology, radiology, surgery, non-surgical oncology and palliative care. This allows the significance of the pathology result to be put clearly in the context of the clinical case and answers any outstanding questions. Appropriate clinical management decisions can then be made.

FURTHER READING

Cotran R S, Kumar V, Collins T, Robbins S L (eds) 2004 Neoplasia. In: Robbins Pathologic basis of disease, 7th edn. W B Saunders, Philadelphia

Underwood J C E 2000 General and systematic pathology, 3rd edn. Churchill Livingstone, Edinburgh

CHAPTER 4

Principles of surgical oncology

Richard Milton and Clive Peedell

INTRODUCTION

Although surgery is the oldest treatment for cancer, it is still the most important and successful treatment modality for most tumour types. In the modern management of cancer, surgical oncology currently encompasses a lot more than simply 'removing the cancer' with very important additional roles in: (1) prevention and screening; (2) diagnosis and staging; (3) palliation; (4) rehabilitation and reconstruction; and (5) follow-up.

Surgery is now very commonly used in combination with radiotherapy and chemotherapy and surgical oncology is therefore heavily focused towards the multidisciplinary approach to cancer management. Today's surgical oncologist not only has to be a good technician, but must also have a sound knowledge of the biology and natural history of cancer, as well as an understanding of the non-surgical specialties (radiation oncology, medical oncology and palliative care).

Over the years, improvements in surgical techniques, anaesthesia and pain control, medical care and infection control have led to greater resection rates, improved functional outcomes, better local control and increased survival from cancer.

THE ROLES OF SURGICAL ONCOLOGY

PREVENTION AND SCREENING OF CANCER

(See also Ch. 10 on cancer screening.)

Some cancers are more likely to be cured if they are detected and treated at an earlier stage. This has worked well for gastric cancer (in Japan) and also cervical cancer and breast cancer, although much debate persists.

There are also some underlying conditions and genetic traits that lead to an extremely high risk of developing a subsequent cancer. One of the best examples is familial adenomatous polyposis, a condition in which nearly all patients will develop colorectal cancer by the age of 30. Prophylactic proctocolectomy is the advised management for these patients, with screening colonoscopies and genetic testing for relatives. Hereditary non-polyposis colorectal cancer (HNPCC) and ulcerative colitis are also high risk conditions for colorectal cancer and regular screening with colonoscopy is required with colectomy offered if indicated. In women with a high risk of breast cancer (e.g. strong family history and the BRCA 1 and 2 genes), estimation of the approximate risk of cancer can be calculated and prophylactic mastectomy may be offered. Careful counselling on the pros and cons of prophylactic surgery is required.

CANCER DIAGNOSIS AND STAGING

The diagnosis of cancer usually relies on histopathological examination of biopsied tissue obtained from the suspected tumour. As well as establishing a diagnosis, biopsy may also be helpful for staging purposes and judging disease response to treatment.

Tissue may be acquired in numerous ways with various levels of difficulty. The main techniques are as follows:

1. Fine needle aspiration (FNA). May be guided by simple palpation or image-guided with ultrasound or CT. It provides material for cytological analysis offering a tentative diagnosis of malignant tissue. In nearly all clinical scenarios, confirmation with histopathological examination of tissue is also required.
2. Core needle biopsy. A core of tissue can be obtained within the hollow of a needle passed into the suspect tissue. The size of tissue removed is adequate for diagnosis of most tumour types, but larger amounts of tissue may be required to diagnose lymphomas, sarcomas and other mesenchymal tissues.
3. Incisional biopsy. A small wedge of tissue is removed from a larger tumour mass. This is useful when a larger amount of tissue is required for diagnosis (e.g. sarcomas), or if the lesion is ulcerated or necrotic.
4. Excisional biopsy. The whole suspected tumour is excised with little normal tissue margin, allowing the pathologist to examine the entire tumour. This is suitable for smaller tumours, if it can be performed without compromising the definitive surgical procedure. Excision is often the preferred method of biopsy and may minimise the risks of disseminating cancer cells. It also guarantees the provision of microscopic sections representative of the material under investigation.

Image-guided and endoscopic biopsy techniques have dramatically reduced the need for major surgical procedures (such as laparotomy) to obtain histological specimens.

Some general surgical principles apply to all biopsy techniques. These include close cooperation with the pathologist to decide on the best technique to use and the amount of tissue required to obtain the most accurate diagnosis (e.g. extra tissue needed for special stains, flow cytometry and electron microscopy). Careful placement of needle punctures or incisions is needed for certain cancers (e.g. soft tissue sarcomas), to allow their excision during the definitive surgical procedure. Contamination of new surgical planes and large haematomas should be avoided. Avoidance of necrotic and infected tissue should be attempted if possible. If necessary, the sample should be marked to help in orientation and the appropriate fixative used.

Despite major technical advances in radiological staging, pathological staging is still very important for many cancer sites and can be obtained either before or during the definitive surgical procedure.

Lymph node dissection in breast and colon cancer surgery not only provides prognostic information that guides decisions on adjuvant therapies, but is also therapeutic if the nodes are involved with metastatic disease. In lung cancer patients, mediastinoscopy or mediastinotomy with biopsy of enlarged mediastinal nodes (greater than 1 cm seen on CT) is crucial before deciding to go ahead with a thoracotomy and major lung resection because positive mediastinal (pN2) nodes generally predict a very poor prognosis.

Lymph node involvement may also be assessed intraoperatively by frozen section, whereby lymph nodes are sent 'fresh' directly to an experienced pathologist. The surgeon can proceed to a definitive resection at the same sitting (i.e. with the patient under the same anaesthetic) when the frozen section result is negative. In oesophageal cancer surgery, for example, frozen section examination of coeliac and para-aortic nodes at operation may help avoid unnecessary oesophageal resection.

In ovarian cancer, examination and biopsy of peritoneal surfaces, or peri-toneal washings and omental biopsy are undertaken as this may influence the decision for giving adjuvant chemotherapy.

TREATMENT OF CANCER

Ideally, the aim of cancer treatment is the complete eradication of all cancer cells resulting in the patient being cured from their disease. Unfortunately, in many instances there are residual undetectable cancer cells, despite complete macroscopic resection of the tumour, and many of these patients will go on to develop recurrent disease. However, some patients will remain free from symptomatic recurrence throughout the remainder of their lifetime and eventually die from other unrelated causes and from the patient's perspective this is equivalent to a cure.

1. Primary cancer

If no metastatic disease is present, then simply removing the tumour can achieve cure. Unfortunately this is often not the case, as approximately 70%

of patients have micrometastatic disease either locoregionally or in distant sites at presentation. Careful selection of local therapy with adequate surgical margins of normal tissue is therefore required. A thorough understanding of the natural history of cancer, as well as the most accurate staging information possible, is vital. Some curative procedures may simply require a wide excision (e.g. early melanoma), whereas others require local nodal dissection (e.g. head and neck cancer).

Sparing function and minimising surgical morbidity are key principles. This may be made easier by combining surgery with radiotherapy and/or chemotherapy. For example, postoperative radiotherapy following surgical excision of soft tissue sarcoma avoids the need for amputation without compromising cure or overall survival. In breast cancer, breast-conserving surgery with postoperative radiotherapy is as effective as mastectomy, and neoadjuvant chemotherapy may render an inoperable breast tumour operable.

Over the years improved surgical techniques have: (i) reduced margins of excision without compromising cure; (ii) improved local control rates (e.g. total mesorectal excision – TME); and (iii) reduced surgical morbidity (e.g. nerve sparing techniques for prostatectomy).

2. Cytoreductive surgery

Removal of all gross local disease is often not possible due to technical reasons and/or the widespread extent of the disease. Removing the bulk of the disease may lead to residual disease that may be controlled with other modalities of treatment. A good example is ovarian cancer, where cytoreductive surgery (to $<2\,cm^3$ of residual disease) followed by chemotherapy has been shown to improve survival. Debulking some brain tumours may also be of benefit.

3. Metastatic disease

Metastatic disease does not always preclude cure. In general, if a patient has a single site of metastatic disease that is technically operable with good postoperative function anticipated, then resection should be considered if there is not a more effective way of treating the disease. A proportion of patients with more than one metastasis in the liver, lung or brain can still be cured. Good prognostic factors are long disease-free intervals, fewer metastases and smaller metastases (see Chs 49, 51 and 59 on brain, liver and pulmonary metastases, respectively).

4. Palliative surgery

Surgery is often useful in the palliative setting for relief of various symptoms. Examples include:

- removal of masses causing severe pain and/or disfigurement and/or at risk of fungation
- relief of bowel obstruction and perforation

- relief of urinary obstruction
- relief of fistulas with bypass procedures, e.g. defunctioning stoma
- relief of airway obstruction and oesophageal obstruction by laser surgery or stenting
- fixation of pathological fractures
- vertebrectomy/laminectomy and spinal stabilisation procedures for acute spinal cord compression
- vertebroplasty (injection of methylmethacrylate cement into vertebral body) for painful spinal metastases
- placement of feeding tubes
- ligation of vessels to treat bleeding
- surgical pleurodesis for pleural effusions
- treatment of biliary obstruction with stenting
- relief of ascites or raised intracranial pressure with shunt procedures
- insertion of epidural pumps for pain relief.

5. Surgical oncology emergencies

Surgical emergencies in the cancer patient may pose a particularly difficult problem, especially if the patient is neutropenic, thrombocytopenic or receiving radiotherapy. Great care is required in assessing the pros and cons of treatment. Typical emergencies that may be managed by surgery include perforation of a viscus, exsanguinating haemorrhage, abscesses, spinal cord compression, and raised intracranial pressure (ICP) from a space-occupying lesion (SOL).

RECONSTRUCTION AND REHABILITATION

Advances in surgical reconstructive techniques and rehabilitation have greatly improved function and cosmetic appearances for patients with cancer. Along with these improvements comes enormous psychological benefit. Head and neck cancer provides some of the best examples, such as bone grafting and free tissue flaps aiding reconstruction of the face with functional gain in speech and swallowing. Surgical prostheses may also improve lost function as well as appearance (e.g. artificial limbs).

FOLLOW-UP

The role of follow-up for cancer patients is poorly understood and controversial. Its aim is to detect recurrent disease and new primaries, but in general if there are no clinical symptoms then routine investigations are probably of little benefit and may be very costly. Monitoring of tumour markers has not been shown to improve survival but may be a helpful tool in making treatment decisions. However, there are some tests that are worthwhile in follow-up, e.g. regular cystoscopies for bladder cancer, colonoscopies for bowel cancer and mammography for breast cancer.

FUTURE PERSPECTIVES

One of the important areas of surgical research at present is the role of sentinel node biopsy in operative staging of melanoma and breast cancer. The sentinel node is the first node that receives drainage from the tumour and it can be identified by the technique of injecting a radioactive colloid or dye around the primary tumour, which is then detected in the sentinel node. Biopsy of this node may obviate the need for extensive nodal dissection if it is negative for metastases. It is now a standard technique in the staging and management of melanoma, but still requires more research in breast cancer.

Research continues on advancing surgical and anaesthetic techniques to improve local control, reduce hospital stay, improve quality of life and reduce mortality. Further integration with the specialties of radiation oncology, medical oncology and palliative care is ongoing.

FURTHER READING

DeVita V T, Hellman S, Rosenberg S A 2001 Principles of cancer management: surgical oncology. In: Cancer: Principles and practice of oncology, 6th edn. Lippincott Williams & Wilkins, Philadelphia

Principles of radiotherapy

INTRODUCTION

Radiotherapy is the practice of treating disease (mainly malignancy) with ionising radiation. The first medical use of radiotherapy was by Emile Grubbe in 1896 just after the discovery of X-rays by Wilhelm Conrad Roentgen in 1895. It is now a major treatment modality in the modern management of cancer and approximately 125 000 cancer patients (40–45% of all cancer patients) in the UK will require radiotherapy at some point during their illness. In two-thirds of these cases radiotherapy is given with curative intent, either alone or in combination with surgery and/or chemotherapy. Palliative radiotherapy may offer many other patients relief from symptoms associated with advanced cancer. As with surgery, radiotherapy is a locoregional treatment modality. The main aim of radiotherapy is to maximise tumour cell kill, whilst minimising damage to normal tissues. Over the last 20–30 years, major technological advances have helped greatly in this aim, by improving the delivery of high doses of radiation to irregular tumour volumes.

BASIC PHYSICS

Radiation is a term for the emission, propagation and absorption of energy in either waves/photons (electromagnetic (EM) radiation) or particulate form.

Radiotherapists use ionising radiation to treat disease, which is defined as radiation with sufficient energy to ionise atoms. This includes high energy EM radiation such as X-rays and gamma rays and particulate radiation such as electrons, protons and heavier particles (e.g. alpha particles).

Ionising radiation produces biological effects when ionised atoms cause breakage of chemical bonds leading to the formation of highly reactive free radicals, which react with and damage biomolecules such as DNA.

X-rays, gamma rays and electrons are the most widely used forms of ionising radiation in the clinical setting and the typical energies used vary from 50 kilovolts (kV) to 25 megavolts (MV). The unit of absorbed radiation dose is the Gray (Gy) (1 Gy = 1 joule per kilogram (J/kg)).

BASIC RADIOBIOLOGY

The most important biological effect of radiation is DNA damage; especially double strand (DS) breaks in DNA. Damage to DNA occurs by both direct and indirect means. Direct damage occurs from ionisation of atoms within the DNA molecule itself, but the majority of DNA damage occurs indirectly by reactions with free radicals produced from the hydrolysis of water molecules (e.g. hydroxyl (OH$^{\cdot}$) free radical). The presence of molecular oxygen (O_2) enhances radiation-induced DNA damage by binding to short-lived reactive free radical sites in cellular DNA, thus chemically fixing the damage. This explains why hypoxic (low levels of O_2) cells are more resistant to radiation.

Cellular events following radiation exposure are complex, but involve activation and expression of many genes. Depending on the amount of damage, cells may die immediately or after several cell divisions, have delayed growth (permanently or temporarily), or continue to divide.

FRACTIONATION

In order to cure a tumour, all cancer cells capable of dividing (clonogenic cells) must be killed. Higher doses of radiation kill more clonogenic cells increasing the chances of tumour cure, but also increase the risks of normal tissue damage. Hence, as tumour tissue is not that different to normal tissue, there is often a small therapeutic window between tumour cure and normal tissue damage. However, it was realised by French radiotherapists in the 1920s that an overall higher dose of radiation could be given to tumours with less damage to normal tissue if it was divided into smaller fractions and given over a longer period of time. This is known as fractionation and the biological factors that influence normal tissue and tumour responses to fractionated radiotherapy can be summarised in the five 'Rs' of radiotherapy.

I. Intrinsic radiosensitivity

This is a measure of the extent of radiation damage caused by a particular dose of radiation. It varies greatly between different types of tumours and normal tissues. The radiosensitivity of some tumours may reflect the radiosensitivity of the normal tissue they were derived from. For example, lymphoid and germ cell tissues are very radiosensitive and so are lymphomas and germ cell tumours. Bone, muscle and neuronal tissue are radioresistant and so are sarcomas and gliomas. Cells are most sensitive to radiation in the M (mitosis) and G2 (second gap before mitosis) phases of the cell cycle and therefore tissues with a high proportion of dividing cells are usually more radiosensitive, e.g. lymphoid tissue, gut and skin.

2. Repair and recovery

The majority of cell damage induced by radiation is sublethal and can be repaired. Repair increases cell survival (recovery). Most of the repair in normal tissues occurs within 6 hours of radiation exposure and if a second dose of radiation is given within this period, there is increased risk of normal tissue damage. By allowing adequate time for repair between doses of radiation, a much greater overall dose of radiation can be given with sparing of normal tissues. Fractionation of treatment leads to much less late radiation-induced tissue damage because repair of DNA prevents genetic errors being passed on to daughter cells. Differences in repair rates between normal tissue and malignant tissue contribute to the therapeutic ratio of effective radiotherapy, i.e. if cancerous cells have less ability to repair damage, there will be far less sparing of cancerous tissue than normal tissue.

3. Repopulation

Prolonged courses of treatment allow time for cellular proliferation, repopulation and recovery of irradiated tissue. However, if the repopulation rate of the tumour is higher than normal tissue, then protracted courses of radiotherapy or delays in treatment may allow time for tumour regrowth, thus decreasing the chances of tumour control. This is most likely to occur in some anaplastic tumours with large growth fractions and short cell cycle times (e.g. head and neck cancer).

4. Reoxygenation

Hypoxic cells are much more radioresistant than well-oxygenated cells (see above). Thus, tumours with inadequate blood supply due to poor vasculature, clotting abnormalities and fast tumour growth are more likely to be radioresistant. Increasing the fraction time allows surviving hypoxic cells to reoxygenate after the better oxygenated (more radiosensitive) cells have died off. The reoxygenated cells are then more radiosensitive to the next fraction of radiotherapy. The exact mechanism of reoxygenation is not clear, but death and damage of the oxic cells reduces the oxygen consumption rate of the tumour and as the tumour shrinks, diffusion of oxygen is also increased.

5. Reassortment/redistribution

This occurs when cells in the more radiosensitive phases of the cell cycle (M/G2) die off and the surviving radiosensitive cells redistribute into the more sensitive phases of the cell cycle. Subsequent fractions of radiation may then be more efficient at killing these cells.

Fractionation regimens

In clinical radiotherapy practice, the dose of radiation given to tumours is determined mainly by the tolerance of surrounding normal tissues. For radical radiotherapy treatments, most centres use once daily fractionation schedules during weekdays without treatment at the weekends. (The usual daily doses are 1.8–2.75 Gy over a 4–6-week period). This is not optimum fractionation according to the above radiobiological principles, but is standard practice for logistical reasons. However, there has been much research into defining the optimal radiotherapy fractionation regimen and the following are examples of altered fractionation regimens in clinical use:

1. Hyperfractionation. This aims to decrease late effects of radiotherapy on normal tissues and improve tumour control by using smaller, more frequent fraction sizes. This allows an overall higher dose to be given over a similar period of time as conventional regimens. Typically, 2–3 daily fractions <1.5 Gy are used.
2. Accelerated hyperfractionation (AH) and continuous hyperfractionated accelerated radiotherapy (CHART). Accelerated hyperfractionation aims to overcome tumour repopulation by reducing overall treatment time. This can be achieved with the same dose and fraction number as conventional treatment by using multiple daily fractions of radiotherapy 6–8 hours apart. CHART is similar, but patients are also treated at weekends to decrease the overall treatment time even further. CHART has recently been shown to improve survival in lung cancer patients compared to standard fractionation. However, both AH and CHART increase acute side effects of treatment and due to logistical problems in terms of implementation, they are not in wide use in the UK.
3. Hypofractionation. A smaller number of fractions are given, but the dose per fraction is higher. The overall dose given must be lower than with conventional radiotherapy, due to the increased risk of late side effects. Hypofractionation is particularly useful in the palliative situation as the overall treatment time is short and the large daily doses can be particularly effective in fast growing, aggressive, symptomatic cancers.
4. Split-course irradiation. Large doses per fraction are used daily, increasing the risk of late side effects; therefore a treatment gap of a few weeks is allowed before continuing. It is mainly used in the palliative setting as it is not as effective as conventional radiotherapy due to the problem of tumour repopulation during the treatment gap.

OTHER WAYS OF IMPROVING THE THERAPEUTIC RATIO

1. Radiosensitisers and radioprotectants

Drugs that enhance tumour radiosensitivity or protect normal tissues from radiation damage have been the focus of much research. Oxygen is the most important radiosensitiser known. Positive results have been seen with hyperbaric oxygen as a radiosensitiser, but logistical difficulties of treating patients in hyperbaric chambers have restricted its use to the experimental setting. Other drugs that can mimic the properties of oxygen have been tried (e.g. misonidazole, nimorazole) but toxicity problems have limited their use. The radioprotectant amifostine is a free radical scavenger and has shown much promise in clinical trials, but also has significant side effects.

2. Hyperthermia

Moderately heating tissues to 42–45°C can destroy malignant and normal cells. The combination of hyperthermia with radiotherapy is particularly attractive because radioresistant tissues with poor blood supply and hypoxia are more responsive to hyperthermic damage than well-oxygenated tissues. In addition, hyperthermia increases tissue radiosensitivity. Many clinical trials have shown hyperthermia alone and in combination with radiotherapy to be effective in a wide variety of malignant diseases, but logistical problems such as the treatment of deep-seated tumours and cost have restricted its use to research institutes. Microwave and ultrasound are the most commonly used heating techniques.

3. Concurrent chemoradiotherapy

Concurrent chemoradiotherapy has become a major treatment modality in the treatment of many cancers including head and neck, cervix, rectum, anus, lung and oesophagus. The simultaneous administration of chemotherapy during a course of radiotherapy may enhance the tumour response by a variety of mechanisms that include inhibition of cellular repair, reduction in the number of hypoxic tumour cells, redistribution of cells into the more radiosensitive phases of the cell cycle and treatment of microscopic systemic disease. Unfortunately, this is often at the expense of increased normal tissue toxicity. Commonly used drugs with radiation include cisplatin, 5FU, gemcitabine and mitomycin C.

PRODUCTION AND DELIVERY OF THERAPEUTIC RADIATION

Clinically useful radiation is produced both artificially and naturally and can be delivered by three main methods – external beam radiation, brachytherapy, and systemic isotope therapy.

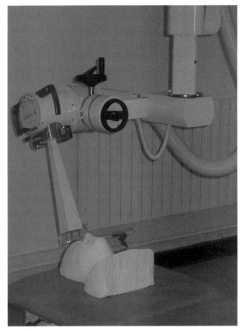

FIGURE 5.1 A superficial X-ray treatment machine with applicator attached. The Gulmay unit (Cookridge Hospital) is capable of delivering 80 kV and 220 kV superficial X-rays. (Courtesy of Leeds Teaching Hospitals NHS Trust.)

EXTERNAL BEAM RADIATION (TELETHERAPY)

This involves delivery of radiation from a unit located external to the body. The most commonly used external beam units are superficial X-ray machines, ^{60}Co machines and linear accelerators.

Superficial X-ray machines (Fig. 5.1)

Differing energies can be produced. X-rays with energies of 10–150 kV are known as superficial X-rays and are useful for treating skin cancers. X-rays with energies of 200–500 kV are known as orthovoltage and can be used to treat thicker skin lesions and superficial bone lesions such as rib metastases.

^{60}Co machines

Gamma rays with energies of 1.17 and 1.33 MeV are emitted from the artificially produced radionuclide cobalt-60. A source of ^{60}Co can be placed within a heavily shielded (lead and uranium) treatment head and moved mechanically over an aperture to produce a beam of radiation that can be

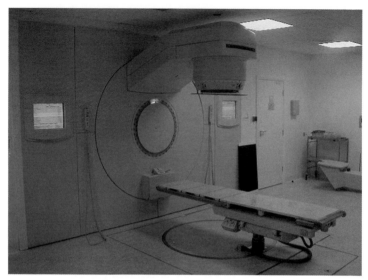

FIGURE 5.2 A linear accelerator: the 'SLC' – Cookridge Hospital. (Courtesy of Leeds Teaching Hospitals NHS Trust.)

aimed at the patient. Some of these machines are still in use, but most have been replaced by linear accelerators.

Linear accelerators (Fig. 5.2)

These machines can produce very high-energy megavoltage X-rays (photons) (4–40 MV) and electrons. The design of the machine allows the treatment head to rotate 360°, allowing treatment of the patient at any angle. This type of high-energy radiation has a advantages of good tissue penetration coupled with a skin-sparing effect. Linear accelerators can also produce electron beams by simply removing a tungsten target and replacing it with thin copper foil, which is virtually transparent to the incident electron beam. Electrons are very useful for treating superficial tumours as they have a rapid fall off in dose and can thereby spare underlying tissues such as lung and spinal cord. The effective treatment depth in centimetres is approximately equal to one-third of beam energy (e.g. 12 MeV electrons have an effective treatment depth of ~4 cm).

BRACHYTHERAPY

This involves placement of radioactive sources within tissues/tumours (interstitial therapy) or body cavities (intracavitary therapy). Very high doses of radiation can be delivered directly to the immediate area where the sources are placed, with a rapid fall off in dose intensity with increasing distance from the sources (inverse square law). Therefore, accurate placement of the radioactive sources is required to achieve an adequate dose distribution to eradicate the tumour and minimise normal tissue damage. Brachytherapy may be used radically with curative intent (e.g. cervical cancer, prostate cancer, tongue cancer), adjuvantly (e.g. breast 'boost') or in the palliative setting (e.g. recurrent head and neck cancer).

Interstitial therapy

This involves implanting radioactive sources into a target volume including the tumour. The implants may be permanent or temporary. Sites that can be treated include the head and neck (tongue, floor of mouth, neck nodes), breast, prostate, vagina, anal canal and skin.

1. Permanent implants include iodine-125 seeds, which are commonly used to treat early prostate cancer. ^{125}I has a half-life of 60 days and emits low energy (27–35 kV) gamma rays, which do not penetrate far into tissue. A very good dose distribution can be obtained by implanting 50–120 seeds under ultrasound guidance. A minimum peripheral (prostate capsule plus a 2–3 mm margin) dose of 160 Gy is usually given.
2. Temporary implants. Iridium-192 is the most commonly used temporary implant. It has a half-life of 74 days and emits gamma rays with a relatively high energy of 300–612 kV. Wires or seeds may be directly implanted into the target volume and then removed at a specified time when the required dose has been given (e.g. tongue and floor of mouth tumours). Afterloading techniques may also be used. This involves inserting hollow tubes/catheters into the target volume and then loading them with radioactive sources either by remote control or manually. This method reduces radiation exposure to the patient and staff.

Intracavitary therapy

This involves placement of hollow applicators into body cavities and then using afterloading techniques to introduce radioactive sources safely. The main use is in gynaecological oncology (see chapters on cervical and endometrial cancer) and various techniques are in clinical use. For treatment of cervical cancer, an intrauterine tube and two vaginal ovoid applicators (Figs 5.3, 5.4) are inserted and connected to a remote afterloading machine. This automatically loads ^{60}Co or ^{192}Ir sources in the appropriate positions within the tubes to achieve the best dose distribution. This is a high dose rate (HDR) system that allows large doses of radiation (up to 7 Gy) to be given within minutes under anaesthetic. Four or five of these treatments are usually given a week apart. Low dose rate systems (e.g. with caesium-137) can also be used but require 2–3 days of hospital admission and bed rest. For endometrial cancer in the adjuvant setting,

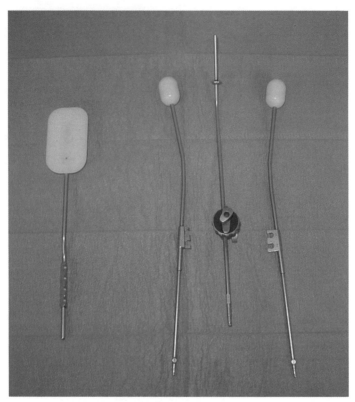

FIGURE 5.3 Vaginal intracavitary applicators before assembly. Note the intrauterine tube with flange, two vaginal ovoids (which are placed up into the vaginal fornices), and the rectal retractor (which helps to reduce the rectal dose by pushing the rectum further away from the radiation source). (Courtesy of Leeds Teaching Hospitals NHS Trust.)

a vaginal applicator (Dobbie) is applied and then connected to an afterloading system.

SYSTEMIC ISOTOPE THERAPY

Involves the oral or intravenous administration of systemic radionuclides. The best example is the use of iodine-131 in the treatment of thyroid cancer (see Ch. 45 on thyroid cancer) and thyrotoxicosis (Fig. 5.5). Other examples include the use of strontium-89 to treat bone metastases, phosphorous-32 for the treatment of polycythaemia and MIBG for neuroblastoma. The use of

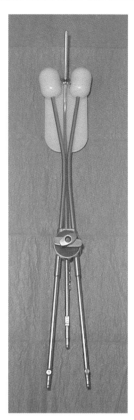

FIGURE 5.4 Assembled vaginal applicators. Following assembly inside the patient, the applicators can be connected to a remote afterloading device to deliver the appropriate dose of radiation safely. (Courtesy of Leeds Teaching Hospitals NHS Trust.)

monoclonal antibodies conjugated with radionuclides for cancer therapy (radioimmunotherapy) is under investigation.

THE RADIOTHERAPY DEPARTMENT

Radiation oncology is a multidisciplinary specialty that requires a skill mix of clinicians (radiotherapists and radiologists), specialist nursing staff, therapy radiographers, physicists, dosimetrists, technicians (workshop,

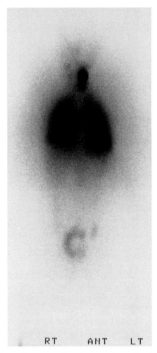

RT   ANT   LT

FIGURE 5.5 Iodine-131 uptake scan of patient with residual thyroid tissue and multiple miliary lung metastases. Note the 'blackout' of the entire lung fields bilaterally. (Courtesy of Leeds Teaching Hospitals NHS Trust.)

electronic, mould room) and IT specialists. A wide variety of technical equipment and machinery is required and includes linear accelerators, superficial X-ray machines, simulators, treatment planning systems, brachytherapy and afterloading facilities, MLC (multileaf collimator) and portal imaging systems, computer networks and software upgrades, CT/MRI linked to planning systems. Linear accelerators need to be housed in bunkers that have high-density concrete walls for radiation protection. The enormous capital costs and specialist staffing mean that radiotherapy departments need to serve a large population to be cost-effective and most centres serve at least a population of a few million. The Royal College of Radiologists recommends that there should be 5 linear accelerators per million population to provide an adequate service (the UK currently has 3.5/million!).

EXTERNAL BEAM RADIOTHERAPY PLANNING

The aim of radiotherapy in the radical setting is to deliver the maximum possible dose of radiation to the tumour to achieve permanent local tumour control, whilst trying to spare surrounding normal tissue. In the palliative setting, the aim is to decrease symptoms and the treatment is usually shorter, simpler and of lower dose for patient convenience and reduced side effects. Therefore varying levels of technical complexity are required depending on the equipment/facilities available, the tumour type and site and the treatment intent. Treatment planning is a multistep process.

1. Pre-planning
This initially involves clinical evaluation and staging of the tumour. The decision to treat with radical or palliative intent is then decided, followed by choice and scheduling of treatment (i.e. surgery, radiotherapy, chemotherapy, etc.).

2. Planning
This is the most crucial part of the radiotherapy process and involves decisions about choice of radiation modality, treatment machine, number and arrangement of beams, dose and fractionation. The tolerance of normal surrounding tissues must be taken into account when deciding on the prescribed dose.

3. Method of patient positioning and immobilisation
Patients must be treated in the same position every day – a position that is technically sound, comfortable and reproducible. This minimises the risk of a geographical miss that may compromise tumour control and increase surrounding normal tissue damage. To help in this process various immobilisation devices are available, which include vacuum moulded bags of polystyrene beads, breast boards, and foam blocks and wedges, which can be used for trunk and limb immobilisation (Fig. 5.6). Higher degrees of precision are required for treatment of CNS and head and neck tumours due to the close proximity of critical structures such as the spinal cord, eyes and optic chiasm. This can be achieved with immobilisation devices such as custom-made Perspex/plastic moulded shells (masks) that can be fixed to the treatment couch (Fig. 5.7).

4. Choice of target volume (Fig. 5.8)
This has been revolutionised with the advent of CT and MRI imaging. The volumes to be irradiated have to include the demonstrated tumour (gross tumour volume – GTV), and the predicted subclinical spread of disease (clinical target volume – CTV). In order to make sure that the entire CTV receives the prescribed dose a further margin is required to account for

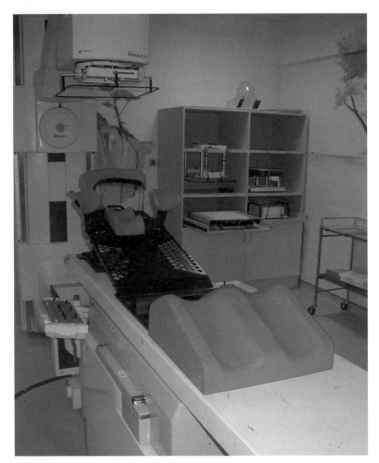

FIGURE 5.6 Breast board and foam block for immobilisation of breast cancer patients. (Courtesy of Nucletron BV and Leeds Teaching Hospitals NHS Trust.)

day-to-day variations due to patient and organ movement (e.g. respiratory movements, bladder filling, bowel emptying, etc.). This is known as the planning target volume (PTV). The palliative treatment of cancer may include the total tumour burden (e.g. T4 bladder cancer) or only the symptomatic areas of widespread disease (e.g. a single painful bone lesion in a patient with multiple bone metastases).

5. Target volume localisation and simulation
In order to accurately treat the required target volume on a daily basis, the target volume needs to be localised within the patient in relation to external

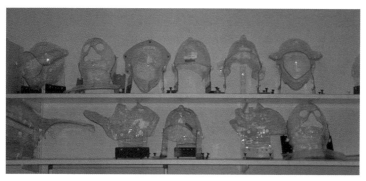

FIGURE 5.7 Various Perspex shells used for immobilisation of patients with brain and head and neck tumours. (Courtesy of Leeds Teaching Hospitals NHS Trust.)

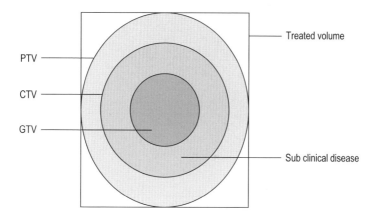

GTV – Gross tumour volume
CTV – Clinical target volume
PTV – Planning target volume

FIGURE 5.8 Treatment planning volumes (International Commission on Radiation Units and Measurements (ICRU) report 62, definitions). GTV, gross tumour volume; CTV, clinical target volume; PTV, planning target volume.

reference points (marked with ink and/or tattoos). This allows the radiographers to set up the patient in exactly the right treatment position every day. Tumour localisation is achieved with diagnostic imaging information (X-rays, MRI, CT, etc.) and the use of a simulator (Fig. 5.9). The simulator is a highly specialised diagnostic X-ray machine that also has the facility for real-time screening with an image intensifier linked to a closed

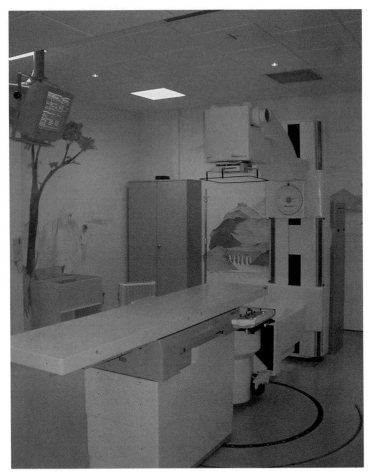

FIGURE 5.9 A simulator (Cookridge Hospital). (Courtesy of Nucletron BV and Leeds Teaching Hospitals NHS Trust.)

circuit TV. It duplicates a radiation treatment unit in terms of its geometrical, mechanical and optical properties. By radiographic visualisation, the position of the target volume in relation to the treatment field on the surface of the patient can be obtained (Fig. 5.10). Appropriate adjustments of field sizes can be made to encompass the target volume. This process can be aided by using metal markers for palpable disease and barium/contrast to define the tumour

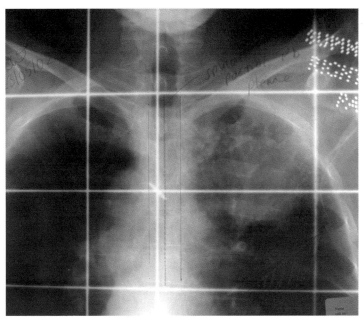

FIGURE 5.10 Conventional simulator X-ray film showing a typical rectangular field for palliative treatment of a lung carcinoma. Note the large tumour in the left upper lobe. (Courtesy of Leeds Teaching Hospitals NHS Trust.)

or critical normal structures (e.g. small bowel). Surface markings and tattoos can then be applied, which help radiographers to reproduce the same field on each day of treatment. Simulation X-rays are taken for each treatment beam to allow verification of the field position and also serve as a permanent record of treatment. These films also allow the clinician to make any changes to the field or mark areas that require shielding.

For some very simple palliative treatments, a simulator may not be required, as a field can be marked directly onto the patient by the clinician. Examples include treatment of skin cancers and whole brain irradiation.

The CT-simulator (also known as the 'virtual simulator') is an exciting new development that allows the clinician to identify the tumour on CT images and mark appropriate radiation fields on screen (Fig. 5.11). A laser system allows radiographers to mark and tattoo the patient for treatment set-up.

6. Dosimetry

The amount of radiation dose absorbed by the patient is calculated. This is known as dosimetry. For simple field arrangements (single fields and parallel opposed fields), beam data for treatment units are available as depth dose

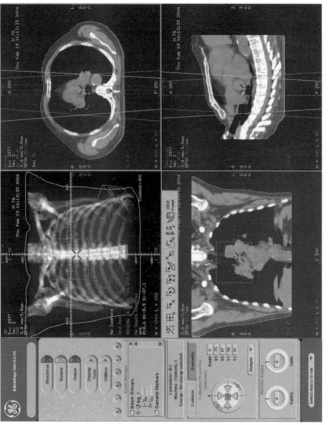

FIGURE 5.11 CT simulator ('virtual simulator') images with radiation fields marked on screen. (Courtesy of Leeds Teaching Hospitals NHS Trust and GE Healthcare.)

charts that allow simple calculation of the required given dose. Radical treatments often require multiple and complex field arrangements to achieve the optimum dose to the tumour with normal tissue sparing, and modern computer planning systems are required to carry out the very complex dosimetric calculations.

7. Treatment delivery

The patient is placed on the couch of the treatment unit in exactly the same position as during simulation with the aid of set-up instructions (produced from simulation) and the reference skin marks and tattoos. The beam parameters are then set (gantry angles, beam collimation to set field size, etc.). Any further modifications with shielding blocks or wedges are also made. The prescribed dose is then checked and the amount of time (number of monitor units) each radiation beam needs to be turned on for to give the required dose is calculated. Treatment can then be given.

8. Verification

To ensure the accuracy of treatment, check X-ray films are taken with the first fraction of radiotherapy treatment. These films show the anatomical landmarks that the radiation beam has passed through and they can be compared to the simulator films to confirm patient positioning is correct. Further check films may be required to confirm reproducibility of the field throughout the course of radiotherapy. Newer machines have portal imaging systems that utilise computer software programs to produce daily images of the treated area to help assess for deviations of the treatment field.

THREE-DIMENSIONAL CONFORMAL CT PLANNING

Most radical radiotherapy planning now utilises this technology. Conformal radiotherapy can help maximise tumour dose and minimise dose to normal surrounding tissue. CT scans are taken of the patient in the treatment position and the images are transferred into the treatment-planning computer. The clinician can then mark on each CT slice the required volume to be treated. The computer generates a 3D image of the volume to be treated and critical structures at risk can be highlighted. This helps define the best beam arrangement and the computer then calculates the optimum dose distribution (Fig. 5.12). A beam's eye view can be generated digitally (digitally reconstructed radiograph – DRR) to give an image of how the simulation film should look and this is also used in treatment verification (Fig. 5.13). Critical structures can be shielded by beam shaping, which can be achieved with customised lead blocks or the use of multileaf collimators (MLCs – computer controlled motorised movable lead leaves within the treatment machine which can block part of the radiation field). The radiation field can therefore be conformed to the shape of the volume to be treated.

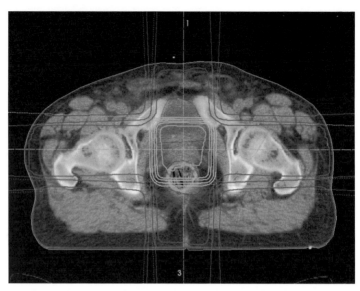

FIGURE 5.12 3D CT conformal radiotherapy plan for radical treatment of localised carcinoma of the prostate. (Courtesy of Leeds Teaching Hospitals NHS Trust.)

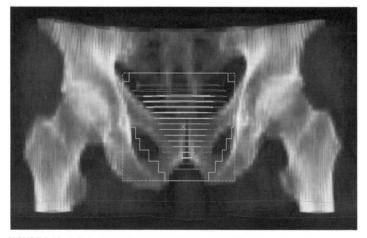

FIGURE 5.13 A digitally reconstructed radiograph (DRR) giving a beam's eye view of an anterior radiation beam in the treatment of a carcinoma of the prostate (3D CT conformal radiotherapy). The inner white volume is the clinical target volume (CTV) and the outer grey volume is the planning target volume (PTV). Note the shielding provided by the multileaf collimators (MLCs). (Courtesy of Leeds Teaching Hospitals NHS Trust.)

INTENSITY-MODULATED RADIOTHERAPY – IMRT

This is an exciting recent development in 3D conformal radiotherapy made possible by technical advances in computer technology. IMRT is based on the concept of inverse treatment planning which means that the clinician defines the treatment volume and surrounding normal tissue volumes and specifies certain dose restrictions on these volumes. The computer then calculates optimisation of beam parameters. With this information the computer is then able to control the shape of the radiation beam and modify its intensity by moving multileaf collimators in and out of the treatment field. This process can produce additional sparing of critical normal tissues, allowing further dose escalation to the tumour, and is especially useful for volumes with concave surfaces.

However, there are disadvantages to IMRT. There is very little room for error in patient set-up and any organ movements or patient movements may drastically alter the dose plan. For these reasons IMRT requires precise patient set-up each day as well as excellent immobilisation techniques. It is used for tumour sites where movements (of the tumour and the patient) tend to be minimal or can be minimised effectively, e.g. brain tumours, head and neck cancer and prostate cancer.

The other main disadvantages are cost (as the technology and equipment is expensive and requires a high level of expertise) and increased treatment time for the patient.

STEREOTACTIC RADIOTHERAPY AND RADIOSURGERY

This modality of treatment is a technique of high precision localised radiotherapy allowing high dose radiation to the target volume with minimal dose to surrounding normal tissue. Its main use is in the treatment of brain metastases. One very large fraction (stereotactic radiosurgery) or 2–3 smaller fractions (stereotactic radiotherapy) are usually given. Proper immobilisation with a stereotactic frame attached to the skull is required to ensure very accurate delivery of the high dose radiation, which can be delivered by the ^{60}Co gamma knife or a linear accelerator with specialised collimators. Both techniques rely on the production of multiple thin (pencil) radiation beams focused on a small volume (maximum tumour size usually 3–4 cm).

CLINICAL USE AND INDICATIONS FOR RADIOTHERAPY

RADICAL TREATMENT

Radiotherapy may be curative as a single modality or when combined concurrently with chemotherapy (Table 5.1).

TABLE 5.1 Cancers potentially curable with single modality radiotherapy or chemoradiotherapy

Radiotherapy alone	Chemoradiotherapy
Anus	Anus
Bladder	Cervix
Prostate	Oesophagus
Penis	Head and neck
Cervix	Lung
Uterus	Vulva
Vagina	
Lung	
Head and neck	
Seminoma (stage IIA)	
Skin cancers	
Lymphoma (stage I/II)	

Radical radiotherapy tends to involve complex planning and a protracted fractionated course of treatment. Most radical treatments are given over 4–6 weeks, in 1.8–2.75 Gy fractions with 20–30 fractions to a total dose of 50–70 Gy. Much lower doses (35–40 Gy) are required for seminomas and lymphomas.

Concurrent chemoradiotherapy requires scheduling of chemotherapy during the course of radiotherapy. Further cycles of chemotherapy before and after the radiotherapy may also be administered. Toxicity is often a significant problem and patients should be monitored closely throughout treatment.

ADJUVANT TREATMENT

Radiotherapy is commonly used in the adjuvant setting following initial surgery or chemotherapy. The aim of treatment is to eradicate locoregional residual microscopic disease. Adjuvant radiotherapy doses are usually slightly less than the doses used for radical treatment of macroscopic disease, but treatment planning may be just as complicated. The following cancers may require adjuvant radiotherapy following surgery: breast cancer, sarcomas, endometrial cancer, and head and neck cancer.

NEOADJUVANT TREATMENT

Radiotherapy or chemoradiotherapy may be given prior to surgery either to increase operability by downstaging the disease and/or to treat locoregional microscopic disease. Examples include the treatment of locally advanced rectal cancer and vulval cancer.

PALLIATIVE TREATMENT

Radiotherapy has a crucial role in the palliative setting and is effective for a variety of symptoms:

1. Pain – especially pain from bone metastases, but also visceral pain
2. Bleeding – haematuria, haemoptysis, PR bleeding, bleeding/fungating ulcers
3. Tumour obstruction of a hollow organ, e.g. bronchus, oesophagus, rectum
4. Superior vena cava obstruction (SVCO)
5. Spinal cord compression
6. Symptoms from brain metastases and leptomeningeal disease
7. Skin metastases
8. Symptomatic nodal disease.

Palliative radiotherapy is given over a shorter period of time with larger fraction sizes but a lower overall dose. Patient set-up and radiotherapy techniques are often very simple. Treatment may be given as a single fraction (e.g. 8–10 Gy) or as a short fractionated course (e.g. 20 Gy in 5 fractions, 30 Gy in 10 fractions).

HIGH DOSE/RADICAL PALLIATION

Sometimes it is appropriate to offer higher doses of fractionated palliative radiotherapy to achieve local control of the primary tumour and possibly improve survival. Radical palliation is most commonly used in head and neck cancer treatment, where control of local symptoms is particularly important. Other examples include locally advanced pelvic cancers, locally advanced lung cancer and brain tumours.

SIDE EFFECTS AND TOXICITY OF RADIOTHERAPY

Radiotherapy causes a broad spectrum of normal tissue reactions that limit the total dose of radiation that can be delivered safely to a tumour. The severity and time course of the reactions depends on the total dose of radiation, the fraction size, overall treatment time, tissue type, the volume of tissue irradiated and the clinical state of the patient. The achievable tumour control rate depends on the radiation tolerance of normal tissues.

Radiation effects on normal tissues can broadly be divided into early/acute, subacute and late reactions.

EARLY/ACUTE REACTIONS (Table 5.2)

These occur during, immediately after or within a few weeks of the end of treatment. Acute effects are due to depletion of stem cells and therefore the tissues most affected tend to be the rapidly proliferating tissues such as skin, mucosal tissue and haemopoietic tissue. The intensity of the reaction reflects the difference between stem cell loss and clonogen renewal. Acute reactions are usually self-limiting and normally settle within a few weeks of treatment completion.

TABLE 5.2 Acute effects of radiotherapy

Tissue	Acute reaction	Management
Skin	Erythemas, hair loss, dry desquamation, moist desquamation, and ulceration	Moisturising creams (with hydrocortisone for severe reactions). Dressings for moist desquamation. Antibiotics for infections
Gastrointestinal tract	Oropharyngeal mucositis	Oral hygiene, antibacterial mouthwashes, analgesia, antibiotics/antifungals for infection
	Oesophagitis/gastritis	Mucaine liquid, analgesia, antacids
	Gastroenteritis	Antidiarrhoeals (e.g. loperamide 2 mg p.r.n.) Antiemetics (5-HT$_3$ antagonists if severe and large volume treated)
	Proctitis	Stool softeners, anti-diarrhoeals, steroid enemas (e.g. Proctofoam)
Lung	Pneumonitis	Steroids. May need prolonged course if severe
Bladder	Cystitis – frequency and dysuria	Fluids, analgesia
Bone marrow	Suppression of erythropoiesis	Appropriate transfusions, growth factors, treat infections
Eye	Conjunctivitis, dry eye	Treat infections, artificial tears
Ear	Acute otitis externa, serous otitis	Treat infections. May need topical steroids or myringotomy

SUBACUTE REACTIONS (EARLY DELAYED)

These reactions usually occur between 1 and 6 months after completion of radiotherapy and are usually self-limiting over a period of a few weeks or months. The commonest examples include:

- Radiation pneumonitis. Often responds well to a course of oral steroids.
- Lhermitte's sign. This is an electric shock-like pain that shoots down the spine and represents a reversible type of demyelination injury following spinal cord irradiation.
- Somnolence syndrome. Usually occurs 2–5 weeks following brain irradiation and manifests as a transient period of severe exhaustion, lethargy and anorexia lasting typically for a few weeks.

LATE REACTIONS (Table 5.3)

The late effects of radiation are usually the dose-limiting effects and tend to affect slowly proliferating tissues such as nervous tissue, lung, kidney, liver and heart. Such effects include tissue necrosis, fibrosis and stricture formation, non-healing ulcers and fistulation, cataracts and retinopathy, neuropathy, nephritis, hepatitis, pericarditis, xerostomia and pneumonitis. Pituitary or thyroid irradiation may cause endocrine dysfunction. These effects develop over months or many years following irradiation and are usually progressive. Late effects are more common and severe with greater total doses of radiation, larger fraction sizes and larger treatment volumes. Damage to stromal tissue (vasculature and connective tissue) and reduced proliferative capacity of stem cells are thought to be the main mechanisms for the late effects of radiotherapy (see Appendix 1 for normal tissue tolerance doses and late effects on tissues).

Carcinogenesis is also a late complication following radiotherapy. The latency period for solid malignancies is around 20 years. Leukaemia may occur between 7 and 12 years following radiotherapy.

FUTURE PERSPECTIVES IN RADIOTHERAPY

Current research in radiotherapy is based around technological and biological optimisation of treatment. IMRT is a focus of much interest because of the potential for dose escalation and hence greater local tumour control. Improvements in imaging techniques and planning software allow much greater planning accuracy and treatment verification. New simulators now have inbuilt CT scanners that aid target volume localisation. Particle therapy with protons does have some clinical application but like heavy particle

TABLE 5.3 Examples of late tissue effects

Tissue	Clinical manifestations of late effects
CNS, spinal cord	Lethargy, cognitive impairment, dementia, seizures and ultimately death. Pituitary dysfunction. Spinal cord and peripheral nerve injury may lead to myelopathy and neuropathies respectively
Eye	Cataracts, retinopathy and dry eye
Gastrointestinal	Strictures, obstruction, perforation, bleeding, diarrhoea, and malabsorption. Surgical intervention may be required
Liver	Veno-occlusive disease, hepatitis, ascites and liver failure
Bladder and urethra	Haemorrhagic cystitis, obstructive uropathy, bladder spasms, reduced bladder capacity
Kidney	Hypertension, renal impairment, renal failure
Lungs	Fibrosis, restrictive lung disease
Heart	Pericarditis, cardiomyopathy, valvular disease (mainly aortic valve), arrhythmias (due to conduction system fibrosis), coronary artery disease and myocardial infarction
Head and neck	Xerostomia, laryngeal necrosis, hypothyroidism, Osteoradionecrosis
Female organs	Early menopause, infertility, vaginal strictures and dryness, fistula formation, lymphoedema, telangiectasias and bleeding
Male organs	Infertility, impotence, low volume ejaculate, lymphoedema, telangiectasia
Skin, muscle, bone	Hair loss, fibrosis, contractures, mobility problems, growth problems (mainly in children), osteoporosis, telangiectasias, lymphoedema, permanent hair loss, dysmorphia

therapy is mainly confined to research centres due to cost and logistics. Altered fractionation regimens such as CHART continue to be evaluated. The use of radiosensitisers and radioprotectants is still under clinical investigation. Chemoradiotherapy (CRT) is now the mainstay of treatment for many cancers, but further research into late toxicity and the optimum dosing and scheduling of CRT regimens is needed. Intraoperative radiotherapy (IORT) has shown promising results in head and neck cancer and GI cancer, but is under further evaluation. The combination of radiotherapy and hyperthermia is very attractive in theory, but technically challenging and thus is mainly being assessed in research centres with the appropriate facilities. Systemic radioimmunotherapy involves coupling of targeted monoclonal antibodies to radioactive isotopes and early clinical trials have shown promise, especially in the treatment of lymphoma. Improvements in molecular cancer pathology and predictive assays for tumour response to radiotherapy may one day allow greater individualisation of treatment.

FURTHER READING

Dobbs J, Barret A, Ash D V 1999 Practical radiotherapy planning, 3rd edn. Arnold, London
Steel G 1997 Basic clinical radiobiology, 2nd edn. Arnold, London
Withers H R 1992 Biological basis of radiation therapy for cancer. Lancet 339:156

CHAPTER 6

Principles of systemic therapy

INTRODUCTION

Although surgery and radiotherapy remain the major primary modalities for treatment of most cancers, the majority of cancer patients (60–70%) still develop metastatic disease and therefore systemic therapy is also a key modality in the multidisciplinary management of cancer. The improved understanding of the molecular biology of cancer has led to novel therapeutic targets and the development of many new anti-cancer agents.

Systemic therapy currently encompasses chemotherapy, hormonal manipulation and biological therapy. The main aims of treatment are cure, prolongation of survival, symptom relief and improved quality of life.

PRINCIPLES OF CHEMOTHERAPY

Chemotherapy involves using cytotoxic drugs to treat cancer. Systemic chemotherapy is most commonly used in the adjuvant and palliative metastatic settings. Some tumours are potentially curable with chemotherapy alone even in the advanced setting (Table 6.1). There is also an increasing trend in combining chemotherapy and radiotherapy concurrently.

Cytotoxic chemotherapy drugs are used at the limits of toxicity and efficacy more than any other group of drugs in clinical practice. Maximising efficacy and safety are the prime consideration in chemotherapy practice and this requires a detailed knowledge of the principles of tumour growth and cell cycle kinetics, pharmacokinetics and pharmacodynamics. The concepts of drug

TABLE 6.1 Potentially curable tumours with chemotherapy

Adult	Paediatric
Germ cell tumours	Acute lymphoblastic leukaemia
Gestational trophoblastic disease	Hodgkin's lymphoma
Hodgkin's lymphoma	NHL
Non-Hodgkin's lymphoma (NHL)	Burkitt's lymphoma
Acute leukaemias	Wilms' tumour
Small cell lung cancer	Ewing's sarcoma
Ovarian cancer	Embryonal rhabdomyosarcoma
	Neuroblastoma
	Germ cell tumours

scheduling, drug administration, dose intensity, combination chemotherapy, and high dose therapy are all based on these fundamental principles.

TUMOUR GROWTH AND CELL CYCLE KINETICS

The proliferation rate of a tumour is not constant throughout its lifetime. As tumours enlarge, there is a decrease in the growth rate and the proportion of proliferating cells, and an increase in cell loss leading to a longer doubling time. This is mainly due to reduced blood supply, leading to cellular hypoxia, decreased cellular nutrition and cell death. Tumour effects on the host may exacerbate these factors. The growth pattern of human tumours can be modelled mathematically by the Gompertz equation, which can be shown graphically as an S-shaped semi-log curve (Fig. 6.1). This shows the tumour growth rate slowing as the tumour becomes larger. Chemotherapy is most effective against actively dividing cells and therefore tumours with a higher fraction of proliferating cells with shorter doubling times (at the steepest part of the Gompertzian curve) are most likely to be chemosensitive. Large tumours at the top of the curve are likely to be more chemoresistant and less likely to be cured. The Gompertzian model also predicts that chemotherapy is more likely to be effective with a small tumour burden when the proliferating fraction is at its highest and this forms the basic concept for the use of adjuvant therapy.

The other main reason why larger tumours may be more chemoresistant is due to the development of resistant clones leading to tumour heterogeneity. The Goldie–Colman model suggests that the genetic instability of cancers leads to spontaneous mutations producing resistant malignant clones. As these events are relatively rare the probability of producing a successful malignant clone is greater in larger tumour cell populations. This is known as genetic resistance and helps to explain the inverse relationship between curability and tumour size. This model suggests that chemotherapy is most effective when the tumour burden is low, and when combinations of drugs are used to overcome tumour resistance (see below).

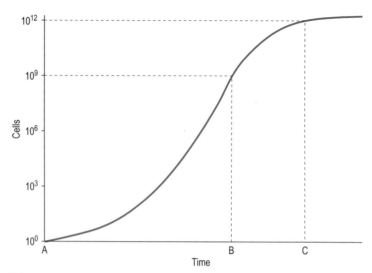

Notes:

B is the point in time that the tumour becomes clinically apparent.

C is the point in time that the tumour causes death.

A–B is the time interval between the development of the first cancerous cell and clinically apparent disease (pre-clinical disease).

B–C is the time interval between clinical detection of tumour and death (clinical disease).

As is clear from the curve, the time interval A–B is much greater than B–C. This helps to explain why tumours have often spread prior to the development of clinical symptoms.

Chemotherapy is most likely to be effective during the steepest part of the curve i.e. before the tumour is clinically detectable.

Chemotherapy is less effective when the curve flattens out and this partially explains why response rates are lower with very large tumours burdens.

FIGURE 6.1 Gompertzian model of tumour growth.

The fractional cell kill hypothesis suggests a certain fraction of cancer cells (not a certain absolute number) will be killed with each course of chemotherapy. According to this hypothesis, chemotherapy can never reduce the number of cancer cells to zero, because the fraction of cells killed is never 100%. However, repeated treatments will continue to decrease the tumour size. This theory assumes all cancers are equally responsive and that drug resistance and metastases do not occur, e.g.

1000 cells ⟶ 100 cells ⟶ 10 cells ⟶ 1 cell
     90% cell kill   90% cell kill   90% cell kill

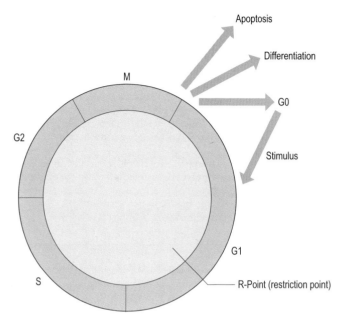

FIGURE 6.2 The cell cycle.

The cell cycle

All dividing cells pass through the cell cycle (Fig. 6.2), which is divided into distinct phases:

G1-phase – gap phase. Enzymes necessary for DNA synthesis are produced. Lasts 0–30 hours.

S-phase – synthesis phase. The total amount of DNA is doubled (DNA is duplicated). Lasts 6–8 hours.

G2-phase – second gap period. Specialised proteins and RNA are synthesised. Lasts 2–4 hours.

M-phase – mitosis stage when cell division occurs. Prophase–metaphase–anaphase–telophase. Lasts <1 hour.

G0-phase – resting phase. The cell is not committed to division, but certain stimuli such as local growth factors can stimulate the cell into the cell cycle.

Most chemotherapy drugs have their greatest effect on cells actively proliferating in the cell cycle and do not cause cellular death in the G0-phase. This is probably due to the fact that cells in the G0-phase have time to repair DNA damage. The proportion of proliferating cells within the cell cycle compared to the total population of cells is called the growth fraction. Most normal tissues have a growth fraction of 20–30%, which is lower than most tumours, and this has important therapeutic implications because chemotherapy will have a greater effect on the tissue with the highest growth fraction, i.e. the tumour. However, some normal tissues such as bone marrow and intestinal epithelium have a very high proliferation rate (often higher than tumours) and some tumours have a very low proliferation rate. Therefore, the chemotherapy doses needed to shrink the tumour may cause severe normal tissue toxicity, e.g. severe myelosuppression. This explains why the therapeutic index (or 'window') is often very narrow in cancer chemotherapy.

Some chemotherapy drugs are also cell cycle phase specific, which means they are more toxic to cells at certain stages of the cell cycle. For example, 5FU is S-phase specific and vincristine is M-phase specific. Drugs are therefore often classified as cell cycle phase specific or non-phase specific. This has important implications for chemotherapy scheduling (see below).

PHARMACOLOGY

As described above, the therapeutic index in the chemotherapy of cancer is narrow, and therefore an understanding of the variability in toxicity and response to treatment is very important. This variability can be divided into two main aspects:

Pharmacokinetics. This describes 'what the body does to the drug'. It is the study of the concentration-time history of drugs in relation to absorption, distribution, metabolism and excretion.

Pharmacodynamics. This describes 'what the drug does to the body'. It is the study of dose–response relationships and describes the therapeutic effects and toxicity of drugs.

The understanding of pharmacokinetics helps to formulate the administration strategy in terms of dose, scheduling and the route of administration. Variations in pharmacokinetic parameters between patients also help to explain some of the inter-patient differences in toxicity and tumour response. The vast majority of cytotoxic drugs are dosed according to body surface area (BSA) because of the relationship between body size and physiological parameters such as renal function. This is an attempt to standardise chemotherapy drug dosing, but evidence for using BSA is very limited. Renal and liver dysfunction may lead to problems with excretion and metabolism of drugs and further dose adjustments are often required to prevent severe toxicity, whilst at the same time trying to maintain tumour drug concentration and exposure time.

Treatment toxicity and efficacy are key pharmacodynamic parameters that require monitoring throughout chemotherapy treatment. Dose adjustments or withdrawal of drugs may be needed if problematic toxicity occurs.

Assessment of symptom relief and measurement of tumour size (and/or tumour markers) are necessary to monitor clinical response to treatment, which will ultimately be key to further treatment decisions.

Scheduling

Chemotherapy is usually given cyclically because this allows recovery of normal tissue (usually the haemopoietic system) between cycles. Chemotherapy will only kill a certain fraction of cells and therefore repeated full dose treatments are required to maximise the effect on the tumour. Pharmacological factors must be taken into account for safe drug scheduling. Cytokinetics also influences specific sequencing of drugs. For example, cell cycle specific drugs generally achieve greater cell kill with continuous infusion or multiple doses. This is because there is more time for the drug to encounter the vulnerable phase of the cell cycle than there would be if it were given as a single bolus.

Combination chemotherapy

Single agent chemotherapy is rarely curative due to the development of drug-resistant malignant clones. Two or more drugs given simultaneously or in sequence will produce a broader range of coverage of resistant clones. This concept has led to cures in leukaemia, germ cell tumours and many paediatric tumours. When designing combination regimens it is important to consider the following principles:

1. Selected drugs should be active as single agents.
2. The drugs should preferably have different mechanisms of action to allow for additive or synergistic effects on the tumour.
3. Combinations of drugs with different resistance patterns minimise cross-resistance.
4. Drugs with different side effect profiles and different dose-limiting toxicities should be used.
5. There should be no known severe drug–drug interactions.

It should be noted that the combination of too many drugs might lead to the regimen being ineffective due to excessive toxicity requiring significant dose reductions and dose delays.

Dose intensity and high dose chemotherapy

Many human tumours show a positive dose–response relationship. This means that the higher the dose the greater the tumour response. However, dose intensification is restricted by normal tissue toxicity.

Dose intensity is an important concept and is usually expressed as the average dose given per week ($mg/m^2/week$). Dose intensity can be increased in the following ways:

1. High dose chemotherapy with haemopoietic rescue. Very high dose chemotherapy that is marrow ablative can be administered followed by

haemopoietic rescue with prior harvested peripheral stem cells or bone marrow allografting. This technique has been very effective in haematological malignancies and is often curative, but has been very disappointing in solid malignancies such as breast cancer and small cell lung cancer.

2. Changing scheduling. Instead of giving 3- or 4-weekly cycles of chemotherapy, a smaller less toxic once-weekly dose can be administered to achieve a higher total dose over the same time period.

3. Local drug administration. Local drug administration by the intrathecal, hepatic-arterial, portal-vein, intravesical and intraperitoneal routes, and isolated limb perfusion can produce very high local drug concentrations. However, with the exception of the proven intrathecal and intravesical routes, most of the techniques require further evaluation in clinical trials.

DRUG RESISTANCE

Despite combinations of drugs and the development of new drugs with different mechanisms of action, drug resistance is still the main reason for treatment failure. There are multiple mechanisms of resistance:

1. Cytokinetic drug resistance. Cellular sensitivity to phase-specific drugs depends on the cell cycle position.

2. Pharmacological resistance. Drug concentrations may be too low due to:
   - anatomical drug barriers – sanctuary sites (e.g. testes and CNS)
   - increased drug inactivation by normal tissues
   - increased normal tissue sensitivity leading to toxicity
   - increased excretion, decreased uptake or 'third spacing' of drugs.

3. Cellular/molecular resistance
   - Multiple drug resistance (MDR) gene. This encodes a cell membrane p-glycoprotein, which pumps drugs out of the cell (mainly anthracyclines, vinca alkaloids, taxanes).
   - Decreased cellular drug uptake.
   - Increased intracellular drug metabolism and detoxification. e.g. increased levels of glutathione, which binds to reactive metabolites preventing DNA damage, are found in resistant tumours.
   - Resistance to chemotherapy-induced apoptosis. Genetic mutations of vital genes involved in the mechanism of apoptosis lead to cancer cell 'immortality'.
   - Decreased drug activation. Many drugs are pro-drugs that require intracellular enzymatic conversion to active metabolites. Reduced expression of activating enzymes is common in tumours (e.g. cytochrome P450).
   - Gene amplification. Some drugs inhibit specific key cellular proteins, but genetic amplification can produce overexpression of these proteins and hence drug resistance.

- Altered expression of target proteins. Drugs with very specific action on a target protein will be less active if the target protein has been mutated.
- Increased repair of DNA damage.
- Immune escape mechanisms, e.g. loss of major histocompatibility complex (MHC) proteins that are vital for the immune response.

CLASSIFICATION OF CHEMOTHERAPY DRUGS

Chemotherapy drugs may be classified according to their mechanism of action (see also Appendix 2: A–Z of commonly used chemotherapy drugs).

1. Alkylating agents

These drugs damage cellular DNA by alkylation, and cell killing is cell cycle phase non-specific. This group encompasses a wide variety of drugs, which have a wide variety of potencies and toxicities. They are classified according to chemical structures and mechanisms of covalent bonding:

- nitrogen mustards – e.g. melphalan, chlorambucil, cyclophosphamide, ifosfamide
- nitrosoureas – e.g. lomustine (CCNU), carmustine (BCNU)
- alkane sulphonates – e.g. busulphan
- aziridines – e.g. thiotepa, mitomycin C
- tetrazines – e.g. dacarbazine and temozolomide.

2. Platinum analogues

Platinum complexes bind to DNA and form adducts/crosslinks between and along DNA strands causing cell death mainly by apoptosis. Cisplatin, carboplatin and oxaliplatin are the main agents in clinical use.

3. Antimetabolites

These agents are structural analogues of normal metabolites involved with DNA and RNA metabolism. They act by competing with or substituting with the normal metabolites, causing key enzyme inhibition or altered function of DNA and RNA. They are most active in the S-phase of the cell cycle, having little effect on cells in G0. They are classified into the following groups:

- antifolates – methotrexate
- fluoropyrimidines – 5-fluorouracil, capecitabine
- cytidine analogues – cytosine arabinoside, gemcitabine
- purine analogues – fludarabine, 6-mercaptopurine, 6-thioguanine.

4. Anti-tumour antibiotics

These agents include a wide variety of natural products of microbial metabolism and their synthetic analogues. There is considerable structural diversity among these compounds and hence a variety of mechanisms of action. Anthracyclines are the most important group in this class and disrupt DNA and RNA synthesis by causing DNA base-pair intercalation resulting in inhibition of the enzyme topo-isomerase II, which is vital to successful DNA replication. They also produce highly reactive free radicals resulting in DNA breakages. The anti-tumour antibiotics can be grouped as follows:

- anthracyclines – doxorubicin, epirubicin, daunorubicin, idarubicin
- non-anthracyclines – bleomycin, actinomycin D, mitoxantrone.

5. Mitotic spindle inhibitors
The vinca alkaloids and taxanes are mitotic spindle inhibitors. The mitotic spindle is composed of microtubules made up of polymerised tubulin subunits and is vital for successful cell division. Interference in the assembly or disassembly of microtubules causes metaphase arrest and therefore inhibition of cell division. The vinca alkaloids are derived from the periwinkle plant and inhibit microtubule assembly by binding to tubulin to prevent polymerisation. The taxanes are derived from yew tree bark and prevent disassembly of the microtubule by promoting stabilisation of the microtubule complex.

- Vinca alkaloids – vincristine, vinblastine, vinorelbine, vindesine
- Taxanes – paclitaxel, docetaxel.

6. Epipodophyllotoxins
Epipodophyllotoxins are derived from the May apple or mandrake plant. Although podophyllotoxin itself is a tubulin binder, its derivates act as DNA topo-isomerase II inhibitors. This important enzyme is vital to DNA replication and transcription. Etoposide and teniposide are the agents in clinical use.

7. Camptothecin analogues
Camptothecin is derived from the Chinese ornamental tree. The semisynthetic analogues irinotecan and topotecan inhibit the enzyme DNA topo-isomerase I, thereby preventing the elongation phase of DNA replication.

8. Differentiation agents
Differentiation agents can induce cells to an irreversible commitment to terminal differentiation, i.e. the cell is fully differentiated and cannot re-enter the cell cycle. The retinoids are the most important member of this group and have been very successful in the treatment of leukaemia, e.g. all-*trans*-retinoic acid (ATRA).

9. Miscellaneous
- Hydroxyurea. Inhibits DNA synthesis by inhibition of ribonucleotide reductase.

- Procarbazine. Monoamine oxidase inhibitor, which inhibits RNA, DNA and protein synthesis.
- L-Asparaginase. Catalyses the breakdown of asparagine, which is an important amino acid already lacking in malignant lymphoid cells.

DEFINITIONS IN CHEMOTHERAPY

Adjuvant   In patients with no evidence of macroscopic disease following successful surgery and/or radiotherapy, several courses of chemotherapy are given with the aim of destroying any microscopic residual cancer cells. This has been a successful approach in breast cancer, colorectal cancer and ovarian cancer. (The term may also be applied to hormonal therapies.)

Neoadjuvant   Chemotherapy is given to patients prior to surgery or radiotherapy. This may shrink or downstage a tumour to increase operability (or allow a smaller radiation field) and also treats metastatic disease. Further adjuvant chemotherapy is sometimes given following the surgery and/or radiation. A good example is the treatment of inflammatory breast cancer.

Primary chemotherapy   Chemotherapy is given with curative intent as the main treatment modality, e.g. germ cell tumours, lymphomas and choriocarcinoma.

Palliative   Chemotherapy is given with the aim of improving/controlling symptoms, improving quality of life and prolonging life.

Salvage   Following failure of another mode of treatment, chemotherapy is given with curative intent. An example includes the use of the BEP chemotherapy regimen following relapse of stage I or IIA seminoma after primary radiotherapy.

Induction   High dose chemotherapy is given to induce a complete remission when initiating a curative regimen. Mostly applies to haematological malignancy.

Consolidation   Following a complete remission to an induction regimen, the treatment is repeated to try to increase the cure rate or the duration of remission.

Intensification   Following complete remission to an induction regimen, higher doses of the same chemotherapy drugs are given to try to increase cure rates or the duration of remission. Mostly applies to haematological malignancy.

Maintenance   Following complete remission, long-term low dose chemotherapy is given to prevent relapse of disease. Mostly applies to haematological malignancy.

SIDE EFFECTS AND COMPLICATIONS OF CHEMOTHERAPY

Chemotherapy is toxic to normal tissues and may cause numerous significant side effects and complications. The most important are discussed below. (For toxicity of individual drugs, see Appendix 2.) Severe toxicity may require dose reductions, delay of chemotherapy, withdrawal of individual drugs (that are most likely to be the cause of the toxicity), or complete withdrawal of the chemotherapy regimen.

MYELOSUPPRESSION AND NEUTROPENIC SEPSIS

Myelosuppression is common to most chemotherapy regimens and is the main dose-limiting side effect. It also results from malignant infiltration of the bone marrow and can be exacerbated by radiotherapy. It is a major cause of cancer mortality due to its main complications of infection and bleeding.

I. Neutropenic sepsis

This is one of the most feared and dangerous complications of cancer and its treatment. Approximately 50–60% of neutropenic patients with a fever will have an infection and ~20% of patients with a neutrophil count less than $0.1 \times 10^9/l$ will have a bacteraemia. The commonest organisms are Gram-positive cocci (e.g. coagulase-negative staphylococci, *Staph. aureus*, streptococci) or Gram-negative bacilli (e.g. *E. coli*, *Klebsiella*, *Pseudomonas*). Fungal infections usually arise after prolonged bouts of neutropenia. Viral infections can also be very severe in the immunocompromised.

Neutropenia is defined as a neutrophil count less than $1.0 \times 10^9/l$. The risk of major infection increases with counts less than $0.5 \times 10^9/l$ and again at $0.1 \times 10^9/l$. The risk is also greater with a rapidly falling count. Fever is defined as a single temperature $\geq 38°C$ or a sustained fever of $37.5°C$ over at least one hour. The diagnosis of neutropenic sepsis should also be assumed in afebrile patients with shock (systolic BP <90 mmHg or decrease of 50 mmHg in hypertensive patients), multi-organ failure, and DIC.

All acute hospitals should have written protocols for investigation and management of neutropenic sepsis. Empirical intravenous antibiotics should be started immediately with appropriate resuscitation measures. If fever persists, antibiotics should be changed and antifungals added as per local protocols. Outpatient oral antibiotic therapy may be indicated for low risk patients, i.e. patients who are well with no associated medical co-morbidity and an expected short period of neutropenia (less than 10 days).

2. Thrombocytopenia

This is defined as a platelet count of $<150 \times 10^9/l$, but the risk of bleeding only significantly increases with platelet counts below $50 \times 10^9/l$ (unless there is an associated coagulopathy). Platelet transfusions aiming to keep the platelet count above $50 \times 10^9/l$ should be offered if there is active bleeding. If there is no bleeding, transfusions are only necessary when the platelet count falls below $10 \times 10^9/l$. Severe chemotherapy-induced thrombocytopenia is rare.

3. Anaemia

Chemotherapy-induced anaemia requiring transfusion is uncommon and if haemoglobin levels fall below $9 \times g/dl$, other causes should be sought. Symptomatic anaemia may respond well to blood transfusions or erythropoietin.

EMESIS (NAUSEA AND VOMITING)

Severe chemotherapy-induced emesis is one of the most distressing side effects of cancer treatment and dramatically affects quality of life. It may compromise potential cure by limiting the dose of chemotherapy and may shorten life in the palliative setting due to nutritional/metabolic problems and general debilitation. Although the development of very effective antiemetic regimens has resolved many of these problems, some patients still have a difficult time. Certain risk factors for chemotherapy-induced emesis are recognised (Table 6.2).

Chemotherapy-induced emesis may be acute, delayed, anticipatory or refractory.

1. Acute

This usually occurs 2–6 hours after treatment, but may happen within minutes of administration. 5-HT$_3$ antagonists (e.g. granisetron or ondansetron) are highly effective and prevent vomiting in 70–90% of patients.

2. Delayed

This is defined as emesis occurring after 24 hours following cisplatin chemotherapy. It may last for several days and occurs in up to 50% of

---

TABLE 6.2 Risk factors for chemotherapy-induced emesis

Female sex
Young age
History of motion sickness or severe pregnancy-associated morning sickness
Anticipatory anxiety
History of alcohol induced nausea and vomiting
Gastritis
Dehydration

cisplatin-treated patients. 5-HT$_3$ antagonists are generally ineffective and the drugs of choice are dexamethasone and cyclizine.

3. Anticipatory

Anticipatory emesis is a psychological state that patients develop prior to chemotherapy administration. Any stimulus that is related to chemotherapy (e.g. sights, smells and even people) may evoke emesis. It occurs in up to 20% of patients and is more likely in those who have had severe emesis with previous cycles of chemotherapy. The best treatment is prevention, i.e. use the optimum antiemetic schedule. Psychotherapy, hypnosis and anxiolytics (e.g. lorazepam) may also help.

4. Refractory

For patients with refractory emesis, a careful clinical evaluation should be made to identify any obvious cause, e.g. pain, infection, bowel obstruction, constipation, raised intracranial pressure and medication. Consider adding metoclopramide, domperidone, haloperidol, methotrimeprazine or cyclizine. Other options include adding anxiolytics such as lorazepam (1 mg) or using syringe drivers with cyclizine (150 mg over 24 hours) or methotrimeprazine (75–150 mg over 24 hours).

Chemotherapy drugs have different emetogenic potentials (Table 6.3). Combinations of drugs and high dose schedules increase emetogenic potential.

Chemotherapy with high risk regimens requires intravenous and oral dexamethasone and 5-HT$_3$ antagonists, pre- and post-treatment. Other antiemetics such as metoclopramide or domperidone may be added. Intermediate risk regimens require dexamethasone plus metoclopramide or domperidone. Low risk regimens may need metoclopramide or domperidone alone.

MUCOSITIS

A common problem, which may be very painful and affect nutrition. Secondary infection and poor dentition worsen the problem. Good mouth

TABLE 6.3 Emetogenic potentials of various chemotherapy agents

High risk	Moderate risk	Low risk
Cisplatin	Cyclophosphamide	Bleomycin
Carboplatin	Etoposide	Chlorambucil
Dacarbazine	Taxanes	Vinca alkaloids
Anthracyclines	Methotrexate	Melphalan
Ifosfamide	Irinotecan/topotecan	5FU
High dose cyclophosphamide	Mitomycin C	Hydroxyurea
Carmustine	Gemcitabine	

care with antiseptic $\pm$ anaesthetic mouthwashes is required. Sucking ice cubes at the time of chemotherapy can also be helpful.

ALOPECIA

This is reversible and usually noticeable 1–2 weeks following chemotherapy and most apparent at 1–2 months. Main causes are anthracyclines, alkylating agents, etoposide, taxanes and vinca alkaloids. Scalp cooling can be effective at preventing hair loss, but should not be used in patients with leukaemia or at risk of scalp metastases.

DIARRHOEA

This is usually mild, but may be life-threatening, especially if it is associated with neutropenic infection. Typhlitis is a life-threatening (30% mortality rate) Gram-negative infection of the caecum that usually occurs in neutropenic patients. Urgent treatment with intravenous fluid resuscitation and antibiotics is required and surgical intervention may be necessary. Life threatening diarrhoea may also result from the cholinergic syndrome seen with irinotecan and also occurs in patients with dihydropyrimidine dehydrogenase (DPD) deficiency receiving 5FU.

CONSTIPATION

Can be caused by chemotherapy drugs and antiemetics (e.g. cyclizine and 5-HT_3 inhibitors). Vinca alkaloids may cause an autonomic neuropathy, which often results in constipation.

CNS TOXICITY

1. Peripheral neuropathy
This is the most common form of neurotoxicity. It is usually sensory in the glove and stocking distribution, but may progress to loss of tendon reflexes, functional impairment and weakness. Usually due to cisplatin, oxaliplatin, taxanes, and vinca alkaloids. Symptoms often improve after discontinuation of the drug, but may sometimes be permanent.

2. Cranial nerve toxicity
Ototoxicity with progressive loss of high-tone hearing and/or tinnitus occurs with cisplatin.

3. Autonomic neuropathy
May cause abdominal pain, paralytic ileus, constipation, urinary retention, postural hypotension and bradycardias. Vinca alkaloids and cisplatin are the usual causes.

4. Cerebellar toxicity

Ataxia and nystagmus can result from administration of cytarabine and 5FU.

5. Encephalopathy

An acute encephalopathy with symptoms of confusion, seizures, agitation, somnolence and coma can be caused by a number of drugs. Ifosfamide is the usual cause and methylene blue is an effective antidote to this drug.

RENAL TOXICITY

Several drugs are nephrotoxic, but cisplatin is responsible for the majority of cases. Adequate saline pre-hydration and a good urine output (>100 ml/h) are crucial to minimise cisplatin's nephrotoxicity. An estimation or measurement of the patient's glomerular filtration rate (GFR) should be performed prior to treatment with any nephrotoxic chemotherapy drug.

LIVER TOXICITY

Chemotherapy-induced liver damage is caused by many drugs and occurs by a variety of mechanisms, including parenchymal injury with fatty change, necrosis, fibrosis, cholestasis, veno-occlusive disease, and vascular injury. Withdrawal of the offending drug is the mainstay of treatment.

PULMONARY TOXICITY

Occurs in 5–20% of patients receiving chemotherapy. Interstitial pneumonitis and pulmonary fibrosis are the usual manifestations with progressive dyspnoea being the predominant symptom. The drugs most commonly implicated are bleomycin, nitrosoureas, mitomycin C, busulphan and methotrexate. Pulmonary irradiation increases the risk of damage. Other pulmonary toxicities include bronchospasm due to hypersensitivity reactions and increased risk of pulmonary thromboembolism.

CARDIAC TOXICITY

This may include arrhythmias, cardiomyopathy, pericarditis, coronary artery disease, cardiac failure and myocardial infarction. Anthracyclines, taxanes, many alkylating agents and 5FU are the most cardiotoxic drugs. Toxicity is potentiated by mediastinal irradiation.

HYPERSENSITIVITY REACTIONS

Any drug can potentially cause a hypersensitivity reaction. The taxanes are responsible for the majority of chemotherapy-related cases and regimens including these drugs should include premedication with steroids and antihistamine drugs.

FEVER

Drug fevers are not uncommon and are most often caused by bleomycin, mitomycin and interferon.

EXTRAVASATION INJURY

Fortunately, extravasation injuries are now very rare due to improved cytotoxic drug administration techniques and greater awareness of the problem. Every chemotherapy unit should have an extravasation kit with treatment instructions. Cytotoxic drugs are classified as vesicants, irritants or non-vesicants (Table 6.4). Extravasation should be suspected if the patient complains of pain, swelling and redness around the injection site, especially if there was venous resistance to drug administration. A severe extravasation injury may cause skin necrosis, tendon injury and neurovascular damage leading to functional compromise. A plastic surgery opinion is needed if the extravasation is large or ulceration occurs as debridement and skin grafting may be necessary. Urgent treatment is therefore paramount to minimise the damage. The drug infusion should be stopped and 3–5 ml of blood aspirated from the cannula, which should then be removed. Further management depends on which vesicant was involved:

- Anthracycline extravasation should be treated with limb elevation and a cold compress to the affected site.
- Vinca alkaloid extravasation tends to be less severe and should be treated with a warm compress and hyaluronidase injections around the affected site to increase drug dispersion.

TABLE 6.4 Chemotherapy agents and extravasation injury		
Vesicants (potential to cause severe tissue damage and necrosis)	Irritants (potential to cause pain, phlebitis or local hypersensitivity reactions)	Non-irritants
Doxorubicin	Mitoxantrone	Bleomycin
Epirubicin	Busulphan	Cyclophosphamide
Daunorubicin	Etoposide	Ifosfamide
Mitomycin C	Docetaxel	Cytarabine
Vinca alkaloids	Cisplatin	Fludarabine
Paclitaxel	Carboplatin	Gemcitabine
Carmustine		Irinotecan
Dacarbazine		

- Paclitaxel extravasation is treated with a warm compress and local infiltration with hyaluronidase and hydrocortisone injections.
- Irritants are treated with limb elevation and cold compresses.

REPRODUCTIVE ORGANS

Chemotherapy can affect the gonadal function of men and women.

In men, the stromal Leydig and Sertoli cells are relatively resistant as they are non-proliferative. Therefore hormonal function is not usually affected. In contrast, seminiferous (germinal) stem cells are highly sensitive and spermatogenesis can be affected. Alkylating agents (e.g. cyclophosphamide, chlorambucil, nitrogen mustards, melphalan) are the most damaging agents to spermatogenesis and may cause transient or permanent azoospermia. Higher cumulative doses are more likely to result in permanent azoospermia. Cisplatin, doxorubicin and etoposide tend to cause transient and reversible azoospermia.

Alkylating agents are also the most gonadotoxic in women. They cause primary ovarian failure leading to oligomenorrhoea/amenorrhoea, hot flushes, vaginal dryness, decreased libido and low levels of circulating oestrogens with compensatory increases in follicle-stimulating hormone (FSH) and luteinising hormone (LH). Loss of maturing follicles and ova also result from treatment with alkylating agents. Recovery of ovarian function may occur after prolonged amenorrhoea, but this is less likely with increasing age.

SECONDARY MALIGNANCIES

Some chemotherapy agents are carcinogenic. Excessive second malignancies are seen with alkylating agents and etoposide. Acute myeloid leukaemia is by far the commonest second malignancy caused by chemotherapy and usually occurs within 10 years of drug exposure. Cyclophosphamide increases the risk of bladder cancer, but the risk of other solid malignancies is low with chemotherapy alone. However, the addition of radiotherapy to chemotherapy may increase the incidence of solid tumours such as breast cancer, lung cancer, sarcomas, melanoma and thyroid cancer, as seen in many patients treated for Hodgkin's disease.

PRINCIPLES OF HORMONE THERAPY

A variety of hormones are well known to affect both the growth and development of tumours and withdrawal or inhibition of their effects has been shown to be effective for a number of tumour types. The main hormone-responsive cancers are breast, prostate and endometrial cancer and the main hormones involved are oestrogens, androgens and progesterones respectively. Thyroid cancer is also a hormone-responsive cancer, and suppression of thyroid-stimulating hormone (TSH) with thyroxine is important in the management of this disease.

There is much current interest in primary prevention of breast cancer and prostate cancer with hormonal agents – an example of chemoprevention. Breast cancer trials with adjuvant tamoxifen have shown a 30% reduction in the incidence of contralateral breast cancer, although there was an increased risk of endometrial cancer and thromboembolic disease. There are ongoing worldwide studies in this area.

Hormonal therapies may also be useful for treatment of paraneoplastic syndromes such as carcinoid syndrome (octreotide), symptoms of advanced cancer such as anorexia (progestogens and corticosteroids) and inflammation and oedema caused by cancer (corticosteroids).

The mechanisms by which hormonal therapies have their effect are as follows:

1. Downregulation of hypothalamic-pituitary axis, e.g. gonadotrophin agonists and antagonists
2. Blockade of hormone receptors, e.g. tamoxifen, non-steroidal anti-androgens
3. Inhibition of steroidogenesis, e.g. hydrocortisone, progestogens, aromatase inhibitors, adrenalectomy
4. Inhibition of peripheral steroidal conversion, e.g. aromatase inhibitors.

BREAST CANCER

1. Ovarian ablation
Surgical ovarian ablation (oophorectomy) was first shown by Beatson in 1896 to be an effective treatment for metastatic breast cancer. In premenopausal women, ovarian ablation causes a fall in circulating oestrogen to menopausal levels. Ovarian irradiation (X-ray menopause – X-RAM) or medical manipulation of the pituitary-gonadal axis with gonadotrophin agonists (GnRH analogues) can achieve the same effect. The different methods are equally effective in both the metastatic and adjuvant settings. Its role in combination with tamoxifen and chemotherapy is still under evaluation.

2. Tamoxifen
Tamoxifen is a non-steroidal oestrogen antagonist with partial agonist activity. Its precise mechanism of action is unknown, but it competitively inhibits oestrogen binding to the oestrogen receptor leading to inhibition of breast cancer cells. It also has anti-angiogenic effects and inhibitory effects on growth factors. Tamoxifen also has partial oestrogen agonist effects, which has both adverse and beneficial effects. The adverse effects include increased risk of endometrial cancer and thromboembolic disease and the beneficial

effects include lowering of cholesterol and improvement in bone mineral density in postmenopausal women.

Tamoxifen is an effective agent in both the adjuvant and metastatic settings in patients with (o)estrogen receptor (ER) and/or progesterone (PR) positive breast cancer. The standard daily dose is 20 mg. Side effects include vaginal bleeding and discharge, hot flushes and mood changes.

There is much current interest in the development of newer selective oestrogen receptor modulators (SERMs) that will hopefully have fewer side effects and greater beneficial effects than tamoxifen.

3. Aromatase inhibitors

The aromatase enzyme is located in peripheral adipose and skeletal tissue and converts steroidal androgens into oestrogens. The aromatase inhibitors comprise non-steroidal inhibitors (anastrozole and letrozole) and steroidal inhibitors (exemestane and formestane). These drugs further suppress oestrogen levels in postmenopausal women. Anastrozole is the most commonly used aromatase inhibitor in the UK. Its main use is in postmenopausal patients with hormone receptor positive metastatic breast cancer as either a first or second line agent. It is now generally preferred to tamoxifen as it has fewer side effects and less risk of endometrial cancer. Mature results are awaited from the ATAC trial before it is accepted as a first line adjuvant therapy in postmenopausal women. It should only be used in premenopausal women following ovarian ablation.

4. Progestogens

The mechanisms of action of progestogens are complex and include suppression of oestrogen receptors and adrenal steroid synthesis, alterations in hormone metabolism, effects on growth factors and direct cytotoxic effects. Medroxyprogesterone and megestrol acetate are the main progestogens in clinical use. They are now much less commonly used in breast cancer treatment due to the development of the aromatase inhibitors. However, they can be used in the third line metastatic setting and are also useful for the treatment of hot flushes and anorexia. Side effects include nausea and weight gain.

PROSTATE CANCER

1. Castration

This may be achieved either surgically by bilateral orchidectomy, or medically with GnRH (gonadotrophin releasing hormone) analogues. Both are very effective in the treatment of metastatic prostate cancer, with up to 80% of patients responding. Goserelin and leuprorelin are the most commonly used GnRH analogues and are given by subcutaneous injection 1- or 3-monthly. They cause an initial increase in gonadotrophin (FSH and LH) release from the pituitary, followed by an inhibition due to loss of the normal pulsatile stimulation of the pituitary. The initial excessive gonadotrophin release is responsible for the tumour flare effect and although rarely clinically significant it is common practice to prevent its occurrence with a non-steroidal anti-androgen. The development of GnRH antagonists will prevent the tumour flare problem and will be commercially available soon. The main side effects are hot flushes, impotence and erectile dysfunction, gynaecomastia, depression and mood swings.

2. Non-steroidal anti-androgens
These drugs are androgen receptor antagonists and block the effect of dihydrotestosterone on prostate cancer cells. Plasma testosterone levels may actually increase and therefore side effects are less severe than with GnRH analogues, except for gynaecomastia. Flutamide and bicalutamide are the two main drugs used in the UK.

3. Steroidal anti-androgens
Cyproterone acetate is the main drug in this class. It has a complex mechanism of action that includes inhibition of the androgen receptor and progestogenic effects. Since the introduction of the non-steroidal anti-androgens its use has declined mainly due to its side effect profile of liver dysfunction and thromboembolic risk.

4. Oestrogens
Diethylstilbestrol (DES) is very effective in the treatment of prostate cancer, but its use has been limited because of its association with excessive deaths from cardiovascular events. It is usually a third line agent and should be combined with aspirin to reduce its prothrombotic effect. DES is now being replaced by ethinylestradiol.

5. Progestogens
Progestogens can be used to treat prostate cancer, but their use has been superseded by other agents. They are useful for the treatment of hot flushes.

6. Hydrocortisone
Often used as a last resort following treatment failure of other hormonal agents. Response rates of 10% have been reported, but are usually short-lived. Low dose dexamethasone 1.5–2 mg may be more effective.

ENDOMETRIAL CANCER

1. Progestogens
Medroxyprogesterone or megestrol acetate can be used to treat patients with hormone receptor positive metastatic endometrial cancer. Response rates are ~30% and duration of response is ~6–10 months. There is no evidence of benefit in the adjuvant setting.

2. Tamoxifen

Tamoxifen has been used to treat metastatic disease, but is less effective than progestogens.

CARCINOID SYNDROME

Octreotide

Octreotide is a somatostatin analogue that has been extremely effective in the palliative symptom management of carcinoid syndrome and pancreatic hormone secreting tumours. Response rates are high and often prolonged for many months or years. It inhibits the somatostatin receptor and decreases secretion of insulin, glucagon, pancreatic polypeptide and gastrin.

PRINCIPLES OF BIOLOGICAL THERAPY

The recent advances in molecular biology have led to a greater understanding of the mechanisms of the cancer process and the body's response to it. Biological therapy produces an anti-cancer effect by either targeting the cancer directly with natural substances or by enhancing the body's own defence responses. Several biological approaches have been developed and are discussed below.

IMMUNOTHERAPY

1. Cytokines

These are substances produced by a variety of cell types that regulate the immune response. The main cytokines are:

1. Interferons. Represent a family of naturally occurring proteins, first recognised for their ability to confer cellular resistance to viral infection. They have anti-proliferative and immunomodulatory functions. There are three main types – alpha interferon, beta interferon and gamma interferon, but alpha interferon is the most useful in cancer therapy, having useful activity in CML, follicular lymphoma, myeloma, renal cancer, melanoma, carcinoid, Kaposi's sarcoma and hairy cell leukaemia. Side effects include a flu-like syndrome that can be severely debilitating.
2. Interleukins. There are numerous interleukins that have been identified, but interleukin-2 (IL-2) is clinically the most important. It stimulates the production of T-lymphocytes, natural killer (NK) cells, and lymphokine-activated killer (LAK) cells. It has mainly been used in the treatment of malignant melanoma and renal cancer, but its use has been limited due to severe side effects at higher doses, e.g. capillary leak syndrome resulting in multi-organ failure.

3. Tumour necrosis factor alpha (TNF-α). Normally produced by macrophages and has shown anti-tumour activity in many human tumour cell lines. Unfortunately it is too toxic to be given systemically at a therapeutic dose, but has been used with some success in isolated limb perfusion for malignant melanoma.

2. Haemopoietic growth factors

These are normally produced by lymphocytes and macrophages and include granulocyte colony-stimulating factor (G-CSF), granulocyte-macrophage colony-stimulating factor (GM-CSF). They stimulate the maturation of granulocyte and macrophages and are very useful for promoting bone marrow recovery following cytotoxic chemotherapy.

3. Monoclonal antibodies (MAbs)

The development of MAbs against tumour antigens is an exciting area in cancer treatment. Tumour cells can be targeted by specific antibodies, which then activate an immune response to cause tumour cell death. Success in the clinical setting has now been achieved with a number of MAbs including rituximab (lymphocyte anti-CD20 antibody) for lymphomas and trastuzumab (antibody to the HER-2/*neu* receptor) for breast cancer. Specific MAbs can also be conjugated with toxins (immunotoxins) or radioisotopes (radioimmunotherapy) to improve cell kill and many of these agents are undergoing clinical trials.

4. Tumour vaccines

The immune response to tumours may be enhanced by exposure to various immunostimulants, which may be specific (e.g. tumour antigens or tumour cells), non-specific (e.g. viral and bacterial proteins), or cell-based. This forms the basis of tumour vaccine-based therapy. The following are examples of vaccine therapy:

1. Adjuvant immunogens. Various immunoglobulins, viral and bacterial proteins have been used in clinical trials to improve immune responses.
2. Tumour antigens and cell-based vaccines. Tumours that have been removed can be lethally irradiated or lysed and infused back into the patient to try and enhance the immune response. This can be similarly attempted with a pool of allogeneic tumour cells. Specific protein vaccines can also be used, e.g. MAGE 1 melanoma antigen. Clinical trials mainly in melanoma are ongoing.
3. DNA-vaccines. Plasmid DNA that produces cancer-specific antigens can be injected into tumour tissue, but this remains investigational.
4. Dendritic cell-based vaccines. Dendritic cells (DCs) are extremely important cells in the immune response because they are the main antigen-presenting cells (APCs). They present antigens to T-lymphocytes and activate them. DCs can be removed and exposed to tumour cells and then

reinfused to stimulate an immune response to the tumour. Encouraging early results have been seen in melanoma patients.

GENE THERAPY

Gene therapy involves the introduction of genetic material into cells for a therapeutic purpose. A variety of different approaches are possible, but all require successful gene transfer and expression. The commonest and most effective mode of gene transfer is with viruses, but other methods involve direct injection into tissue, liposomal delivery and DNA-coated gold bead pellet guns ('gene guns'). Potential therapeutic approaches include the following:

- Enhancing immune response, e.g. by introducing cytokine genes or specific antigen genes into tumours.
- Enhancing immune cells; e.g. introduce IL-2 gene to improve survival of T-cells or TNF gene to increase killing effect of T-cells.
- Replacing defective tumour suppressor genes in tumour cells, e.g. p53 gene.
- Introduce suicide genes into tumour cells.
- Antisense oligonucleotides. These are short DNA sequences that prevent expression of vital genes within the tumour cell.
- Introduce multidrug resistance genes into normal tissues, e.g. haemopoietic stem cells. This will allow more toxic therapies to be given safely.

Gene therapy is still in its infancy. The difficulty of successful gene delivery and expression without producing the associated risks of insertional mutagenesis (i.e. may cause cancer if gene inserted in the wrong place) and viral infection remains a major obstacle.

ANGIOGENESIS INHIBITORS

A tumour's growth is dependent on its blood supply. Tumours produce a number of different molecules that promote angiogenesis. These include the vascular endothelial growth factor (VEGF) family, angiogenin, TNF-α, platelet-activating factor, nitric oxide, prostaglandins, transforming growth factor-β etc. Inhibitors of angiogenesis are also produced (e.g. thrombospondin, angiostatin) and there is normally a balance between inhibition and promotion. The multitude of mechanisms involved in this process offers several targets for therapeutic intervention and many anti-angiogenesis agents are currently being investigated in clinical trials. Some drugs in clinical use are known to have anti-angiogenic properties. These include thalidomide, interferon-α, tamoxifen and trastuzumab (Herceptin).

INHIBITORS OF METASTASIS

In order to spread, tumours first need to invade through the basement membrane and into blood vessels and lymphatics. This process is aided by tumour production of matrix metalloproteinases that break down the extracellular matrix. Inhibitors of these proteins have been used in clinical trials, but results are very disappointing at present.

FURTHER READING

Chabner B A, Longo D L (eds) 1996 Cancer chemotherapy and biotherapy: principles and practice, 2nd edn. Lippincott Williams & Wilkins, Philadelphia
Pratt W B, Ruddon R W, Ensminger W D, Maybaum J (eds) 1994 The anticancer drugs, 2nd edn. Oxford University Press, Oxford

CHAPTER 7

Principles of radiology

Rhidian Bramley

INTRODUCTION

Radiology has an important role in modern oncology practice and all clinicians should have a basic understanding of the range of imaging modalities and examinations available. A more detailed knowledge of individual imaging tests is required to determine the optimum choice and timing of investigations, particularly when a number of complementary imaging techniques are available. This choice depends on several factors including the relative sensitivity and specificity of the tests, specific cautions and contraindications, radiation dose considerations, and local factors such as availability of the technique, waiting times and local radiological expertise. Radiologists can assist clinicians with this decision-making process and, where possible, imaging protocols should be devised and agreed within a multidisciplinary team environment.

In UK oncological practice, clinicians are also required to interpret radiological images. Plain films may be viewed in the clinic and on the ward before a formal radiological report has been issued. Radiotherapy planning scans also largely go unreported by radiologists, and may provide the only locoregional staging assessment of disease. Cross-sectional imaging is increasingly a prerequisite to surgical intervention and surgeons should be able to correlate the radiology with their operative findings. As treatment planning techniques evolve, oncologists require an ever more detailed understanding of the imaging modalities that apply to their clinical practice.

The main applications of imaging in oncology are:

1. Screening for cancer and diagnosing disease at clinical presentation
2. Providing a formal staging assessment
3. Radiotherapy treatment planning
4. Assessment of treatment response

5. Identifying recurrent disease at follow-up (including radiology surveillance)
6. Determining the various complications of the disease and its treatment.

Radiologists also undertake interventional (invasive) techniques to:

1. Provide further diagnostic information (e.g. angiography)
2. Obtain specimens for cytological and histological assessment (e.g. FNA or core biopsy)
3. Assist in therapeutic management (e.g. nephrostomy, gastrostomy, superior vena cava (SVC) stenting, central line placement, tumour embolisation).

CANCER SCREENING AND SURVEILLANCE PROGRAMMES

The national breast cancer screening programme was introduced between 1988 and 1991 and is the only universal population-based radiology screening programme in the UK. Currently, all women over the age of 50 are offered mammography every 3 years until the age of 70, with the aim of detecting and treating breast cancer at an earlier stage. It is estimated that 30% of the recent fall in breast cancer mortality rates is due to the screening programme. Targeted screening is under evaluation for populations at risk for ovarian cancer (CA125 and pelvic ultrasound), prostate cancer (PSA and transrectal ultrasound), and lung cancer (low dose spiral CT). (See Ch. 10 on cancer screening for more details.)

Imaging is also being used increasingly in the surveillance of asymptomatic treated oncology patients to assess for disease relapse. There are recommended radiology surveillance protocols for treated lymphoma, testicular tumours, sarcomas, lung cancer and colorectal cancer. In general, however, the evidence to support such surveillance programmes is lacking and further studies are required to determine the optimum timing and frequency of investigations. A recent meta-analysis has shown a 9–13% improvement in absolute survival in patients randomised to intensive clinical and radiological follow-up after resection of colorectal cancer, although the relative contribution of the radiology surveillance to outcome is unclear.

CANCER STAGING

An important role of imaging is to determine the locoregional tumour extent and identify metastatic disease spread. This information is central to all management decisions, and provides a prognostic indication of likely outcome. Accurate stratification of patients by tumour type and stage is also a prerequisite of cancer research, enabling valid comparison of outcomes among treatment groups.

The most commonly used staging system is the Tumour Node Metastasis (TNM) classification, which has common stratification groups for each tumour type. The TNM cancer staging classifications are reviewed regularly by the International Union against Cancer (Union Internationale Contre le Cancer, UICC) with contributions from associated national and international organisations. Additional staging systems are in existence, which usually predate the TNM classifications and have fewer stratification groups. In gynaecological malignancy, the main alternative staging system is the Fédération Internationale Gynécologie et Oncologie (FIGO) classification. Colorectal cancer is commonly staged by the Dukes classification (principally in the UK).

ASSESSMENT OF TREATMENT RESPONSE

Serial measurements of tumour size and extent on imaging provide an objective assessment of treatment response. Until recently, the main system used was the World Health Organisation (WHO) criteria, which established a standard of bi-dimensional measurements of marker lesions, and defined surrogate endpoints for complete response (CR), partial response (PR), stable disease (SD) and progressive disease (PD). In 2000, an attempt was made to simplify and standardise radiological measurement for trials with the Response Evaluation Criteria in Solid Tumors (RECIST) guidelines published jointly by the NCI and EORTC. These are more stringent than the WHO criteria, and include specifications on the imaging technique and maximum number of lesions that should be measured (up to 5 lesions in a single organ and 10 in total). An important difference with RECIST is that only uni-dimensional measurements are recorded (the longest diameter of marker lesions), and these are summed to give an overall RECIST score. Endpoints for treatment response also differ to take account of the uni-dimensional measurement, and it should be noted that these are not directly equivalent to the WHO definitions. The basic definitions of response criteria in solid tumours using WHO and RECIST criteria are listed in Table 7.1.

TABLE 7.I Response evaluation criteria in solid tumours		
	WHO (bi-dimensional measurements[a])	RECIST (uni-dimensional measurements)
Complete response (CR)	Resolution of all disease	Resolution of all disease
Partial response (PR)	50% decrease in sum of areas	30% decrease in sum of longest diameters
Stable disease (SD)	Between PR and PD	Between PR and PD
Progressive disease (PD)	25% increase in sum of areas	20% increase in sum of longest diameters

[a]WHO: lesion area = product of longest diameter × greatest perpendicular diameter.

IMAGING MODALITIES

The rest of this chapter will review the main imaging modalities available, highlighting some general principles and techniques that can help in selecting the appropriate investigation, and image interpretation. An overview of the basic terminology used in describing imaging appearances on different imaging modalities is given in Table 7.2.

PLAIN RADIOGRAPHY

Plain radiography provides a relatively cheap and convenient method of assessing disease status, particularly in evaluating chest and bone pathology. Waiting times are minimal and the imaging can be reviewed as soon as the films emerge from the processor or, with modern systems, as soon as the digital (DICOM) images are stored on the picture archiving and communication system (PACS). Plain radiography is generally less sensitive than cross-sectional imaging (CT, MR and ultrasound), but can provide more specific diagnostic information in certain circumstances, e.g. in the evaluation of primary bone tumours. Plain films are also more sensitive in the investigation of myeloma, whereas isotope bone scans are more sensitive for other types of metastatic bone disease.

Chest radiography is the most frequently performed radiological examination, and clinicians should be aware of the more common errors made by those interpreting images outside the radiology department. These are:

1. Partially obscured pulmonary lesions. Pulmonary pathology may be overlooked where the lungs are partially obscured by overlying structures (e.g. overlapping the ribs and clavicles at the lung apices, in front of and behind the pulmonary hila, behind the heart, and behind the dome of the diaphragm). These areas require special attention and are termed the review areas on the chest radiograph. If a rounded nodule is projected over any of these structures, then it is likely to be surrounded by air, and lie

TABLE 7.2 Basic terminology used in describing imaging appearances on different imaging modalities

	Conventional image settings	
	Bright areas on the image	Dark areas on the image
Plain film and CT	High attenuation (high density)	Low attenuation (low density)
Ultrasound	High echogenicity (hyperechoic) Increased reflectivity	Low echogenicity (hypoechoic) Reduced reflectivity
MR	High signal	Low signal
Nuclear medicine	Low activity	High activity

within the lung (in front or behind the overlying structure). This is called the silhouette sign.

2. Pulmonary collapse. Isolated collapse of a lobe or segment of lung usually indicates compression or occlusion of the supplying bronchus, and is thus an indirect sign of proximal disease. Complete collapse can be difficult to identify on plain radiographs. The hallmarks are volume loss in a hemi-thorax and displacement of adjacent structures (pulmonary fissures and hila).

3. Mediastinal lesions. Look for the common sites of lymphadenopathy (right paratracheal, hilar and subcarinal). You should be able to make out both sides of the right tracheal wall.

4. Bone lesions. Consciously trace the course of the ribs. It may help to rotate the film or image through 90° as rib lesions and pneumothoraces may become more conspicuous. Assess the spine on the frontal and lateral view for skeletal metastases and pathological fractures.

A lateral chest radiograph can help localise lesions and identify occult pathology and, for these reasons, many cancer centres perform a lateral projection routinely. Lesions above the aortic arch are usually better seen on separate apical views. The review areas on the lateral chest radiograph are:

1. The anterior clear space – superior to the heart (opacified in anterior mediastinal lymphadenopathy and upper lobe collapse).

2. The posterior clear space – behind the heart. This should be more exposed, 'blacker', as you progress down the vertebral column (opacified with posterior mediastinal masses, lower lobe collapse and pleural effusions).

3. The pulmonary hila.

FLUOROSCOPY

Modern fluoroscopy techniques use an image intensifier to display a 'real time' X-ray image on a monitor screen. Image quality is poor compared to conventional radiographs, but comparable spot images can be obtained by temporarily increasing the dose rate (fluence) and storing the resultant image (exposure).

Fluoroscopy is used in many diagnostic and interventional procedures. When moving the patient or X-ray tube, it is often desirable to confirm correct positioning prior to exposure; this is termed 'screening for position'. It may also be useful to screen during movement to help determine the relationship of structures within the beam, e.g. overlapping bowel loops during a barium follow-through examination. These same basic principles apply to radiotherapy planning practice using a simulator.

Fluoroscopy can also demonstrate the flow of contrast after routine administration (e.g. barium swallow) or following dynamic injection (e.g. angiography). Fluoroscopic imaging is used to guide the radiologist during interventional procedures, such as in positioning a biopsy needle, an angiographic catheter, or a drainage tube etc. Specialised equipment (e.g. C arm rotating fluoroscopy tubes) and functions (e.g. background image subtraction) have been developed to assist with these procedures.

ULTRASOUND (US)

Like fluoroscopy, ultrasound is a dynamic examination and as such, it is generally easier to identify lesions in 'real time' on the monitor than on hard copy images. Static hard copy images can also be misinterpreted and should therefore be reviewed with caution. A formal report is essential.

Ultrasound is ideal for superficial structures (close to the probe) where resolution is better than on CT or MR. Examples include neck imaging (thyroid and the lymph nodes) and scrotal imaging, as well as transvaginal and a transrectal scanning. Ultrasound is generally better than CT in distinguishing cystic from solid lesions (e.g. in equivocal hepatic or renal lesions). Ultrasound can also obtain images in multiple planes, which can overcome limitations with axial CT (e.g. in distinguishing a renal mass lesion indenting the liver from a hepatic lesion displacing the kidney). In general, however, CT and MR are more sensitive at demonstrating intra-abdominal pathology. Ultrasound contrast agents using microbubbles improve ultrasound sensitivity but are not widely used.

Doppler ultrasound is the preferred method for assessing deep venous thrombosis and has a role in evaluating mesenteric and hepatic vessel flow in suspected veno-occlusive disease. Tumour vascularity can be assessed although angiography is considered to be the gold standard technique in the work-up for tumour embolisation.

The 'real-time' imaging of ultrasound is particularly useful for directing interventional procedures such as image-guided biopsy and drainage procedures, and is sometimes used in conjunction with fluoroscopy.

COMPUTED TOMOGRAPHY (CT)

CT is the staging examination of choice for most thoracic and abdominal neoplasms. In both diagnostic CT and radiotherapy CT planning, the main aims are to identify locoregional disease extent and assess for evidence of metastatic disease.

Technique
Spiral scanning is preferable to conventional CT as it avoids inter-slice gaps. Spiral scanning also enables overlapping images to be reconstructed, improving the definition of small lesions. Images may be reformatted in different planes, albeit at a lower spatial resolution (e.g. sagittal and coronal images). The faster scan times of spiral CT also minimise movement artefact.

Oral contrast (e.g. 2% gastrograffin) should be administered in all abdomino-pelvic imaging to help distinguish bowel loops from lymph nodes and other sites of disease. Routine administration of contrast improves diagnostic certainty and avoids the need to rebook equivocal cases. Negative contrast agents (e.g. carbonated water) are sometimes preferred in the assessment of proximal gastrointestinal tumours.

Intravenous contrast helps distinguish blood vessels from lymph nodes, and improves the sensitivity for detecting organ metastases (e.g. liver and brain). Contrast enhancement can be optimised by imaging at predefined intervals during passage of a bolus of contrast (e.g. separate arterial and portal phase imaging of the liver).

Hepatic metastases are usually best demarcated in the portal venous phase of enhancement, although highly vascular tumours (e.g. neuroendocrine tumours and hepatoma) may be more conspicuous in the arterial phase.

Slice thickness is an important consideration, and in general thin section CT is preferred to reduce partial volume averaging. This occurs when a lesion is smaller than the slice thickness. The attenuation of the lesion is then averaged with the surrounding 'normal' tissues within the slice, resulting in reduced conspicuity of the lesion on the final image. There is a trade off, however, as at the same exposure, thin section images contain more *noise* (quantum mottle), and this can also obscure lesions. In practice, slice thickness is limited by scanner design. With improvements in technology, there has been a trend to reduce slice thickness from 10 mm to 5 mm in routine body imaging. New multi-slice CT machines can now achieve 2.5 mm sections throughout the body in a single acquisition.

High resolution CT (HRCT) is a technique used principally to characterise pulmonary interstitial disease. In oncology practice it may help distinguish lymphangitis carcinomatosa from pulmonary oedema, infection and drug-induced pulmonary interstitial changes. Ultra-thin conventional CT sections (1–2 mm) are obtained at intervals (usually 10 mm or more) through the abnormal area of lung. It should be noted that HRCT only 'samples' the abnormal lung and can miss metastases, as there is a large inter-slice gap.

Viewing

CT images should be viewed on a monitor (soft copy) using four different window settings (abdomen, lung, liver and bone). Each window setting is optimised to demonstrate pathology in the specified organ/system. Hard copy images are usually printed on only one or two window settings. Soft copy viewing has several other advantages including being able to view images in stack mode (on top of each other), which assists in distinguishing tubular structures such as vessels from discrete lesions such as lymph nodes.

Problem solving

Various techniques can be employed when there is uncertainty about the significance of a lesion. Additional CT images may be obtained by rescanning the patient (e.g. delayed or decubitus scans) or by reformatting image data (e.g. as overlapping images). HRCT images may be obtained to characterise pulmonary interstitial disease (see above). Other options include using different imaging modalities (ultrasound, MR or nuclear medicine), image guided biopsy, or adopting a wait-and-see policy. A radiologist will help assist with this decision.

MAGNETIC RESONANCE IMAGING (MRI)

Magnetic resonance techniques can be confusing due to the complex physics and multiple imaging sequences, many of which are known by vendor specific acronyms. The basic principles are well established, however. The main advantages of MRI over CT are the multi-planar capability, greater soft tissue contrast, and use of non-ionising radiation. The main disadvantages are longer scan times (producing movement artefact) and claustrophobia (in up to 10% of patients).

MRI is generally superior to CT in imaging the CNS, head and neck, pelvis and limbs (musculoskeletal imaging). Movement artefact in thorax (heart and lungs) and abdomen (respiration and bowel peristalsis) has traditionally limited the use of MRI in these areas. However, modern MRI systems have high performance gradients enabling shorter scan times and breath hold imaging. Movement artefact can also be reduced with cardiac and respiratory gating.

The main pulse imaging sequences used in oncology are:

Spin echo. Good quality images (high signal to noise ratio) but prolonged acquisition times. Turbo spin echo sequences are similar but with faster acquisition times.

Gradient echo. Fast acquisition times but noisier images (lower signal to noise ratio, SNR). More susceptible to imaging artefacts (e.g. chemical shift and susceptibility artefacts), although this can be used to benefit (e.g. in detecting haemosiderin deposition following haemorrhage).

Inversion recovery. These sequences are most commonly used to suppress signal from fat (STIR – short tau inversion recovery) or fluid (FLAIR – fluid attenuated inversion recovery). In STIR imaging, fat (which has relatively high signal on T1 and T2 weighted images) is suppressed appearing dark (low signal). This can help distinguish cellular tumour from surrounding fat-containing tissues (e.g. in bone marrow). STIR imaging can also help characterise fat-containing tumours (e.g. well-differentiated liposarcomas). FLAIR imaging is used in brain imaging, and is a sensitive indicator of disease.

Each type of sequence may be *weighted* by changing the timing of the radiofrequency pulses and signal acquisition.

T1 weighted images are generally good for identifying normal anatomy. Free water (urine, ascites, effusions) appears dark (low signal).

T2 weighted images are generally good for distinguishing pathology from a normal tissue. Free water, tumour and oedematous tissue usually appear bright (high signal).

Proton density images have properties in between T1 and T2 weighted images.

Other MR imaging techniques include:

1. 3D imaging. Data is obtained as a volume of tissue, as opposed to individual slices. This allows images to be reformatted in any plane after the examination is complete, and improves SNR on high resolution reformatted images. 3D imaging also gets round the potential problem of the small inter-slice gap left between images obtained by other sequences. It is thus better for imaging very small lesions (e.g. in the pituitary). Other uses include magnetic resonance angiography (MRA) and magnetic resonance cholangiopancreatography (MRCP).
2. Vascular imaging (e.g. time of flight and phase contrast imaging). Identifies flowing blood, and is used in MRA. Intravenous contrast is not required, although it may be administered to acquire large field flow angiograms (enhanced MRA).
3. Fat saturation suppresses the signal from fat in a different way from STIR, and unlike STIR can used with intravenous contrast (gadolinium DTPA). This property is particularly useful in musculoskeletal imaging.
4. Intravenous contrast (gadolinium DTPA) is used routinely in evaluating CNS and head and neck tumours, and variably in sarcoma imaging. Both positive (gadolinium DTPA) and negative (SPIO – superparamagnetic iron oxide) contrast agents are used in hepatic imaging. Contrast is not widely used in pelvic imaging although it can help in problem solving.

NUCLEAR MEDICINE

Nuclear medicine, unlike most other forms of imaging, provides functional as well as anatomical information. All radioisotopes used in imaging emit gamma rays, which may be detected with a gamma camera.

The most commonly used isotope in conventional nuclear medicine imaging is technetium-99m. The physiological uptake of tracer usually depends not on the isotope, but on the biologically active ligand. Functional information is acquired, as within the body, the biologically active ligand becomes bound to membranes and taken up by active cell transport mechanisms. Further functional data can be acquired by plotting time activity curves (e.g. the isotope renogram). The main tracers used in oncoradiology practice are listed in Table 7.3.

Lymphoscintigraphy

This is a technique that is being used increasingly in the routine staging of melanoma and breast cancer. Intradermal injection of radiolabelled human serum albumin (HSA) around the lesion/scar tracks to the sentinel node,

TABLE 7.3 The principal nuclear medicine tracers used in oncoradiology

Tracer	Scan name	Main use
^{99m}Tc MDP or ^{99m}Tc HDP	Isotope bone scan	Cancer staging
^{99m}Tc MAG3	Isotope renogram	Assess renal function prior to chemotherapy
^{99m}Tc DTPA or ^{51}Cr EDTA	Glomerular filtration rate (GFR)	Assess renal function prior to chemotherapy
^{99m}Tc labelled red blood cells (RBC)	MUGA scan	Assess cardiac function (LVEF) on anthracycline therapy
^{99m}Tc MAA	Perfusion lung scan	Assess for pulmonary emboli
^{99m}Tc Technegas or ^{81m}Kr	Ventilation lung scan	Assess for pulmonary emboli
^{111}I Octreotide	Octreotide scan	Localisation and staging of neuroendocrine tumours
^{123}I MIBG	MIBG scan	Staging, e.g. neuroblastoma; assess for MIBG therapy
^{123}I and ^{131}I	Radioiodine thyroid scan	Investigation and treatment of thyroid cancer
^{99m}Tc human serum albumin (HSA)	Sentinel node imaging (lymphoscintigraphy)	Melanoma, breast and vulval cancer staging

which is the first node to receive drainage from the tumour and the most likely node to contain micrometastases on histological examination. The sentinel node can be localised either on imaging, or with handheld gamma probe at surgery.

Immunoscintigraphy

This is a technique where a radioisotope is bound to a monoclonal antibody, raised to a specific cell surface antigen. The antibodies used in oncological practice are targeted at known tumour markers (e.g. CEA, PSA).

Positron emission tomography (PET)

PET imaging is a relatively new innovation and is currently only available in a few centres in the UK. Most research has concentrated on 2-[F-18] fluoro-2-deoxy-D-glucose (18-FDG), which is retained by metabolically active tumour due to a combination of increased uptake and reduced elimination. It holds promise in detecting hitherto occult disease, such as in normal size lymph nodes and scar tissue following treatment. In the USA it is approved for the diagnosis, staging and restaging of various cancers, including lung, oesophageal, colorectal, lymphoma, head and neck, breast and thyroid cancers.

Plain isotope images may show relatively poor anatomical information, but correlation with other imaging techniques can assist with interpretation.

Cross-sectional nuclear medicine imaging techniques (SPECT and PET) give better resolution, and scans can be superimposed on CT and MR images to provide even better anatomical localisation (fusion imaging). PET imaging provides the best spatial resolution by utilising the properties of positron emission. In this process, two gamma rays are emitted at exactly the same time, but in diametrically opposite directions. By detecting the simultaneous emissions, a direct line can be plotted to intercept precisely the site of decay. Although PET images may be obtained with dual head gamma cameras, dedicated PET machines have been designed with multiple detectors optimised to detect the higher energy gamma radiation produced.

FURTHER READING

Husband J, Resnick H (eds) 2004 Imaging in oncology. Taylor & Francis, Oxford

Sobin L H, Wittekind Ch (eds) 2002 TNM Classification of malignant tumours, 6th edn. Wiley-Liss, New York

Therasse P, Arbuck S G, Eisenhauer E A et al 2000 New guidelines to evaluate the response to treatment in solid tumours. Journal of the National Cancer Institute 92(3):205–216

CHAPTER 8

Principles of symptom management in oncology and palliative care

Suzanne Kite

INTRODUCTION

Most cancer patients present with symptoms, which will resolve, fluctuate or progress depending on the underlying course of the cancer. The commonest symptoms in hospital-based palliative care practice are pain, neuropsychiatric symptoms, nausea, constipation, vomiting, dyspnoea, tiredness, anorexia and low mood (Potter et al, 2003). Some of these symptoms are more amenable to pharmacological therapy and other interventions than others, for example pain, nausea and vomiting and dyspnoea. However, symptoms such as lethargy and fatigue may be as distressing, if not more so, and may only be volunteered on careful questioning.

The therapeutic focus gradually shifts from treating the root causes of the symptoms in earlier disease, to addressing the consequences and impact of symptoms as cancer becomes advanced and progressive. The significance and meaning of symptoms may change with advancing disease but the same underlying principles and approach apply.

The goals of symptom management are to improve quality of life as much as possible, and, where necessary, to enable a good death for the patient in a place of their choosing. The natural history of cancer-related symptoms is often known, enabling realistic goals to be set, and future care planned. Such planning can make a huge difference to how and where the last months, and days, of life are spent. Whilst most people state that they wish to die at home, only about a quarter of cancer patients achieve this. The majority die in hospital (55.5%) and 16.5% in a hospice (Office for National Statistics, 2002).

In the remainder of this chapter a general approach to symptom management is presented.

GENERAL PRINCIPLES OF SYMPTOM MANAGEMENT

These are the same as those underlying any medical problem, i.e.:

- Assessment: history, examination, appropriate investigations – tailored to the patient's condition and likely prognosis.
- Diagnosis of most likely cause/s based on what is known of the underlying pathology and physiology.
- Assessment of psychological, sociological, spiritual and physical aspects which may be contributing to the symptom/s, or arising as a consequence.
- Implementation of a management plan with the patient, and team.
- Review and revise the above.
- Review again, revise again.

The notes below assume patient-centred care, acknowledging the central role of families, and those close to the patient, and in the context of multidisciplinary care. Many palliative care patients will be receiving care from medical social workers, physiotherapists, occupational therapists, dieticians and other allied health professionals, in addition to the care provided by physicians and the nursing team. Each member of the extended multiprofessional team, which forms around each individual patient, will be able to see and manage different aspects of the overall picture. Communication and liaison, and understanding of the differing professional roles, are vital.

KEYS TO SYMPTOM MANAGEMENT SUCCESS IN PALLIATIVE CARE

CAREFUL ASSESSMENT

Use whatever information is available from the patient, family, carers, medical notes and investigation results, to build up as complete a picture as possible (without exhausting the patient). Aim for a four-dimensional model, incorporating the physical with the psychosocial/spiritual. An understanding of the significance of the symptom to the patient may help bring fears out into the open and may even, at times, give the diagnosis.

Are symptoms:

- Due to the cancer?
- Related to cancer treatment?
- Unrelated to cancer (e.g. asthma, angina, scabies)?
- All of the above?

There are often multiple causes and multiple symptoms – all of which will evolve with time and treatment. Yesterday's cause may not be today's. Causes of nausea and vomiting in advanced disease are often multifactorial, and many patients with cancer have more than one pain.

ESTABLISHMENT OF A REALISTIC MANAGEMENT PLAN WITH THE PATIENT AND TEAM AT THE OUTSET (WITH REVISION AS NECESSARY)

What actual options are available for this particular patient, at this particular time, and what is the likelihood of success with each? Success is measured in terms of likelihood of achieving the patient's goals, and a balance in favour of benefits over burdens for any chosen action plan.

A key consideration will be whether the underlying cause is treatable (with oncological treatment, surgery, antibiotics etc.), and, if so, whether the advantages of treatment outweigh the disadvantages.

Where treatment of the underlying cause is unduly burdensome, inappropriate or impossible, palliation should be directed at improving symptoms by modifying the pathological mechanism, and in improving the patient's general level of comfort, and psychological and physical functioning.

If a firm cause cannot be established, because the patient is too frail or because results are inconclusive, then treatment should be started on a probability basis for the most likely cause. Assessing response to this initial treatment and the opportunity for further observation may clarify the situation.

The patient should be actively involved in planning and evaluating symptom management whenever possible. He/she will need to know the likely timescale in which improvement should take place, and the degree of improvement that can be expected. Reassurance should also be given that if initial strategies are ineffective then other options are available or will be explored. This is particularly true when symptoms have already proved difficult to control. For example, for pain which has proved difficult to manage, reassurance can be given in the form of stepwise goals: for pain to be controlled at night, then at rest during the day, and then (where possible) on mobilisation. For vomiting due to an irreversible mechanical cause, the goal may be to treat nausea, and to reduce the volume and frequency of vomits, rather than to stop the vomiting altogether. The skill is in engendering realistic hope without undue pessimism.

ROUTES OF ADMINISTRATION

The oral route is the simplest but may not always be the best. Tablet burden may be a problem, the patient may not be able to swallow, or nausea and/or vomiting may reduce drug absorption. Medication should be reviewed and rationalised regularly. (Think: what is this drug for? Is it still working? Is it needed?), and ask whether tablets, capsules or suspensions are preferred where a choice is available. Alternative routes of drug administration should be considered:

- Rectal route may be acceptable to the patient where appropriate preparations exist (e.g. diclofenac, laxative, domperidone, paracetamol).
- Transdermal route may be appropriate for stable symptoms (time to steady-state blood levels means that they are not indicated for acute symptom management). Examples include fentanyl, buprenorphine and hyoscine hydrobromide.
- Transmucosal forms of lorazepam, prochlorperazine and fentanyl may be useful.
- Subcutaneous route, for one-off injections or as continuous infusions delivered by a syringe driver. Continuous subcutaneous infusions permit a wide range of palliative care drugs to be given parenterally with minimal burden to the patient. Some drugs can be combined for administration and compatibility charts are available (Twycross and Wilcock, 2001). There are different syringe driver models with different rate settings, so care is needed. Note that syringe drivers have acquired some mythical baggage because the need for them is greatest when patients are dying, and so the public and some professionals may see a causal link. However, they are merely a useful mode of administering the same doses of oral medication, or new symptom management medication, as an alternative to the oral route when swallowing or absorption is difficult or impossible.

REGULAR REASSESSMENT

Reassess with a time interval determined by the severity of the symptom. If symptoms persist, consider:

- Has the cause changed?
- Has successful treatment of one symptom unmasked another? This is particularly true of pain. It is common for patients with cancer to have several pains of varying severity, and successful treatment of the most severe pain may allow the patient to become aware of others.
- Is this due to evolution of the underlying disease?
- Do psychosocial factors require more attention? Are depression/anxiety being overlooked? Has enough emphasis been placed on coping strategies, environmental adaptation, time for psychological adjustment?

- Are the drugs being given by the right route? Is the medication being administered? (Check for: drug 'not available'; patient not taking; poor adherence, e.g. transdermal fentanyl patch.)

If a strategy is not working, it should be changed. A patient's goals may change with time, and in response to treatment. If drugs are not working, then they should be stopped. Reassessment and refinement of treatment should continue as necessary.

ANTICIPATE PROBLEMS

A key component of effective symptom management is pattern recognition. Some problems can be anticipated with scope for pre-emptive management. For example, decisions can be made regarding the future management of a patient with recurrent hypercalcaemia or anaemia, or persistent bleeding, including when not to treat actively.

MECHANICAL PROBLEMS NEED MECHANICAL SOLUTIONS

The analgesic of choice for a fractured bone is fixation or immobilisation, and without these the pain will respond poorly to conventional painkillers – although there may be a role for anaesthetic techniques. Likewise, antiemetics are of limited efficacy in vomiting due to gastric outlet obstruction, and laxatives will not cure constipation due to completely occlusive rectal tumours. Ideally, symptoms with mechanical causes need mechanical solutions.

EMERGENCIES IN PALLIATIVE CARE

Symptoms are debilitating and should always be addressed with a sense of urgency. However, some situations, 'emergencies', are such that very urgent attention is required to address symptoms, promote comfort and plan future care. Often these can be foreseen, and pre-empted, or some preparation made. When they do occur they can be devastating for everyone, and maintaining a calm demeanour is therapeutic to all concerned.

Oncological emergencies are covered in the third section of this book. More specific palliative care emergencies include overwhelming pain, severe agitation, respiratory panic, massive haemorrhage, acute psychiatric distress, and urgent discharge so that a patient can die at home. How such emergencies are managed will be strongly influenced by whether patient, family and healthcare team are in agreement, and accept that death is imminent. Where this is the case, care is directed at providing as comfortable and calm a mode of death as possible, rather than in averting death per se (as in other medical emergencies). Where imminent death was not previously recognised and accepted, some urgent decisions will need to be made regarding goals of care. However, as with all medical emergencies, the immediate aim is to stabilise the patient and the situation, pending more definitive action. A series of assessments, discussions and interventions may be required. An overall approach is as follows:

- Do not panic. This will prevent further escalation of anxiety.
- Reassure the patient and carers whilst making a brief overall assessment of the situation. Such reassurance can include, for example, 'I'm going to stay with you until you're comfortable and settled'.
- Immediate steps to ensure greater comfort for the patient, e.g. analgesia, repositioning, anxiolytic, oxygen etc.
- Family members or those close to the patient may need to be called in. Collect thoughts before making the phone call. Introduce yourself calmly, and establish that you are talking to the right person. It may be appropriate to ask whether the person you are talking to is alone, and to give a warning shot before proceeding. Be straightforward and supportive.
- Reassess the situation again and decide what to do next depending on the response to the immediate steps above, and in the context of the overall goals of care. Where such goals are uncertain, they need to be established. Call for more expert help if necessary. Ensure that someone stays with the patient and has a means of signalling for help.
- Once the patient settles, take stock. Plan for recurrence of the emergency if this is likely, e.g. advise patient/family/healthcare team, prescribe p.r.n. medication, alter previous prescriptions, reconsider CPR (cardiopulmonary resuscitation) status if necessary.
- If the patient does not settle, e.g. has overwhelming pain, agitation or breathlessness, repeat the early steps, and make sure nothing has been over-looked such as any underlying physical or psychological causes. Consider also whether it is necessary to treat the associated anxiety and distress with sedatives. Everyone should be in agreement with goals of care.
- Debrief. Those involved should be able to express distress as necessary. At a later date, reflection on whether things could have gone differently/better can sometimes highlight learning points, and allow recognition that everyone did their best in a very distressing situation. The timing of debriefing sessions needs sensitive thought – too soon and emotions may be too raw, and if too delayed the opportunity may be missed. Within a week is probably ideal, and some teams find it helpful to have an empathic outsider to facilitate the session.

THE LAST HOURS/DAYS OF LIFE

The groundwork for care in the last days of life will usually have been laid over the preceding weeks or months. Careful advance consideration of the patient's wishes in relation to location and circumstances of death, including who they wish to be present, what care they wish to receive, and cultural/spiritual requirements, will pay dividends. Many patients are able to contemplate their deaths in this way, but many are not. Death may also come hastily, if not always unexpectedly, particularly when hospital-based treatments are being offered very late in disease, and there may be precious little time to adapt to the changing goals of care. Consideration can usefully be given to this when such treatments are being offered in the first place.

General guidance on the management of symptoms and emergencies applies. Some units may have instituted 'The Liverpool Integrated Care Pathway for the Dying', which provides a multiprofessional care pathway with necessary joint documentation and prompts (Ellershaw and Wilkinson, 2003). This pathway is based around the general principles of terminal care:

1. Recognition that death is imminent. As death approaches, cancer patients often experience increasing weakness and immobility, loss of interest in food and fluid, difficulty swallowing and drowsiness, on a background of gradual deterioration in functional status (Ellershaw and Ward, 2003).
2. Encouragement of participation by patient, family and friends in decision-making and in physical care, according to their views and wishes. What facilities are available to support those close to the patient in staying with them? What information do they need?
3. Continuation of collaborative multiprofessional working. Refer early to specialist palliative care if problems are anticipated.
4. Assessment of patient's needs – from the patient's perspective. Tailor questions to the patient's condition asking specifically about symptoms such as discomfort and pain as these tend to be under-reported. 'Is there anything else we can do to make you more comfortable?' Non-verbal clues of distress may be present. Gentle examination of any site of pain, the mouth, pressure areas, and other areas where clinical assessment suggests that there may be a problem. Exploration of fears, misunderstandings and misapprehensions as appropriate.
5. Comfort measures and symptom management.
   - Discontinue unnecessary medication, investigations and routine observations which no longer contribute to the patient's comfort.
   - As swallowing deteriorates, essential palliative medication should be prescribed via an alternative route, e.g. continuous subcutaneous infusion (syringe driver). Prescription of p.r.n. medication for antici-pated symptoms, e.g. pain, anxiety, agitation, convulsions or for retained oropharyngeal secretions.
   - Dry mouth is the norm rather than the exception for a variety of reasons including mouth breathing, medication and previous treatment. Thirst may or, more usually, may not, be associated. Good mouthcare, and the regular offer of sips of fluid to those who can swallow is sufficient for most. Parenteral fluids are rarely required.

- Mouthcare is vital. Family may wish to help.
- Skincare includes careful positioning and regular turning depending on the patient's general condition, gentle massage, and the choice of an appropriate mattress.
- Urinary catheterisation may be necessary or aid comfort.
- The patient should be spoken to gently and any actions explained. Even when comatose, patients' hearing may persist.
- Relatives' needs. Time spent talking to relatives is much appreciated, to offer reassurance that the patient is comfortable and is being well cared for. Relatives may take the opportunity to ask questions that they otherwise feel reluctant to ask.
- Continued psychosocial support.
- Care in different settings. Many people wish to die at home; this requires careful planning, with family and community services needing as much time as possible to prepare.

6. Continue to visit the patient regularly.

CONCLUSION

The effective application of symptom management guidelines is dependent upon the recognition of where a patient is in their illness trajectory. Clarification is necessary to ensure that all parties involved in decision-making share a mutual understanding of goals of care, and when important transition points have been reached. Assumptions are common and need to be identified and explored.

However, even with the knowledge and skills available, symptom prevalence remains high in oncology settings (Fallon, 2003). Further research is necessary to inform future symptom management strategies, and research interests need to be extended further beyond the physical and pharmacological. For example, oncology outpatients may not volunteer troublesome symptoms if they perceive that valuable clinic time will be spent exploring these at the expense of discussion of active oncological treatments (Dr Marie Fallon, personal communication 2003). So, there is work to be done in applying what we already know more effectively, and in developing strategies for the research and management of more intransigent symptoms such as weakness and fatigue.

ACKNOWLEDGEMENT

Parts of this chapter were previously published in Kite and O'Doherty (2002) and are reproduced with permission of Taylor & Francis.

REFERENCES AND FURTHER READING

There are excellent symptom management guides available, from comprehensive introductions (Twycross and Wilcock, 2001; Regnard and Hockley, 2003; Faull et al, 1998) to reference books (Doyle et al, 2003). More specialised texts are also highly recommended (Twycross et al, 2002; Dickman et al, 2002).

Dickman A, Littlewood C, Varga J 2002 The syringe driver: continuous subcutaneous infusions in palliative care. Oxford University Press, Oxford

Doyle D, Hanks G, Cherny N, Calman K (eds) 2003 The Oxford textbook of palliative medicine, 3rd edn, Oxford University Press, Oxford

Ellershaw J, Ward C 2003 Care of the dying patient: the last hours or days of life. BMJ 326:30–34

Ellershaw J, Wilkinson S 2003 Care of the dying: a pathway to excellence. Oxford University Press, Oxford

Fallon M 2003 Palliative Care Research Society Meeting, Edinburgh, June 2003

Faull C, Carter Y, Woof R 1998 Handbook of palliative care. Blackwell Science, Oxford

Kite S, O'Doherty C 2002 Palliative care. In: Rai G S, Mulley G P (eds) Elderly medicine. Martin Dunitz/Taylor & Francis, London

Office for National Statistics 2002 Annual review of the Registrar General on deaths in England and Wales, 2000. ONS, London

Potter J, Hami F, Bryan T, Quigley C 2003 Symptoms in 400 patients referred to palliative care services: prevalence and patterns. Palliative Medicine 17:310–314

Regnard C, Hockley J 2003 A guide to symptom relief in palliative care, 5th edn. Radcliffe, Oxford

Twycross R, Wilcock A 2001 Symptom management in advanced cancer, 3rd edn. Radcliffe, Oxford

Twycross R, Wilcock A, Charlesworth S, Dickman A 2002 Palliative care formulary, 2nd edn. Radcliffe, Oxford. See also www.palliativedrugs.com

CHAPTER 9

Clinical trials in oncology

D.P.H. Stark and Clive Peedell

INTRODUCTION

In the field of oncology there is constant research and development of new anti-cancer treatments. After the initial preclinical in vitro studies on tumour cell lines and in vivo animal testing of new treatments, high quality clinical trials in humans are needed to establish safety, efficacy and effectiveness before a new treatment is accepted into standard clinical practice.

CLINICAL TRIALS OF CANCER TREATMENT

New agents that are shown to be promising in preclinical studies may progress to clinical trials in cancer patients. Clinical trials of new agents proceed in three phases.

PHASE I TRIALS

The main aim of this first stage in evaluating new agents in people with cancer is to identify the toxicity and the maximum tolerated dose (MTD) of the new agent so that appropriate dose levels, as close as possible to the agent's therapeutic window, are selected for use in future trials. The MTD is defined as the dose at which a predefined proportion of patients experience severe but reversible side effects from a drug using a given schedule and route of administration. Other important information, notably pharmacokinetic and pharmacodynamic data, is also collected. What would be considered significant side effects, as measured by standardised grading systems, are defined by the researchers in the trial protocol, and agreed by peer review and ethics committees.

Patients are only selected for phase I trials if no other standard therapy is available for their type of tumour. Most have been heavily treated already. To be eligible to enter the trial, the patient must have a good performance status, good renal, hepatic and haemopoietic function, no significant medical co-morbidity, and no severe toxicity from previous treatments.

Phase I trials have a dose escalation design. Three patients receive an initial dose of the new agent, often 10% of the lethal dose/kg in mice (LD10). If tolerated, the next three patients will be treated at a higher dose level and so on until significant side effects are seen in one of the three patients. At this point three further patients will receive that dose, before any further escalation. If more than one of the six patients at this level had serious side effects, then this dose is considered as too toxic and dose escalation is stopped at this point. The dose level below this point is defined as the MTD.

The dose escalation scheme may be calculated in various ways, but the modified Fibonacci formula is commonly used. This method involves using an initial steep escalation of dose followed by progressively smaller increases as the MTD is approached. The number of patients in these trials is usually small, there is no use of placebo, and they are not randomised.

PHASE II TRIALS

The aim of phase II trials is to determine the anti-tumour activity of the new agent against a particular type of cancer and therefore the primary endpoint is tumour response. Therefore patients selected for phase II trials usually have disease that can be measured accurately by clinical or radiological assessment. Patients who have received no previous similar treatment or at least have not been heavily pretreated will afford the greatest chance of detecting anti-tumour activity.

Most phase II trials recruit 40–60 patients who will usually receive treatment at the MTD (from the phase I trial). Phase II trials are designed to terminate early if there is minimal or no new agent activity. If the agent is a new drug, given alone, a response rate of 20% is usually required for the new agent to undergo further evaluation, as a single agent in randomised trials, or in combination with other standard agents in phase I and II trials.

Phase II trial results are very variable, even using the same drug at the same dose in the same cancer type. This is because patient selection is a critical determinant of response, such that subtle differences between trials in the extent of pretreatment, its timing, and performance status can make big differences. Therefore there is a trend towards randomised phase II trials, to include a comparator group receiving a standard treatment where one exists. These randomised phase II trials can be quite small (50–100 patients), as they only aim to compare response rate not survival. If there is no alternative to the new agent then placebos may be needed, although this is unsatisfactory for many patients.

PHASE III TRIALS

The aim of phase III trials is to assess the relative efficacy of the new treatments (shown to have had efficacy in phase II trials) compared to the standard treatment (control arm). Differences in efficacy between the treatments are likely to be small, and therefore large prospective randomised controlled trials involving hundreds of patients recruited in multiple centres are required for the trial to be statistically significant. The main endpoints should be overall survival and quality of life, and occasionally progression-free survival. To make the comparison between the arms scientifically valid, randomisation and stratification are used. Randomisation helps to prevent or minimise bias in factors that cannot be measured accurately. For example, if another prognostic factor is discovered the year after the trial, as treatment was allocated by randomisation there is a good chance the two arms were the same by that factor, even though it was not measured.

Stratification of the randomisation procedure may further balance the comparison groups by deliberately balancing study groups matched for important prognostic factors. Phase III trials also generate additional safety and efficacy data.

CLINICAL TRIAL DESIGNS

If important questions are to be answered, clinical trials need to be very carefully designed with clear objectives. A well-written protocol, which is strictly adhered to, is crucial. The protocol should include the following:

1. Outline summary. This gives an overview of the trial, with its goals, basic schema/design and endpoints.
2. Introduction. This should give the relevant background information to the trial with an overview of the scientific facts known about the disease and the previous relevant research. It should explain the rationale of the proposed study based on the information provided.
3. Objectives/aims. The scientific hypothesis of the study should be stated.
4. Endpoints. The measurement of the success or failure of the trial is assessed by precisely stated criteria known as endpoints. The endpoint of greatest clinical importance is known as the primary endpoint. Secondary endpoints include local recurrence-free survival, progression-free survival, response rates, toxicity and economic implications.

5. Trial entry and eligibility. The trial population must be defined. Inclusion and exclusion criteria are defined. The randomisation procedure is only performed after the subject gives informed signed consent. Examples of inclusion criteria include: histological confirmation, measurable disease, good performance status, acceptable liver and renal function. Examples of exclusion criteria include: history of previous malignancy, old or often young age, associated medical conditions, and non-compliance. The criteria for removal from the trial (e.g. disease progression, unacceptable toxicity, patient's wishes) are also defined.

6. Treatment protocol. This should contain information on treatment regimens, scheduling and time frameworks. Any evaluations during treatment are described. The role of additional treatment and salvage treatments should be addressed.

7. Follow-up. Post-treatment evaluation and follow-up policies should be defined.

8. Toxicity criteria. Well-recognised grading criteria are used to record the toxicity of treatment (e.g. the WHO Common Toxicity Criteria).

9. Statistical considerations and analysis plan. This should include information about the sample size, expected time for accrual, and study duration. As studies vary in size, their power is said to vary. No two trials will have identical results, as no two trials will include exactly the same patients. As trial results vary, even for the same treatment in the same cancer type, some may not show a difference between treatments even if there really is one – a false negative. Others may suggest a difference when in fact there is not one – a false positive. These variations can be seen in meta-analyses (see below). The larger the study, the less likely it is to give a false result. The power is a measure of how likely the study is to show the difference the researchers think they will find. An analysis plan sets out the way the data is to be presented and interpreted. This can also include an economic evaluation of effectiveness.

10. Ethical considerations. All UK medical research requires ethical committee approval. Patient information leaflets should be produced and proper consent procedures followed.

11. Appendix. Definitions of response criteria, performance status, toxicity criteria, patient information and clinical forms are included.

IMPORTANT SURVIVAL ENDPOINTS USED IN CLINICAL TRIALS

Overall survival. The time interval between entry into the clinical trial and death from any cause.

Cancer-specific survival. The time interval between entry into the clinical trial and death from cancer. Deaths not attributable to the cancer are handled differently.

Disease-free survival. The time interval between trial entry and development of recurrent disease or death due to any cause.

Progression-free survival (relapse-free survival in adjuvant studies). The time interval between the end of initial treatment, when there is still residual disease, and clinical progression of disease or death due to any cause.

META-ANALYSES OF RANDOMISED CLINICAL TRIALS

Meta-analyses combine the results of randomised clinical trials that were designed to answer the same questions, in order to evaluate small differences in treatment effects. This increases the sample size and therefore statistical power of the data. A meta-analysis is generally used when individual trials yield inconclusive or conflicting results or when several trials asking similar questions have been conducted and an overall estimate of treatment efficacy is required. Over the past 20 years, the number of published meta-analyses has increased dramatically. This is because treatments for solid tumours in adults have only moderate benefits and large numbers of patients are required to detect small differences in efficacy.

The meta-analysis should include: (i) identification of all relevant trials including non-published data, (ii) evaluation of trial quality, (iii) description of the trials, (iv) quantification of the treatment effect, (v) a study of variations of the overall treatment effect between the trials, (vi) identification of subgroups that may benefit more from the treatment.

A high quality meta-analysis provides the best overall summary of a treatment's efficacy and therefore can be very influential and change clinical practice. However, the quality of a meta-analysis is limited by the quality of the trials included – an inappropriate meta-analysis that studies a very heterogeneous group of poorly conducted studies can be misleading. A particular problem with radiotherapy trials is variability in dose, fractionation and techniques between studies, as well as inadequate reporting of acute and late toxicities.

QUALITY OF LIFE

Quality of life (QoL) is a particularly important concept in the treatment of cancer patients. There is often a fine balance of benefit and detriment to the patient from a cancer treatment. For example, palliative chemotherapy may improve survival by a few months, but at the expense of significant side effects. Alternatively treatment may improve symptoms, but not prolong survival. Methods for measuring QoL in clinical trials have been scientifically developed in groups of thousands of patients, although there is still debate about the range of techniques available. Measures address physical, psychological, cognitive and social functioning as well as overall well-being, and usually common symptoms. All these are recorded as the patient reports them, rather than proxy reports by relatives or doctors. Trials now need to assess QoL if they want to demonstrate a new treatment is genuinely preferable, and to do this using validated questionnaires. Examples include the WHOQoL instrument, and the EORTC-QoL C30.

FURTHER READING

Girling D J, Stewart L A, Parmar M K B, Stenning S P 2003 Clinical trials in cancer: principles and practice. OUP, Oxford

Green S, Benedetti J, Crowley J 2002 Clinical trials in oncology, 2nd edn. Chapman and Hall/CRC, London

Principles of cancer screening

INTRODUCTION

In general, treating cancer early in its course will increase the chances of cure. Unfortunately, by the time many tumours become clinically apparent the cancer has already spread and become incurable. If cancers can be detected before they become symptomatic, the chances of cure should be greater as the tumour burden will be less. This forms the basis of the concept of cancer screening to detect asymptomatic cancers.

Certain principles are key to the development of a successful cancer screening programme:

1. The cancer should be common and an important public health problem.
2. The natural history of the disease should be well understood.
3. There should be a long pre-invasive or non-metastatic stage of the disease.
4. The treatment of the disease should be highly effective and facilities for treatment widely available.
5. There should be an agreed policy on the target population to be screened.
6. There should be a diagnostic test able to detect the disease at an early curable stage.
7. The test should ideally be simple, cheap, easy to perform and be widely available and acceptable to the population to be screened.
8. The test should also be sensitive (i.e. give low false-negative results) and specific (i.e. give low false-positive results) to the disease.
9. The test should be well publicised to ensure compliance of the population.
10. The whole process should save lives and be cost-effective.

The potential advantages of a successful screening programme include the following:

1. Reduction in cancer mortality.
2. Less radical treatment is required to achieve cure. This also translates into financial savings for the health service.

3. Reassurance is given by a negative test.
4. Psychological benefit to the population as a whole.

The potential disadvantages of screening include:

1. Increased anxiety and morbidity if no effective intervention is possible.
2. Over-investigation of false-positive cases.
3. Over-investigation and overtreatment of borderline cases that do not require treatment.
4. Exposure to the risks of the screening test.
5. False reassurance of a false-negative test.
6. High resource implications (e.g. increased workload and cost implications).

Some of the disadvantages can be reconciled by limiting screening through targeting at-risk populations (e.g. only screen smokers for lung cancer etc.). This will increase sensitivity and specificity as well as improve compliance and reduce costs. The development of an effective infrastructure involving primary care groups, support groups, and the hospital sector will ensure increased awareness and better uptake of screening with at-risk populations.

Despite many of the common cancers fulfilling most of the criteria for adopting potentially very effective screening programmes, cancer screening remains one of the great controversies of modern medicine. This is in part due to the obvious political, economic, public health and logistical problems of implementing successful cancer screening. However, the main problem has been the difficulty of demonstrating a clear cost-effective mortality reduction in the screened population. Very large randomised controlled clinical studies over many years are needed to demonstrate mortality reduction. Even if benefits are clearly shown, they may not translate from the study population to the target population, as the professional expertise used in the study may not be available to the target population. In addition, three main types of bias may confound the results of a screening programme – lead-time bias, length bias and selection bias.

Lead-time bias. The time of diagnosis is brought forward, but the patient will die at the same time regardless of whether earlier treatment is given, because the tumour has already metastasised at the time of screening. This gives the appearance of longer survival in the screened patient.

Length bias. Faster growing, more aggressive, poorer prognosis cancers are less likely to be detected by screening because they are more likely to become symptomatic during the screening interval than slow growing tumours. Therefore a lower proportion of aggressive cancers may be seen in the screened group.

Selection bias. Those who comply with the screening programme may have different characteristics from the non-compliant population, i.e. they may be more health conscious, better educated and in a higher social group.

This phenomenon has clearly been demonstrated in the NHS breast cancer screening programme.

CANCER SCREENING PROGRAMMES

Despite the controversies over cancer screening, the NHS has endorsed national screening programmes for breast and cervical cancer, which currently screen over 5 million women each year.

BREAST CANCER SCREENING

This national screening programme was introduced between 1988 and 1991. Screening is currently offered every 3 years to all women over 50. At present women receive invitations between the ages of 50 and 70 years and are entitled to request screening every 3 years thereafter. In 1998/9 the breast screening programme detected 8000 cancers, 40% of which were less than 1.5 cm. Two-view mammography will further increase detection rates. It is estimated that 30% of the recent fall in breast cancer mortality rates is due to the screening programme.

CERVICAL CANCER SCREENING

Screening was first introduced in the 1960s, but it was not until 1988 that a comprehensive recall system was introduced. All women aged 20–64 are invited for a Papanicolaou smear test at least every 5 years. The cervical cancer death rate has been falling by 7% a year since the introduction of the screening programme. Changes have recently been announced to the national programme following a recommendation from the National Institute of Clinical Excellence (NICE) that liquid based cytology should replace the traditional Papanicolaou smear and a recommendation from Cancer Research UK scientists that women should be screened from age 25 years at 3-yearly intervals until 49 years and then at 5-yearly intervals until 64 years. HPV testing continues to be evaluated.

COLORECTAL CANCER

Screening is still under evaluation. The main screening tests are faecal occult bloods and flexible sigmoidoscopy. Research in the UK and Denmark has demonstrated that screening for colorectal cancer may produce 15% mortality reduction. High risk patients such as those with a previous primary tumour, polyps, ulcerative colitis and/or a strong family history of colorectal cancer should be screened with regular colonoscopies.

PROSTATE CANCER

Screening for prostate cancer with PSA testing and transrectal ultrasound remains controversial and is subject to large European clinical trials.

OVARIAN CANCER

Screening for ovarian cancer with transvaginal ultrasound and CA125 levels is also the focus of large clinical trials.

LUNG CANCER

Previous trials in lung cancer with chest X-ray and sputum cytology showed no survival benefit to mass screening. However, there is currently much interest in using low dose spiral CT scanning in targeted high risk populations.

FUTURE PERSPECTIVES

The publication of large studies in ovarian cancer, prostate cancer and colorectal cancer are awaited with interest. New, more sensitive and specific tests for early cancer are being developed. One of the most exciting and controversial areas is in the development of genetic screening tests for identification of underlying familial cancer syndromes, e.g. BRCA 1 and 2 for breast cancer and ovarian cancer. The identification of these at-risk populations will allow more effective, targeted screening programmes.

CONCLUSION

The cancer screening debate continues, but the NHS cancer plan stresses the importance of cancer screening in the UK and there is also a national screening committee that is dedicated to ensuring that appropriate measures are taken to introduce national screening programmes on the basis of high quality evidence from clinical trials.

FURTHER READING

Souhami R L, Tannock I, Hohenberger P, Horiot J-C (eds) 2002 Cancer screening. In: The Oxford textbook of oncology. Oxford University Press, Oxford
Wilson J 1968 Principles and practice of screening for disease. Public Health Papers, 34, WHO, Geneva

SECTION TWO

A–Z OF CANCERS

Adrenal cancer

BACKGROUND INFORMATION

Adrenal tumours are very common, but the vast majority are benign and non-functioning and usually diagnosed incidentally following abdominal imaging (CT, MRI, ultrasound). Adrenal cancer accounts for less than 1% of all adrenal tumours and has an incidence in the UK of 0.6/100 000 population. In 1997, there were only 143 new cases of adrenal cancer registered in the UK.

Adrenal carcinoma arising from the adrenal cortex is the commonest primary cancer of the adrenal gland and has a particularly poor prognosis with overall 5-year survival of 35%. It occurs in all age groups, but has a bimodal age distribution with a peak before the age of 5 years and a second peak in the fourth and fifth decades. Approximately 60% are functional, secreting various hormones leading to associated endocrine clinical syndromes (Table 11.1). Polycythaemia, hypoglycaemia and hypercalcaemia can also occur.

Over 90% of adrenal carcinomas are greater than 6 cm in diameter and 60% have spread beyond the gland at diagnosis (stage III and IV disease). The disease spreads contiguously to the kidney and liver and the most common sites of metastases are the peritoneum, lung, liver and bone.

TABLE 11.1 Endocrine clinical syndromes associated with adrenal cancer

Endocrine effect	Hormone secreted
Cushing's (30–40%)	Cortisol
Virilisation and precocious puberty (20–30%)	Androgens
Feminisation (6%)	Oestrogens
Conn's (2.5%)	Aldosterone
Mixed – virilisation and Cushing's (25%)	Cortisol and androgens

Other primary cancers of the adrenal gland include phaeochromocytomas (arising from adrenal medulla – 10–20% are malignant), sarcomas and lymphomas. Phaeochromocytomas are discussed at the end of this chapter.

Metastatic lesions are by far the commonest malignant lesions of the adrenal gland and usually occur in patients with disseminated cancer. The primary tumours that metastasise most often to the adrenals are lung, breast, colon, kidney, lymphoma and melanoma. If the adrenal metastasis is a solitary lesion, then resection may offer the chance of cure.

PRESENTATION

Most patients with functioning adrenal carcinomas present with endocrine symptoms and signs associated with the secreted hormone, e.g. Cushing's (centripetal obesity, muscle wasting, striae, acne and hypertension) and virilisation (hirsutism, oligomenorrhoea).

Patients with non-functioning tumours usually present with abdominal pain and a palpable abdominal mass. Other features include weight loss, malaise, fever, anorexia, myalgia, and symptoms and signs of metastatic disease. Many patients also present with an incidental finding of an adrenal mass (incidentaloma).

DIAGNOSIS AND STAGING

Investigations should include full history and examination; baseline FBC, renal and liver function tests; CXR. Hormonal studies should include screening for possible phaeochromocytoma, as there is a risk of lethal

TABLE 11.2 TNM staging of adrenal cancer	
T1	Tumour diameter smaller than or equal to 5 cm with no local invasion
T2	Tumour diameter larger than 5 cm with no local invasion
T3	Tumour any size with local extension but not involving adjacent organs
T4	Tumour any size with local invasion of adjacent organs
N0	No regional lymph node involvement
N1	Positive regional nodes
M0	No distant metastasis
M1	Distant metastasis
Stages	
Stage I	T1, N0, M0 (20% of patients)
Stage II	T2, N0, M0 (20% of patients)
Stage III	T1–2, N1, M0 or T3, N0 (20% of patients)
Stage IV	Any T, any N, M1 or T3, N1 or T4 (40% of patients)

hypertensive crisis following biopsy or resection. CT abdomen is the initial imaging modality of choice for adrenal masses. Malignant lesions tend to be greater than 5 cm in size with blurred margins, irregular shape and show heterogeneity with contrast. MRI may provide further information to help distinguish carcinomas from adenomas and phaeochromocytomas, and is also better for assessing renal vein/vena cava involvement.

Due to the difficulty of histologically differentiating benign from malignant tumours, CT guided fine needle aspiration or core tissue biopsies are not generally recommended except for possible metastatic deposits.

Staging is by the TNM system (Table 11.2).

MANAGEMENT OF ADRENAL CARCINOMA

Complete surgical excision of all tumour offers the only chance of cure, but is only possible in ~55% of patients. Five-year survival for this group of patients is approximately 40%. There is no proven effective adjuvant therapy, although the adrenolytic agent mitotane has been used.

In unresectable patients, mitotane has also been used to try and downstage tumours to allow resection with limited success. Median survival for patients with unresectable disease is 3–9 months.

Most patients have metastatic disease at presentation. Useful palliation can be achieved with mitotane, which has produced objective response rates of 19–34% and improvement in hormonal symptoms for many patients. However, mitotane is generally ineffective in prolonging survival and has significant side effects including nausea, anorexia, weakness, somnolence, confusion, lethargy, headache, ataxia and dysarthria. Cisplatin-based regimens have also been used with limited success (response rates of ~30%). Radiotherapy may be used to palliate bone metastases.

Lifelong follow-up is recommended for survivors as late relapses after 10 years have been reported.

PROBLEMS IN ADVANCED DISEASE

1. Endocrine syndromes.
   - Cushing's may respond to mitotane, ketoconazole, metyrapone, or aminoglutethimide.
   - Conn's may respond to spironolactone, amiloride and antihypertensive medication.
   - Feminisation can respond to anti-oestrogens such as tamoxifen and danazol.

- Virilisation may respond to anti-androgens such as flutamide, cyproterone acetate, bicalutamide, and megestrol acetate. Other options include ketoconazole, spironolactone, cimetidine and aromatase inhibitors.
2. Bone metastases (see Ch. 48 on bone metastases).

PHAEOCHROMOCYTOMAS

Phaeochromocytomas arise from chromaffin cells of the adrenal medulla. Ninety per cent are sporadic, with 10% being associated with MEN 2A/B, neurofibromatosis or Von Hippel–Lindau syndrome. Only 10% are malignant. They secrete catecholamines such as adrenaline, noradrenaline and dopamine and may therefore produce symptoms such as headache, sweating, palpitations, abdominal pains, anxiety, tremor, dizzy spells and collapse. Patients may have severe episodes of hypertension, which may be exacerbated by stress, infection, drugs and anaesthesia leading to a hypertensive crisis.

Diagnosis is based on demonstrating elevated urinary catecholamines along with imaging (CT/MRI) confirmation of the tumour.

Surgical excision under expert anaesthesia is the treatment of choice. Preoperative alpha-adrenergic blockade is required to allow expansion of the blood volume. Beta-blockers can then be used to treat tachycardias.

Metastatic disease usually runs an indolent course and 5-year survival is just under 50%. Therapeutic options include surgical debulking, chemotherapy or radionuclide therapy with iodine-131 MIBG (which concentrates in chromaffin cells).

FURTHER READING

Ng L, Libertino J M 2003 Adrenocortical carcinoma: diagnosis, evaluation and management. Journal of Urology 169:5–11

CHAPTER 12

AIDS-related cancer

BACKGROUND INFORMATION

The acquired immunodeficiency syndrome (AIDS) was first described in 1981 and definitions of the disease at that time included associations with malignancy, especially Kaposi's sarcoma and CNS lymphomas. The following malignancies are AIDS-defining conditions:

- Kaposi's sarcoma
- non-Hodgkin's lymphoma (intermediate, or high grade B-cell NHL)
- cervical squamous cell carcinoma.

Other tumours reported to have a higher incidence in this population are Hodgkin's disease, anal cancer, testicular cancer, lung cancer, head and neck cancer, non-melanoma skin cancer, plasmacytoma and leukaemia.

Over the last few years there has been significant progress in the management of HIV/AIDS. The use of combinations of at least three antiretroviral drugs, known as highly active antiretroviral treatment (HAART), has led to a dramatic decrease in opportunistic infections, AIDS-defining illnesses (including malignancies) and mortality.

Despite the advances made with HAART, AIDS-related cancers still pose difficult management problems because of the following factors:

1. Compromised bone marrow function due to HIV/AIDS itself and the antiretroviral drugs used to treat it
2. Enhanced sensitivity of HIV-infected patients to irradiation
3. Medical co-morbidity, e.g. due to opportunistic infections.

EPIDEMIC OR AIDS-ASSOCIATED KAPOSI'S SARCOMA (KS)

Kaposi's sarcoma has been reported in 20–50% of the AIDS population, making it the commonest AIDS-related malignancy. However, the incidence of KS has fallen since the introduction of HAART.

KS is particularly seen in homosexual men with HIV-1 infection, suggesting an infectious co-factor is involved. It is now clear that the primary and necessary factor in the development of all forms of KS is the presence of the Kaposi's sarcoma herpes virus (KSHV). It appears that KSHV has spread from epicentres of AIDS in the US to homosexual groups in Canada and Europe. The disease affects skin and lymph nodes (often causing debilitating lymphoedema), mucous membranes (predominantly the palate), and the lungs. The clinical course is variable with some patients having indolent disease and others suffering highly aggressive and fatal disease.

Patients are treated with antiretroviral therapy, which may halt the progression of the disease or induce tumour shrinkage. More than 50% of patients with cutaneous KS will respond to HAART alone. Local and systemic treatments are also used. Radiotherapy, cryotherapy and intra-lesional vinblastine or interferon alpha are all useful options for limited cutaneous lesions that have not responded to HAART. Due to the increased radiation sensitivity of AIDS patients, radiotherapy may cause severe side effects, especially in sites such as the oral cavity and soles of feet. This can be minimised by lower dose modified fractionated radiotherapy schedules and careful skin care with moisturisers. Strontium-90 eye applicator brachytherapy can be used for eyelid and conjunctival lesions.

Systemic disease can be treated with chemotherapy such as liposomal doxorubicin or daunorubicin, which produces response rates of 25–60% with little associated toxicity. Paclitaxel may be used as a second line agent. Vincristine, bleomycin and etoposide are also active agents. Systemic interferon alpha given subcutaneously or intravenously is also a useful option. The use of thalidomide and retinoids is experimental, but promising. Despite these treatments, the outlook is poor for patients with more aggressive forms of the disease, where median survival is measured in months. Poor prognostic features include CD4 counts $<300/mm^3$, presence of B symptoms (see Table 25.1), pulmonary disease and history of opportunistic infections.

Three other variants of KS that are unrelated to HIV/AIDS are also recognised:

1. Classic – multiple firm purplish/pink/red skin nodules/plaques seen in elderly men of Eastern/Mediterranean origin. Tends to be multifocal and recur despite treatment with surgical excision, local radiotherapy and chemotherapy. However, the prognosis is very good, with median survival measured in years or decades.
2. Endemic – seen in African children and adults. Lymph nodes are commonly involved and the prognosis is less good.
3. Immunosuppression/transplant associated – occurs in 0.5% of organ transplant recipients. Tends to be aggressive, involving lymph nodes, mucosae, and visceral organs in 50%, but regresses when immunosuppressive treatment is withdrawn or modified. This is feasible for renal transplant

patients (as dialysis can be used), but more of a problem with liver/heart transplants. Other options include local radiotherapy and chemotherapy.

NON-HODGKIN'S LYMPHOMA (NHL)

Unlike KS, AIDS-related NHL occurs at similar rates in all groups of HIV-infected patients. The annual incidence of NHL in HIV-infected patients is 1.6–2%. The majority of patients (90%) present with extranodal disease in contrast to non-HIV NHL patients. The common extranodal sites are CNS, bone marrow, gastrointestinal tract and liver. It may also present as primary effusion lymphoma (PEL) involving a body cavity. Systemic B symptoms are common (70–80%) and so it is important to exclude underlying opportunistic infections. Pathologically, AIDS-related NHL are almost exclusively B-cell in origin and high or intermediate grade. These include diffuse large cell lymphoma, immunoblastic, and Burkitt's or Burkitt's like lymphomas. Treatment generally consists of low dose chemotherapy, although patients with a good performance status and CD4 count $>100/mm^3$ may tolerate full dose CHOP (cyclophosphamide, doxorubicin, vincristine, prednisolone). Prognosis is poor, with median overall survival of 6–9 months.

Primary cerebral lymphomas (PCL) are usually a late manifestation of AIDS and patients have traditionally fared very poorly, with a median survival of only 2–3 months, despite high dose steroids and whole brain radiotherapy. The poor survival rates were mainly due to deaths from opportunistic infections rather than progressive lymphoma. However, since the introduction of HAART, survival has improved for these patients and new treatment modalities for PCL need to be explored.

CERVICAL SQUAMOUS CELL CARCINOMA

Cervical dysplasia and cervical squamous cell carcinoma are associated with HIV and human papilloma virus (HPV). Cervical cancer is considered an AIDS-defining malignancy. Treatment is generally similar to that for patients who do not have HIV, but the clinical stage tends to be higher at presentation and the outlook less good.

HODGKIN'S, ANAL CANCER AND OTHER NON-AIDS-DEFINING MALIGNANCIES

Hodgkin's lymphoma is reported as occurring with increased frequency in HIV/AIDS, but it has not been accepted as part of the definition of AIDS as yet. It presents in a more aggressive manner and advanced stage than non-HIV Hodgkin's, often with extranodal disease or bone marrow involvement. Treatment strategies are similar to the HIV-negative population. Median survival is 8–20 months.

Cancers of the anus are more common in homosexual HIV-infected patients. The human papilloma virus (HPV) appears to be the causative agent. Standard treatment approaches with chemoradiation may offer high response rates and long-term survival. Patients with low initial CD4 counts should start HAART.

The survival benefits of HAART have made HIV a chronic immuno-suppressive disease and this will lead to an increasing number of HIV patients with non-AIDS-defining tumours such as lung cancer, skin cancer and myeloma.

FURTHER READING

Antman K, Chang Y 2000 Kaposi's sarcoma (review). New England Journal of Medicine 342:1027–1038

Cottrill C P, Bottomley D M, Phillips R H 1997 Cancer and HIV infection. Clinical Oncology 9:365–380

Lukawska J, Cottrill C, Bower M 2003 The changing role of radiotherapy in AIDS-related malignancies. Clinical Oncology 15:2–6

Scadden D T, Howard W W 1998 AIDS-related malignancies. Oncologist 3:119–123

Wool G M 1998 AIDS-related malignancies. Oncologist 3:279–283

CHAPTER 13

Anal cancer

BACKGROUND INFORMATION

Anal cancer is an uncommon malignancy accounting for around 2% of gastrointestinal system cancers with 637 registered cases in the UK in 1999. The exact aetiology is unknown, but risk factors include: infection by the human papilloma virus (notably HPV type 16), history of anal intercourse, history of sexually transmitted disease, multiple sexual partners, history of cervical/vulvar/vaginal cancer, immunosuppression (e.g. organ transplantation), HIV infection and smoking. Chronic inflammatory anorectal disorders pose little or no increased risk.

Anatomically, the anus is divided into the mucosal-lined anal canal and the epidermis-lined anal margin (Fig. 13.1).

The anal canal, which extends from the anal verge to the rectal mucosa, is lined by squamous epithelium and hence squamous cell carcinoma (SCC) is by far the commonest histology (>90%). They are usually non-keratinising and poorly differentiated. Tumours arising from the upper part of the anal canal, around the dentate line, show mixed patterns of adenocarcinoma and squamous cell carcinoma and are termed basaloid carcinomas (also known as cloacogenic or transitional carcinomas). Adenocarcinomas in the anal canal are rare (5–10% of cases). They behave like rectal cancer and should be treated as such.

Anal margin squamous cell carcinomas are usually keratinising and well differentiated and are much less common than anal canal SCCs. In fact many cancers seen at the anal margin have actually arisen from the anal mucosa or extend from the anal canal, and these are managed as anal canal cancers.

Other rare anal tumour types include melanoma, adenoid cystic carcinoma, mucoepidermoid carcinoma, small cell carcinoma, sarcomas and lymphomas.

The majority of patients with anal canal SCCs can be cured by concurrent chemoradiotherapy, with preservation of sphincter function. Overall 5-year survival is now ~70%.

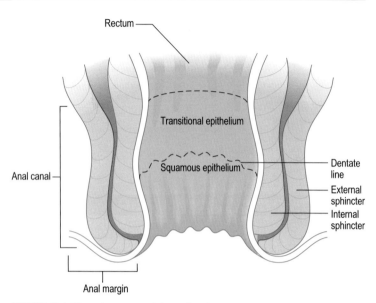

FIGURE 13.1 Normal anatomy of the anal region.

PRESENTATION

Rectal bleeding is the commonest presenting symptom. Around a third of patients have pain or sensation of a mass. Other symptoms include change in bowel habit, rectal discharge, pruritus ani, and tenesmus. An anal lump may be visible or palpable. In advanced disease there may be symptoms and signs of fistulation, palpable groin nodes or a palpable liver.

DIAGNOSIS AND STAGING

Investigations used in the diagnosis of anal cancer include history and examination, including careful digital rectal examination (DRE) and palpation of inguinal and femoral nodes; routine bloods (FBC, renal/liver function tests); calcium; CXR; CT of the chest and abdomen; MRI scan of the pelvis; examination under anaesthetic (EUA) and biopsy of lesion; and fine needle aspiration (FNA) of palpable groin nodes. Endo-anal ultrasound may offer additional information regarding the local extent of the tumour. Consider HIV test and CD4 count if appropriate.

Staging is by the TNM 2002 system (Table 13.1).

TABLE 13.1 2002 TNM staging of anal canal SCC (simplified)

T1	Tumour ≤ 2 cm
T2	Tumour > 2 cm to 5 cm
T3	Tumour > 5 cm
T4	Tumour invades other organ (vagina, urethra, bladder, sacrum)
N0	No nodes
N1	Perirectal nodes
N2	Unilateral internal iliac and/or inguinal nodes
N3	Perirectal and/or bilateral internal iliac or inguinal nodes
M0	No distant metastases
M1	Distant metastases

MANAGEMENT

CANCER OF THE ANAL MARGIN

Small T1, N0 lesions may be treated by local excision or local radiotherapy. Patients with locally advanced disease are generally treated with concurrent chemoradiotherapy.

CANCER OF THE ANAL CANAL

Carcinoma in situ

Carcinoma in situ may be treated with local excision alone if adequate margins are obtained. Re-excision should be offered to patients with positive resection margins.

Invasive disease

Primary chemoradiotherapy is now the mainstay of treatment for invasive cancer as it offers high cure rates without the need for mutilating surgery. Salvage surgery with anorectal excision and colostomy (abdominoperineal resection – APR) is reserved for patients with persistent or locally recurrent disease with no evidence of distant metastases.

In selected patients with early small well-differentiated tumours (<2 cm), local surgical excision, external beam radiotherapy or interstitial brachytherapy are treatment options with high cure rates (70–90%). However, most patients with anal cancer are treated with concurrent chemoradiotherapy, which offers local control rates of ~70%+ and overall 5-year survival of ~65%. The optimum chemoradiotherapy schedule has yet to be defined, but a minimum dose of 45–50 Gy over 5–6 weeks is commonly used concurrently with two cycles of 5FU and mitomycin C given on day 1 only.

A low dose schedule (e.g. 30 Gy in 15 fractions (3 weeks) with one cycle of 5FU) may be used for frail elderly and medically unfit patients with all stages of locoregional disease (any T, any N). This schedule is also suitable for HIV/AIDS patients.

Acute toxicity of chemoradiotherapy can be severe and includes painful perianal skin reactions, diarrhoea and myelosuppression. Late effects include painful necrosis of the anus, skin ulceration, bleeding, anal stenosis, fistula formation, pelvic insufficiency fractures and chronic diarrhoea. Up to 5% of patients have complications severe enough to require a permanent colostomy.

Management of inguinal nodes
Node-negative patients Clinically node-negative patients with T1 tumours do not require elective treatment of the inguinal region. However, those with T2-4 tumours have a significant risk of nodal microscopic disease and prophylactic elective radiation may be offered (e.g. 30 Gy in 15 fractions over 3 weeks – 'phase 1'). The radiation field should include the pelvic and the inguinal nodes. The primary tumour alone then receives a further 'boost' dose of radiotherapy (e.g. 20 Gy in 10 fractions over 2 weeks – 'phase 2'). Some clinicians opt for a watch and wait policy, offering salvage surgery and radiotherapy for inguinal node relapse.

Inguinal node-positive patients Patients with positive inguinal nodes require full dose radical chemoradiotherapy to the primary tumour and the involved nodes.

Recurrent disease
Local recurrence occurs in 10–30% of patients following chemoradiation and may be salvageable by APR in approximately 60% of cases. Around 50% of these patients will enjoy long-term disease control. Isolated inguinal recurrence may be salvaged by block dissection of the groin and radiotherapy depending on previous treatment.

Metastatic disease
Palliative cisplatin-based chemotherapy (e.g. cisplatin and 5FU) may be offered to patients with metastatic disease, but little data exists regarding its benefits.

FUTURE PERSPECTIVES

The role of cisplatin in concurrent chemoradiation is being addressed in phase III trials. For example, the MRC ACT II trial is assessing whether the addition of mitomycin C or cisplatin to 5FU and radiotherapy will produce a better complete response rate. In addition, the trial is also assessing the role of maintenance cisplatin/5FU chemotherapy versus no chemotherapy.

PROBLEMS IN ADVANCED DISEASE

See Chapter 58 on problems in advanced pelvic malignancy.

FURTHER READING

Ryan D P, Compton C C, Mayer R J 2000 Medical progress. Carcinoma of the anal canal. New England Journal of Medicine 342:792–800
START oncology group 2001 Cancer of the anus. Available at: www.startoncology.net

Bladder cancer

BACKGROUND INFORMATION

Bladder cancer is the fifth commonest malignancy in the UK with 11 080 new cases in 2000. The incidence has been increasing in almost all European countries. It is three times commoner in men than women and over 70% of patients are aged over 65 years. In 2002, there were 4910 deaths from bladder cancer in the UK.

Approximately 80% of patients present with superficial bladder cancer (Ta, T1, carcinoma in situ), which generally has an excellent prognosis. However, 20% of patients present with muscle-invasive disease (penetration beyond lamina propria – T2–4) and this group have an overall 5-year survival of only 40–50%. Unfortunately, even after 5 years many continue to die due to the recurrent nature of the disease.

Exposure to arylamines such as benzidine and naphthylamine formerly used in the textile dye industry is associated with a 20-fold increased risk of bladder cancer. These substances have been banned in many countries so are not an important contributor any more. In contrast, smoking increases risk only about two-fold, but has a much greater global impact. The association with smoking also explains the serious medical co-morbidity often seen in bladder cancer patients. Other risk factors include schistosomiasis (causes squamous cell carcinoma), use of cyclophosphamide (10-fold risk after 12 years), neuropathic bladders and NSAIDs.

Pathologically, 90% of bladder cancers are transitional cell carcinomas (TCCs), 8% are squamous cell carcinomas and 2% are adenocarcinomas or rare tumours such as sarcomas. Grossly, tumours may be papillary polypoid lesions, plaque-like flat lesions, non-invasive mucosal thickening or invasive lesions. Histologically bladder tumours are graded 1–3, where grade 1 lesions are well differentiated, grade 2 lesions are moderately differentiated and grade 3 lesions are poorly differentiated. Bladder cancer is often associated with a field defect of the urinary mucosa and the entire lining of the urinary tract may be at risk for developing malignancy.

Superficial bladder cancers often recur following resection (up to 70% recurrence rate), but progression to invasive disease is fortunately uncommon. Progression to muscle invasive disease is more likely in grade 3 tumours, carcinoma in situ (CIS) and T1 lesions.

CIS is a flat lesion replacing the entire thickness of the urothelium with high grade malignant tissue and is an important precursor to invasive bladder cancer.

Muscle-invasive bladder cancer may spread locally to the prostate, seminal vesicles, rectum, uterus, vagina, retroperitoneal soft tissue and sacrum. Metastases occur to the lymph nodes, lungs, liver, skin, peritoneum, and bones and sometimes the brain.

PRESENTATION

Painless haematuria, frequency, dysuria and urgency are the commonest presenting symptoms. Pelvic pain, bony pain, leg oedema and symptoms and signs of uraemia and hydronephrosis are indicative of advanced disease.

DIAGNOSIS AND STAGING

Investigations include full history and examination including pelvic and rectal examination; renal and liver function tests; FBC; and CXR. EUA and

TABLE 14.1 2002 TNM staging of bladder cancer (simplified)	
Tx	Primary tumour cannot be assessed
Ta	Non-invasive papillary tumour
Tis	In situ 'flat tumour'
T1	Tumour invades subepithelial tissue only
T2	Tumour invades muscularis
	2a superficial muscle
	2b deep muscle
T3	Tumour extends beyond muscularis
	3a microscopically
	3b extravesical mass
T4	4a Tumour invades prostate, uterus or vagina
	4b Tumour invades pelvic wall or abdominal wall
N1	Single node $\leqslant 2$ cm
N2	Single node >2 to 5 cm, multiple nodes $\leqslant 5$ cm
N3	Any node >5 cm
M1	Distant metastases
Stage I	T1, N0, M0
Stage II	T2a/b, N0, M0
Stage III	T3a/b, T4a, N0, M0
Stage IV	T4b, N0, M0; any T, N1–3; any T, any N, M1

cystoscopy with transurethral resection of bladder (TURB) is the investigation of choice to obtain histological diagnosis. Other investigations include CT scan of the abdomen and pelvis (MRI offers no clear advantage over CT) to assess for local extent of disease, lymph node spread and other organ involvement. Intravenous urogram (IVU) may reveal a filling defect in the bladder and also allows visualisation of the entire urothelium. Ultrasound is sometimes used to assess the bladder wall and to evaluate the kidneys and ureters. Urine cytology is an easy and cheap way to obtain a diagnosis with a high specificity and sensitivity of 80% in grade 3 tumours, but is not so helpful for grade 1 or 2 tumours. A bone scan can be performed if there is suspicion of bone metastases. There is currently no screening programme for bladder cancer in the UK.

Bladder cancer is staged by the 2002 TNM system (Table 14.1).

MANAGEMENT

SUPERFICIAL BLADDER CANCER (Ta,TI, CARCINOMA IN SITU (CIS))

Most of these tumours are low risk and may be treated with transurethral resection (TURB) and/or fulguration. TURB involves removal of the tumour and the underlying detrusor muscle. A single instillation of intravesical chemotherapy (e.g. epirubicin or mitomycin C) is usually administered following resection of low grade tumours, but regular cystoscopic follow-up is recommended due to high recurrence rates (50% recur within 6–12 months). Patients with grade 3 superficial tumours, T1 disease, or multiple recurrences are at higher risk of progressing to muscle invasive disease and should receive intravesical BCG immunotherapy, which halves the recurrence rates. Long-term cystoscopic follow-up is required. The overall prognosis in this group is very good. Cystectomy or sometimes radiotherapy are options for patients with multiple high grade recurrences, or multifocal high grade disease.

Carcinoma in situ

CIS should be thought of as potentially aggressive disease and needs treatment, as 55% will develop invasive disease at 5 years and 90% within 14 years without intervention. Intravesical therapy with BCG is standard treatment. It is usually administered as three separate weekly treatments every 6 months and response rates are over 80%. A radical cystectomy is the treatment of choice for CIS resistant to BCG therapy.

MUSCLE INVASIVE BLADDER CANCER (T2–4b)

The primary treatment options for muscle invasive bladder cancer are surgery or radiotherapy. Unfortunately, no comparison in a prospective randomised trial has been made between radical radiotherapy and radical surgery. Local control is almost certainly greater with surgery, but whether overall survival is better with surgery is more contentious due to patient selection bias (i.e. patients selected for surgery tend to be fitter and younger with less co-morbidity), lack of surgical staging for radiotherapy patients and the fact that selected radiation failures have the option of salvage cystectomy.

Surgery

Surgery is considered to be the primary treatment of choice for muscle invasive bladder cancer in most of Europe and the USA, but this has not tended to be the case in the UK, where the use of radiotherapy has traditionally been higher.

Surgery is favoured in younger patients (less than 70 years) with good performance status, and minimal co-morbidity. Radical cystectomy (removal of bladder, prostate, seminal vesicles/anterior vaginectomy and meticulous lymph node dissection) with ileal conduit formation is the usual surgical intervention. Surgical mortality rates are 1–3%. Surgical morbidity includes haemorrhage, urinary leakage, impotence, sepsis, wound infection, urinary tract infection, and thromboembolism. Newer techniques such as nerve sparing cystectomy, the Koch ileal reservoir (with cutaneous reservoir) and the orthoptic ileal reservoir anastomosed to the urethra have improved patient morbidity (e.g. impotence rates improved from 95% to 70%) and quality of life, but require a high level of surgical skill and are not available in many centres. Partial cystectomy is possible in highly selected patients with solitary tumours and no evidence of CIS.

Five-year survival rates following radical cystectomy are 60–75% in T2 disease and 20–40% in T3–4 disease. Overall surgical 5-year survival rates are of the order of 40–50%. Patients with positive lymph nodes have a poor outlook with 15–20% 5-year survival.

A recent MRC meta-analysis has suggested that neoadjuvant platinum-based combination chemotherapy improves absolute 5-year survival by 5% (increased from 45 to 50%) and this approach should be considered for patients fit enough to receive it. The role of postoperative adjuvant chemotherapy is less clear.

Radiotherapy

Radical radiotherapy (55–65 Gy over 4–6 weeks) produces overall 5-year survival rates of around 35–40%, which may be improved with salvage cystectomy, although relatively few patients are suitable for this. Its main advantages are bladder conservation (70% retain normal bladder function) and low rates of impotence. Radiotherapy should be delivered using modern 3D conformal techniques. Acute side effects including diarrhoea and cystitis are common. Late effects including radiation proctitis, bladder neck obstruction and haematuria secondary to telangiectasia have traditionally occurred in 10–25% of patients, but may be less common with conformal techniques. Follow-up with regular cystoscopy is required. Patients with residual disease at check cystoscopy (usually performed 3–6 months after radiotherapy) have a very poor prognosis.

Palliative radiotherapy, e.g. 30–35 Gy in 10 fractions, is useful for relief of symptoms in patients with locally advanced disease (especially haematuria). Shorter regimens such as 20 Gy in five fractions, 21 Gy in three fractions, or a single 8 or 10 Gy fraction may be more appropriate for patients with poor performance status. The role of neoadjuvant chemotherapy and concurrent chemoradiotherapy is still under evaluation.

METASTATIC BLADDER CANCER

Untreated, the median survival is 3–6 months and the 5-year survival less than 5%. Patients with local symptoms such as pain and bleeding or bony metastases should be offered palliative radiotherapy. Chemotherapy with MVAC (methotrexate, vinblastine, doxorubicin and cisplatin) has response rates of 40–70% with complete responses of 18%, but long-term survival is rare (<4%). This regimen has substantial toxicity with high rates of neutropenic infections, mucositis, and nausea and vomiting. The toxic death rate with MVAC is 3–4%. Recently, a new chemotherapy combination with cisplatin and gemcitabine produced response rates and survival that were similar to MVAC but with less toxicity, and this has become the treatment of choice in many centres. Median survival of over 12 months can now be expected. Patients with good performance status, nodal disease and TCC histology have a better prognosis. Those with liver and bony disease and or adenocarcinoma/squamous cell histology do particularly badly.

FUTURE PERSPECTIVES

In superficial bladder cancer, there is much interest in the role of local microwave hyperthermia in combination with intravesical chemotherapy.

In muscle invasive disease, there is currently much research focusing on multimodality bladder preservation with clinical trials of neoadjuvant chemotherapy and concurrent chemoradiation. The identification of molecular markers to predict radiotherapy response may help in the selection of patients for bladder preservation therapy or cystectomy and is a key area of current research interest. The taxanes are being evaluated in the metastatic setting. Novel agents such as EGFR (epidermal growth factor receptors) inhibitors are currently being assessed in clinical trials.

PROBLEMS IN ADVANCED BLADDER CANCER

See also Chapter 58 on problems in advanced pelvic malignancy.

1. Frequency, dysuria and incontinence. May be side effects of radiotherapy. Can be treated with an anticholinergic, e.g. oxybutynin. A urodom sheath or long-term catheterisation is sometimes required.
2. Bladder spasms. Usually due to irritation at the trigone, causing attacks of severe suprapubic pain radiating into the urethra and perineum. Treatment options include NSAIDs, oxybutynin 5 mg t.d.s., Buscopan s.c. infusion 180 mg/24 hours, flavoxate 200 mg t.d.s. or instillation of 0.5% bupivacaine 20 ml for 20 minutes.

FURTHER READING

Juffs H G, Moore M J, Tannock I F 2002 The role of systemic chemotherapy in the management of muscle invasive bladder cancer. Review. Lancet Oncology 3(12):738–747.

Petrovich Z, Baert L, Brady L W (eds) 1998 Carcinoma of the bladder. Springer-Verlag, Berlin.

Sengelov L, von der Masse H 1999 Radiotherapy in bladder cancer. Review article. Radiotherapy and Oncology 52:1–14.

CHAPTER 15

Brain tumours

BACKGROUND INFORMATION

The incidence of primary brain tumours is 7/100 000 per year in the UK with 4660 new cases registered in the year 2000. There were 3370 deaths attributable to brain tumours in 2002, representing 2% of all cancer deaths. Brain tumours also represent the second commonest type of childhood cancer.

Unfortunately, the incidence of these tumours is increasing, and although there are new treatment strategies, the improvements in overall survival figures remain very disappointing. Brain tumours have a devastating effect on both patients and their loved ones. There is little knowledge of their aetiology.

In adults, gliomas (tumours of the supporting cells) account for about 60% of primary brain tumours. Astrocytomas account for 80% of gliomas. The other types are ependymomas and oligodendrogliomas. Most (70%) occur supratentorially. The other primary brain tumours include meningiomas, lymphomas, medulloblastomas (PNET – primitive neuroectodermal tumours), acoustic neuromas, pituitary tumours, pineal tumours and other rarer tumours (WHO classification).

Pathologically, tumours are graded according to the 2002 WHO classification, which grades tumours between 1 and 4. Grade 1 represents a well-differentiated tumour and grade 4 represents a very poorly differentiated and highly malignant tumour. Grade 1–2 astrocytomas are simply called low grade astrocytomas; grade 3 astrocytomas are anaplastic astrocytomas (AA); grade 4 astrocytomas are called glioblastoma multiforme (GBM). The grade of the tumour is very strongly correlated to prognosis: 5-year and 10-year survival of grades 1 and 2 is 65% and 35%, but 5-year survival of grades 3 and 4 is less than 10%. The median survival for treated glioblastomas is between 6 and 9 months. Unfortunately, most adult brain tumours are high grade.

PRESENTATION

Brain tumours are not always easy to diagnose. Symptoms may be generalised or focal. Mass effect leads to raised intracranial pressure (ICP), which produces generalised symptoms of headache, nausea, vomiting and drowsiness that are worse in the mornings, and this is a common mode of brain tumour presentation. Small lesions may also cause raised ICP if they interfere with the flow of CSF (e.g. tumour near fourth ventricle). The type of focal symptoms will obviously depend on the site of the tumour, e.g. frontal tumours produce personality changes, cerebellar tumours will produce ataxia, tremor and nystagmus. Symptoms also depend on the time scale in which the tumour is growing – some patients remain asymptomatic despite huge tumours that have been slow growing over many years. Epileptic seizures occur in about 30% of patients with supratentorial tumours and may take many forms, giving clues to the site of the tumour, e.g. olfactory attacks imply a lesion of the temporal lobe. Seizures may predate onset of other neurological symptoms by many years in slow growing tumours. Around 10% of adults with late onset epilepsy (>25 years of age) will have a brain tumour. Very occasionally patients may have symptoms resulting from endocrine disturbance due to the involvement of the pituitary or hypothalamus.

DIAGNOSIS

CT and MRI with contrast are the most commonly used imaging methods. MRI is superior at defining lesions in the posterior fossa and some low grade astrocytomas.

CT-guided biopsy may be performed by making a small twist drill opening in the skull and passing a needle into the tumour under CT guidance. Stereotactic CT-guided biopsy can obtain specimens from small tumours in difficult areas with high precision. This is achieved by using a frame fixed to the skull with an attached guidance system allowing any two points in 3D space to be traversed.

Positron emission tomography (PET) and single photon emission computed tomography (SPECT) help delineate areas of metabolic activity which may distinguish tumour from oedema or radiation necrosis. This is particularly useful for differentiating recurrent disease from radiation necrosis in pre-treated patients, which is difficult with both CT and MRI.

MANAGEMENT

GENERAL MEASURES – ACUTE MEDICAL PROBLEMS

Patients presenting with symptoms and signs of raised ICP should start immediate high dose dexamethasone (e.g. 16 mg) (favoured steroid because of potent anti-inflammatory effects, low mineralocorticoid effects and greater bioavailability to brain). Mannitol 20% (1 g/kg) over 20–40 minutes is also used. Lying the patient flat with head elevated to 20–30°, analgesia for pain and loosening clothes around the neck are simple measures that may also help to lower ICP. Any fever should be treated with antipyretics. Hypotonic fluids should not be given as they may increase free water in the brain interstitium. If acute hydrocephalus is evident on CT/MRI a ventriculo-peritoneal shunt can be inserted. Seizures should be managed with anticonvulsants.

GENERAL MEASURES – LONG TERM REHABILITATION

Many patients require help from a multidisciplinary team. Patients may require physiotherapy, speech therapy, pain control, psychological help (e.g. cognitive, behavioural, pharmacological) and occupational and social support. Family members and other carers may also need support.

LOW GRADE ASTROCYTOMAS, OLIGOASTROCYTOMAS, OLIGODENDROGLIOMAS

The role of surgery is controversial. Complete surgical excision of grade 1 pilocytic astrocytomas is usually curative and should be attempted if technically feasible with minimal risk to eloquent areas of the brain. However, curative surgery is not possible in grade 2 tumours due to diffuse infiltration of surrounding brain parenchyma. Radical resection does reduce mass effect and may improve symptoms, but does not prolong survival and is therefore only justified if tumour removal is likely to improve symptoms. Postoperative irradiation for this group of patients is also controversial because they are often young and may develop late radiation sequelae. Currently, radiotherapy is offered at disease progression because delaying RT until disease progression does not affect overall survival. However, upfront RT should be considered for poorer prognosis patients who may benefit from temporary disease control. Poorer prognostic factors include: (i) tumours >6 cm; (ii) tumours crossing the midline; (iii) neurological deficit prior to surgery; (iv) age >40 years; and (v) astrocytoma histology. Radiotherapy is usually given over 6 weeks at a dose of 54 Gy in 30 fractions. Median survival for patients with grade 2 gliomas is 6–10 years and is even longer for grade 1 tumours.

The use of adjuvant chemotherapy in adults is controversial and not used in routine practice. However, chemotherapy for recurrent disease is sometimes beneficial. Drugs used include nitrosoureas (e.g. BCNU, CCNU), procarbazine, methotrexate, vincristine and carboplatin.

HIGH GRADE ASTROCYTOMAS (GBM, AA) AND ANAPLASTIC OLIGODENDROGLIOMAS

Radical tumour resection has not been proven to prolong overall survival compared to biopsy alone. However, debulking surgery for tumours producing mass effect is very useful in reducing symptoms of raised ICP.

Radical radiotherapy (60 Gy in 30 fractions over 6 weeks – conformal or non-conformal) for GBM improves median survival from 14 weeks to 36 weeks and produces clinical improvement in 25–50%. Patients with good performance status, young age (<45 years), and resectable tumours with no dexamethasone dependency have a more favourable outcome with median survival between 11 and 26 months, but they represent only 15% of all GBMs. Approximately 10% of all patients will survive for 2 years.

A recent phase III trial showed that oral temozolamide used concurrently with RT and for up to six cycles afterwards, compared to RT alone, improves median survival of GBM patients by 3 months and 2-year survival from 8% to 28%. This is likely to become the new standard of care for good PS patients aged <70 years.

Six weeks of radiotherapy for poor prognosis patients is often seen as excessive in view of their short life expectancy, and so therefore many centres use shorter courses (e.g. 30 Gy in 10 fractions over 2 weeks, 30 Gy in 6 fractions over 2 weeks) with median survival of around 5–6 months. Anaplastic astrocytomas have a better prognosis with around 50% alive at 1 year.

Anaplastic astrocytomas respond much better to chemotherapy than do GBMs. Response rates vary between 10 and 30% in AAs, with median times to progression of 6 to 15 months. Response rates in GBM are much lower, varying from 5 to 20% depending on response criteria. In the UK the first line regimen is PCV (procarbazine, CCNU and vincristine). Temozolamide has relatively low toxicity and can be taken at home by the patient. In the UK, the National Institute of Clinical Excellence (NICE) has approved its use in patients with progressive disease who have failed first line chemotherapy, but its benefits are marginal.

The role of second debulking surgery for recurrent high grade gliomas is unclear, but may be an option for selected patients with a longer progression-free interval, good performance status, and tumours in non-eloquent areas.

EPENDYMOMAS

Total surgical excision of low grade tumours often results in long-term survival. Postoperative radiotherapy (54 Gy in 30 fractions over 6 weeks) is routinely offered in the UK. If there is evidence of leptomeningeal spread, the whole craniospinal axis is irradiated. Overall 5-year survival is 50–60%.

ANAPLASTIC OLIGODENDROGLIOMAS (see also above)

Chemotherapy can be used for recurrent disease (e.g. PCV) and response rates are high (>70%) because this group of tumours are unusually chemosensitive.

BRAINSTEM GLIOMAS

Often present with cranial nerve palsies, ataxia and long tract signs. The majority are diffuse pontine gliomas. They are rarely amenable to surgery, and radiotherapy (e.g. 54 Gy in 30 fractions over 6 weeks) is the mainstay of treatment. Median survival is 9 months for patients with diffuse pontine gliomas and 80% die within 18 months.

MEDULLOBLASTOMAS (see Ch. 35 on paediatric oncology)

These tumours are commoner in children and represent only 1–2% of adult brain tumours.

MENINGIOMAS

Meningiomas represent about 20% of adult brain tumours. Benign grade 1 lesions are the commonest type (>90%), with atypical grade 2 lesions (5%) and malignant grade 3 lesions (2%) making up the rest. Primary treatment is with surgery. Radiotherapy is indicated if: (1) the histology is grade 3 (even with complete resection) – e.g. 60 Gy in 30 fractions over 6 weeks; (2) there is incompletely excised grade 1 or 2 disease – e.g. 54 Gy in 30 fractions over 6 weeks; (3) there is recurrent disease.

Observation only is an option for asymptomatic elderly patients with a benign grade 1 meningioma in a non-eloquent area.

RT offers local control rates of 90% for incompletely resected grade 1 tumours. The overall prognosis is excellent.

Malignant meningiomas have a very poor prognosis – median survival is less than 1 year.

PITUITARY TUMOURS

Pituitary tumours represent ~10–15% of all intracranial tumours. The vast majority are benign epithelial neoplasms, but they are clinically important because 75% produce inappropriate amounts of hormones and local extension may cause compression of the optic chiasm leading to visual field defects. Most patients present with symptoms and signs of excess hormone secretion (see below), headaches, visual field defects, and hypopituitarism either alone or in combination.

Many of the clinical features are related to the type of hormone produced. Prolactinomas (~30%) are the commonest functioning tumours and lead to hyperprolactinaemia, which causes galactorrhoea and amenorrhoea in women and poor libido, impotence and infertility in men. Acromegaly results from excess growth hormone production and Cushing's syndrome results from excess ACTH secretion. Thyrotrophin-secreting adenomas are rare, but aggressive and may cause thyrotoxicosis. Gonadotroph adenomas are usually inactive, but may present rarely with premature puberty or postmenopausal bleeding.

Investigations should include visual field assessment, CT/MRI and appropriate hormone function testing.

Treatment options include medical therapy, surgery and radiotherapy. Prolactinomas are usually treated medically with dopamine agonists (e.g. bromocriptine). In addition, tumours causing mass effect and/or excessive hormone secretion should be treated surgically with trans-sphenoidal pituitary resection. Radiotherapy is often given postoperatively if there is residual disease (e.g. 45 Gy in 25 fractions over 5 weeks). Acromegaly can be treated medically with somatostatin analogues.

PRIMARY CNS LYMPHOMA

Accounts for ~1% of all intracranial neoplasms. It is a type of non-Hodgkin's lymphoma (NHL) and is a high grade lymphoma of B-cell origin in 75% of cases. It is the commonest intracranial malignancy in AIDS patients. There are multiple masses in the brain in 25%, leptomeningeal involvement in 25–49% and eye involvement in 20% (bilateral 80%). Treatment is by chemotherapy but the optimum regimen is unknown. High dose methotrexate regimens, with cyclophosphamide, adriamycin, cytarabine and vincristine, or IDARAM (idarubicin, arabinoside, methotrexate), have been used with some success. The role of whole brain radiotherapy following chemotherapy is controversial due to a high incidence of neurological toxicity side effects, especially in older patients. Recent results with combination chemotherapy and radiotherapy have shown 5-year survival rates of 30–40% and median survival of 2 years. The role of surgery is limited to diagnostic purposes (i.e. brain biopsy).

PROBLEMS IN ADVANCED DISEASE

1. Neurological deficits. May cause immobility, speech problems, blindness, incontinence, neuropsychiatric problems etc., leading to increased dependency.
2. Seizures. Can be focal or generalised and are frequently refractory to medical treatment. Commonly used anticonvulsants include phenytoin, sodium valproate and carbamazepine. Metabolic abnormalities such as hyponatraemia and hypocalcaemia should be corrected.
3. Symptoms associated with raised ICP (see above).
4. Steroid side effects. Prolonged use may lead to Cushing's syndrome with central obesity, fluid retention, bruising and skin thinning, diabetes, hypertension and proximal myopathy. Risk of thrush increased. Psychiatric side effects include mania, anxiety, euphoria, frank psychosis, psychomotor agitation and depression. Some of the psychiatric symptoms can be helped by dividing the dose, reducing dose and avoiding night-time doses.
5. Neuropsychiatric problems. Extremely common and include depression, anxiety, delirium, emotional lability, psychosis and dementia. Psychotherapy and pharmacotherapy with antidepressants, anxiolytics and antipsychotics may all play a useful role.

FURTHER READING

Levin V A (ed) 1995 Cancer in the nervous system, 2nd edn. Churchill Livingstone, Edinburgh
Short S C, Brada M 2000 The treatment of malignant cerebral tumours. Hospital Medicine 61(11): 772–777

CHAPTER 16

Breast cancer

BACKGROUND INFORMATION

The UK has some of the highest incidence and mortality rates for breast cancer in the world. Around 40 000 new cases of breast cancer are diagnosed annually and in 2002 there were 12 930 deaths, making it the commonest cause of cancer death among women. It is the leading cause of death in women aged 35–54 years. Despite these figures the 5-year survival rate has improved to 65% over the last 20 years.

The aetiology of breast cancer is complex. Age is the greatest risk factor, with an incidence of 150/100 000 at 50 years and 300/100 000 at 80 years. Women with a first-degree relative with breast cancer have a 3-fold increase in risk, with additional risk if the cancer occurred premenopausally. If a second-degree relative was affected, the risk is also increased but to a lesser extent. Only about 5–10% of cases are familial and about half of these can be attributed to the BRCA 1 and BRCA 2 genes. Patients with BRCA 1 have an 80% lifetime risk of breast cancer. Other postulated risk factors include early menarche and late menopause, postmenopausal obesity, prolonged use of HRT and the oral contraceptive pill, high socioeconomic status, high alcohol intake, atypical ductal hyperplasia and previous benign breast disease.

Pathologically, invasive ductal carcinomas (IDC) account for 90% of breast cancers. They generally present as hard, poorly defined lumps due to increased production of dense fibrous tissue stroma. Involvement of ligaments and ducts leads to dimpling and pitting of skin and nipple retraction. Variants of IDC include medullary carcinoma (6%), colloid carcinoma (2.5%) and Paget's disease (2.3%). Invasive lobular carcinomas (ILC) account for most of the rest and tend to be multicentric and are more often bilateral than IDC with a 40% lifetime risk of cancer in the contralateral breast. They are often mammographically silent due to their diffuse nature and relative radiolucency.

Pre-invasive carcinomas also occur and are known as ductal/lobular carcinomas in situ (DCIS, LCIS). These represent malignant epithelial cells with no evidence of invasion. DCIS progresses to invasive disease in 25–50% of cases. It accounts for 20–30% of malignant lesions detected at screening. It may also present as a mass, nipple discharge or Paget's disease of the nipple. LCIS has an estimated 5–10-fold increased risk of developing invasive disease. It is not detectable by mammography and is usually an incidental finding on biopsy.

The discovery of the epidermal growth factor receptor, HER-2/*neu* (or c-erbB2), has been one of the most exciting developments in molecular oncology. Following its discovery in the late 1990s, it has moved from being a laboratory prognostic indicator to a therapeutic target of the monoclonal antibody trastuzumab (Herceptin). HER-2/*neu* is overexpressed in about 25% of all breast cancer cases and is associated with oestrogen receptor negative (ER −ve) and poorer prognosis tumours.

The natural history of breast cancer is extremely complex and not fully understood. There is a very wide spectrum of behaviour. Some cancers may disseminate very early and cause death even before the primary is clinically apparent, whereas other patients may live for decades untreated with indolent disease. It is not uncommon to have recurrent disease 20–30 years after initial treatment. Unfortunately, very young women (less than 35 years) tend to develop aggressive disease with less than 50% 5-year survival. The disease may spread via the lymphatics and the bloodstream and it is now known that bloodborne disease can be independent of direct lymphatic spread.

The principal prognostic indicators are nodal status, tumour size, histological grade and hormone receptor status. The Nottingham Prognostic Index (NPI) uses histological grade, tumour size and lymph node status to predict the probability of survival (Table 16.1).

$$\text{NPI} = (0.2 \times \text{tumour size in cm}) + \text{grade} + \text{lymph node stage.}$$

(Lymph node stage 1 is no nodes, stage 2 is 1–3 nodes, stage 3 is ≥4 nodes.)

The NPI is a useful tool for helping to select patients most likely to benefit from adjuvant systemic therapy. However, it should be remembered that the NPI does not take into account the hormone receptor status or HER-2/*neu* status of the tumour. These factors must also be considered in the decision-making process.

TABLE 16.1 Nottingham prognostic index scores

NPI	15-year survival (%)
<3	90
3.01–3.4	80
3.41–4.4	50
4.41–5.3	30
>5.4	8

PRESENTATION

A painless lump in the breast is the commonest presenting symptom of breast cancer. It is usually hard and irregular in shape. Most lumps are benign fibroadenomas and cysts, but all discrete or suspicious lesions should be referred to a breast surgeon with the exception of young women with tender lumpy breasts and older women with symmetrical nodularity. Other symptoms include breast pain, bleeding from nipple, nipple inversion/retraction, skin dimpling, changes in size/shape and contour of breast, lymphoedema, axillary mass, skin ulceration and symptoms of metastatic disease. Occasionally a woman may present with an acutely inflamed, red tender swollen breast, which represents diffuse infiltration through the breast and skin lymphatics, referred to clinically as inflammatory carcinoma. This type of breast cancer has a much worse prognosis since the incidence of metastases at diagnosis is high.

Many patients are now mammographically screen detected. The NHS screening programme in the UK is offered to women between the ages of 50 and 70 years every 3 years.

DIAGNOSIS AND STAGING

All patients with suspected breast cancer should have a triple assessment, which includes physical examination, FNAC (fine needle aspiration cytology) and core biopsy, and bilateral breast imaging (mammography/ultrasound). Routine bloods including FBC, renal and liver function, and calcium should be taken and a CXR is also required. Further investigations such as bone scans, CT scans and liver ultrasound in asymptomatic patients with operable tumours are unnecessary. For patients who are screen detected with no clinically palpable lump, ultrasound-guided FNAC or core needle biopsy is necessary.

The oestrogen and progesterone receptor status of the tumour should always be requested on pathological specimens. The HER-2/*neu* status may also be requested.

Breast cancer is staged according to the TNM 2002 classification (Table 16.2).

MANAGEMENT

DCIS

Treatment of this condition remains controversial. Extensive (over 4 cm) or multifocal disease should be treated by mastectomy. For other lesions, local excision with or without radiotherapy is considered adequate. Patients who should be considered for adjuvant radiotherapy include those with close

TABLE 16.2 TNM 2002 breast cancer staging (simplified)

T0	
Tis	(DCIS), (LCIS), (Paget)
T1	Tumour ≥2 cm
	T1mic ≤0.1 cm
	T1a >0.1 ≤0.5 cm
	T1b >0.5 ≤1 cm
	T1c >1 ≤2 cm
T2	Tumour >2 cm ≤5 cm
T3	Tumour >5 cm
T4	Chest wall/skin
	T4a Chest wall
	T4b Skin oedema/ulceration, satellite lesions
	T4c Both 4a and 4b
	T4d Inflammatory carcinoma
TNM clinical nodal staging	
N0	No nodes
N1	Mobile ipsilateral axillary nodes
N2a	Fixed ipsilateral axillary nodes
N2b	Internal mammary nodes
N3a	Infraclavicular nodes
N3b	Internal mammary and axillary nodes
N3c	Supraclavicular nodes
TNM pathological staging of nodes	
pN1mi	Micrometastases, >0.2 mm ≤2 mm
pN1a	1–3 axillary nodes
pN1b	Internal mammary nodes with microscopic metastasis (by sentinel node biopsy – (sn))
pN1c	1–3 axillary nodes and internal mammary nodes with microscopic metastasis (sn)
pN2a	4–9 axillary nodes
pN2b	Internal mammary nodes without axillary nodes
pN3a	≥10 axillary nodes or Infraclavicular node(s)
pN3b	Internal mammary nodes with axillary node(s), or >3 axillary nodes with microscopic internal mammary nodes (sn)
pN3c	Supraclavicular node(s)
M0	No distant metastases
M1	Distant metastases

excision margins, high nuclear grade and comedo necrosis. The role of adjuvant tamoxifen is still under evaluation.

LCIS

Estimated 5–10-fold increased risk of developing invasive cancer. There is no recommended therapy and the role of mammographic or clinical surveillance is unclear. Annual or biennial mammography is usually offered, though. Tamoxifen is under evaluation.

OPERABLE INVASIVE BREAST CANCER (T1–3, N0, N1, M0)

Surgery is the mainstay of treatment, with or without radiotherapy, chemotherapy and hormonal manipulation.

The two main surgical options are mastectomy or breast conserving surgery. There is no difference in overall survival between mastectomy and breast conservation plus radiotherapy.

Mastectomy

Mastectomy is indicated for large tumours, multi-focal cancer or if radiotherapy is contraindicated. The decision is also based on patient preference, fitness for operation, the age of the patient (young women (less than 35 years) are at increased risk of local recurrence) and the ratio of the size of the tumour to the size of the breast (i.e. smaller tumours in large breasts are more suitable for conservation). Breast reconstruction either at the time of (immediate), or after mastectomy (delayed) should be discussed with the patient as it may offer psychological benefits. Immediate reconstruction should not be offered if the patient has a high chance of requiring post-mastectomy radiotherapy.

Radiotherapy to the chest wall following mastectomy should be offered to patients judged at high risk of recurrence (tumour >5 cm, four or more nodes positive, involvement of deep margins). Its role with lower risk cancers is less well established and subject to local radiotherapy centre protocols.

Breast conserving surgery

Breast conserving surgery should normally be followed by radiotherapy to the breast, which reduces local recurrence rates. The supraclavicular fossa is also irradiated if four or more axillary lymph nodes are positive.

Axillary node surgery

Axillary clearance (block dissection of axillary nodes) is often performed when mastectomy or breast conserving surgery is carried out. This provides important prognostic information and also treats any nodal disease if present. Axillary sampling (dissection of at least four nodes from the lower axillary fat) stages the axilla, but is not a form of treatment. Sentinel lymph node biopsy (first node to receive drainage from a tumour which has been injected with dye or radioactive substance) is still under evaluation and has the potential to raise the level of sophistication and accuracy of breast cancer staging, obviating the need for extensive dissections of the axilla.

Axillary radiotherapy after axillary clearance should normally be avoided because of the increased risk of lymphoedema. After axillary sampling, axillary radiotherapy should only be given if nodes are positive. If four or more nodes are positive then the supraclavicular fossa is also irradiated.

Systemic therapy

All women with invasive breast cancer should be considered for adjuvant systemic therapy that includes endocrine therapy and chemotherapy.

Endocrine therapy

Tamoxifen reduces the annual odds of death by 17% and recurrence by 25%, with a 6% improvement in absolute survival at 10 years. These benefits are found in oestrogen receptor positive patients (ER +ve); therefore women with ER +ve or ER unknown tumours should routinely receive tamoxifen 20 mg/day. Patients who are ER −ve, but PR +ve also gain some benefit from hormonal therapy and should therefore be offered treatment. Side effects can be significant and include hot flushes, mood disturbance, increased risk of thromboembolic disease, and increased risk of endometrial dysplasia and endometrial cancer.

Aromatase inhibitors

In postmenopausal women, the aromatase inhibitor anastrozole has recently been shown to improve disease-free survival in the adjuvant setting compared to tamoxifen (ATAC trial), but these results are premature and the long-term survival and safety data from this trial are awaited. Switching tamoxifen to exemestane after 2–3 years (IES 031 trial), and 5 years of letrozole after 5 years of tamoxifen (MA17 trial) have also confirmed disease-free survival benefits over 5 years of tamoxifen alone. In addition, aromatase inhibitors have a better side effect profile than tamoxifen.

Ovarian ablation

Some studies have shown that ovarian ablation is of similar efficacy to chemotherapy in premenopausal women with ER +ve tumours, with a reduction in annual death and recurrence rates of approximately 25%. Ablation can be achieved by surgery (bilateral oophorectomy), radiotherapy (XRAM – X-ray menopause), or now more commonly, pharmacologically (LHRH agonists) and may be considered for premenopausal women with high risk and node-positive and ER +ve tumours in addition to polychemotherapy. The side effects of this treatment are those of a premature menopause.

Polychemotherapy

The recent Early Breast Cancer Trialists Collaborative Group (EBCTCG, 2000) meta-analysis has confirmed the benefits of adjuvant polychemotherapy for most breast cancer patients. In summary, it showed that women under 50 benefit the most, with a 27% mortality risk reduction corresponding to a 10-year absolute survival benefit of 11% in node-positive patients and 7% in node-negative patients. In the 50–69-year-old age group, the corresponding mortality risk reduction is 11% with absolute survival benefit of 3% in node-positive patients and 2% in node-negative patients. The survival benefits in patients over 70 years were not significant, but more data is needed in this group of patients. The most commonly used combination is six 3-weekly cycles of the anthracycline-based regimen FEC (5FU, epirubicin, and cyclo-phosphamide). Another commonly used regimen is six 4-weekly cycles of CMF (cyclophosphamide, methotrexate, 5FU). However, FEC offers superior disease-free and overall survival in node-positive premenopausal women. Regimens containing taxanes are under evaluation in clinical trials.

The decision to offer adjuvant chemotherapy is not always straightforward, but most oncologists offer treatment if the expected absolute survival benefit is 3% or more. The potential absolute survival benefit can be calculated from prognostic tables based on the EBCTCG data and the use of the Nottingham prognostic index.

Hormone receptor positive patients who are to receive chemotherapy should not start hormonal therapy until the chemotherapy is completed. This is because a recent large North American trial has shown a detrimental effect (the benefits of treatment are reduced by 50%) when tamoxifen is given concurrently with chemotherapy.

Selection of adjuvant therapy

Premenopausal women who are ER +ve and intermediate or high risk (node-positive and/or high grade/T3 cancers) should be offered chemotherapy and tamoxifen. Those who are ER −ve and intermediate or high risk should be offered chemotherapy.

Postmenopausal women who are ER +ve and intermediate or high risk should be considered for chemotherapy and/or tamoxifen. Those who are ER −ve and intermediate or high risk should be considered for chemotherapy. It is known that the benefits of chemotherapy decrease with age and toxicity increases with age and so many oncologists use less toxic regimens or hormonal treatment only, in older and poorer performance status patients.

High dose chemotherapy should only be used in the context of clinical trials.

LOCALLY ADVANCED DISEASE (T4 TUMOURS AND INFLAMMATORY CANCER)

These patients should have further staging investigations including a bone scan and liver CT or ultrasound. Systemic therapy (usually anthracycline based chemotherapy regimen or endocrine treatment in older patients with ER +ve tumours) improves local control and survival (response rate 65–95%, complete response 15%). Those with a good response may then be considered for mastectomy followed by radiotherapy. Those with a poor response may have radiotherapy, possibly followed by surgery depending on response. With combination treatment the 5-year survival in patients with inflammatory breast cancer is less than 50%.

LOCAL RECURRENCE

Recurrence in the conservatively treated breast can be salvaged with mastectomy and survival is similar to patients without recurrence. Recurrence in the post-mastectomy chest wall is most common in the first 2 years and decreases thereafter. Many of these patients will either have, or go on to develop, metastatic disease (up to 80% have metastatic disease within 5–10 years) and so all need to be restaged with CXR, bone scan and liver ultrasound. If there is isolated disease then radical treatment may achieve long-term local control, e.g. resection of nodules and/or radiotherapy (if not previously used). Tamoxifen may benefit some patients and has been shown to improve disease-free but not overall survival. Systemic chemotherapy may also be an option. Axillary recurrence is rare as an isolated event. It may be treated with salvage surgery or radiotherapy.

METASTATIC BREAST CANCER

Patients with metastatic breast cancer are a heterogeneous group whose prognoses and clinical courses vary according to patient factors such as performance status and age, and tumour factors such as hormone receptor status, grade, HER-2/*neu* status and the site and burden of disease. Median survival is of the order of 2–4 years, but subsets of patients have prolonged survival.

All patients should be considered for some form of systemic therapy, which has been shown to improve symptom control. However, no overall survival benefit has clearly been shown in randomised trials.

Endocrine therapy

Endocrine therapy is usually the first line treatment of choice for ER +ve patients with a long disease-free interval and soft tissue metastases.

For postmenopausal women, anastrozole 1 mg o.d. is now the first line therapy of choice as recent trials have confirmed its superiority over tamoxifen (clinical benefit 59% anastrozole versus 46% tamoxifen). Tamoxifen can still be used as a second line agent if not used before.

Premenopausal women may receive tamoxifen 20 mg o.d. Another option is ovarian ablation followed by an aromatase inhibitor.

Progestogens such as megestrol acetate and medroxyprogesterone and other aromatase inhibitors such as exemestane are used as second and third line agents.

Chemotherapy

Chemotherapy is used as first line treatment in patients with more aggressive disease, ER −ve tumours and advanced visceral disease. Those with hormone refractory disease may receive chemotherapy as second line therapy. No particular regimen has been proven to be superior in terms of survival. In the UK, patients receive anthracycline-based equivalents or CMF as first line therapy. Overall response rates for first line chemotherapy are around 60–70%, with a median time to relapse of 6–10 months. Newer agents including the taxanes (docetaxel and paclitaxel) and vinorelbine have now been licensed by the National Institute of Clinical Excellence (NICE) for use in the second and third line setting, where initial anthracycline therapy has failed or is inappropriate. In patients with HER-2/*neu* positive metastatic breast cancer, paclitaxel in combination with trastuzumab is licensed for use by NICE. Trastuzumab can also be used as a single agent. In patients with advanced disease and poor performance status, single agent drugs such as weekly epirubicin and vinorelbine can be used. Oral capecitabine is another second or third line option.

High dose chemotherapy with bone marrow transplantation (BMT) has not been shown to improve survival and should only be offered in the context of a clinical trial.

Bisphosphonates

Prevention of skeletal morbidity may be achieved with bisphosphonates, which have shown significant reductions (25–50%) in skeletal fractures, bone pain and hypercalcaemia. There is conflicting evidence that bisphosphonates may also prevent the development of bone metastases and further trials are needed.

MALE BREAST CANCER

Approximately 1 in every 200 cases of breast cancer are seen in men. In general, the natural history of male breast cancer is similar to that of female breast cancer and therefore treatment is based on the female approach including the use of surgery (mastectomy), radiotherapy, chemotherapy and hormonal therapy. However, the overall prognosis in men tends to be poorer as it usually presents at a later stage and in an older age group.

FUTURE PERSPECTIVES

In breast screening, the role of MRI imaging for younger (35–50 years), higher risk patients is being evaluated.

An exciting area of research in molecular pathology is cDNA microarray technology. This process profiles gene expression in cancer tissue and offers the hope of identifying genes that may provide important prognostic information and accurate prediction of response to therapies. More importantly this could lead to identification of new targets for treatment.

In surgery, the role of the sentinel lymph node biopsy is an active area of research.

In radiotherapy, the role of partial breast irradiation, internal mammary node irradiation and intensity modulated radiotherapy (IMRT) are the focus of clinical studies.

The role of various combinations of systemic therapy in both the adjuvant and metastatic setting continues to evolve. The use of aromatase inhibitors in the postmenopausal adjuvant setting is likely to increase as data from the ATAC, MA17 and IES 031 trials matures. The role of the taxanes in the adjuvant setting is subject to large ongoing trials. New approaches with immunotherapy, signal transduction inhibitors, angiogenesis inhibitors, tumour vaccines and gene therapy are being evaluated. Bisphosphonates continue to be evaluated in both the adjuvant and metastatic setting.

In the follow-up and monitoring of breast cancer patients, serum levels of the HER-2/*neu* protein can now be measured and this may become a useful tool for assessing prognosis, predicting response to therapy and detecting early recurrence of breast cancer.

Finally, the role of chemoprevention using tamoxifen, raloxifene, aromatase inhibitors and COX-2 inhibitors is under investigation.

PROBLEMS IN ADVANCED BREAST CANCER

1. Bone metastases (see also Ch. 48 on bone metastases). Radiotherapy (single 8 Gy fraction or 20 Gy in five fractions) is effective for relieving localised pain with response rates of 70–80%. Pain in multiple sites should be treated with systemic therapy, intravenous bisphosphonates or strontium-89. Hemi-body irradiation is also used but may compromise subsequent chemotherapy due to bone marrow toxicity. An orthopaedic opinion should be sought if there is any degree of cortical erosion in weight-bearing bones as this may be an indication for fixation.
2. Spinal cord compression (see Ch. 60 on spinal cord compression).
3. Hypercalcaemia (see Ch. 56 on metabolic problems in cancer).
4. Lymphoedema. Can cause pain and loss of function of the arm. Requires good skin care. Mainstay of treatment is massage, compression therapy with bandaging, compression pumps, elastic support and exercises. Try to avoid venesection and cannulation in the affected arm because of increased risk of infection (e.g. cellulitis).
5. Brain metastases (see Ch. 49 on brain metastases). May respond well to systemic therapy or intrathecal methotrexate, but this is unpredictable. Radiotherapy produces improvement in 40–70% (e.g. 30 Gy in 10 fractions over 2 weeks). A solitary brain metastasis may occasionally be recommended for surgical resection followed by postoperative radiotherapy (usually when there has been a long disease-free period). Average survival is 3 months; 10% survive over 1 year.
6. Choroidal metastases. Present with deteriorating vision. Pain may result from secondary glaucoma. Diagnosed on fundoscopy. Treatment with radiotherapy (e.g. 40 Gy in 15 fractions, 30 Gy in 10 fractions or 20 Gy in

5 fractions depending on overall prognosis) benefits 60–70% of patients. Vision returns to pre-symptomatic levels in one-third. Referral to ophthalmologist is also advised.

7. Skull base metastases. May produce cranial nerve palsies; 50–80% respond to radiotherapy (e.g. 20 Gy in five fractions).

8. Brachial plexopathy. Metastatic spread of tumour and radiation injury are the main causes. Around 85% of patients with tumour infiltration experience pain, usually in the shoulder, elbow, medial forearm and fourth and fifth fingers. Weakness in the C-7, C-8 and T-1 distribution occurs in 75%; paraesthesias occur in 15%; lymphoedema in 10%. Radiation injury produces progressive and irreversible symptoms: pain is less common (20%), but paraesthesias (50%) are prominent. Proximal weakness in the deltoid distribution is present in all patients. MRI is the investigation of choice. If the cause is tumour related, then systemic therapy and local radiotherapy are potential treatment options. Pain management should begin with non-opioid and opioid analgesics with further addition of adjuvants such as amitriptyline and gabapentin. Nerve blocks and ablation may be required.

9. Fungating tumours. Often very distressing and painful, with foul-smelling odour, discharge and bleeding. Requires skilled nursing. Odour may be controlled with metronidazole orally (400 mg t.d.s.) or topically with gel. Activated charcoal dressings may help. Analgesia may be required, especially before dressing changes. Bleeding may be controlled with adrenaline (1 : 1000) soaked dressings. Palliative radiotherapy may occasionally produce a dramatic improvement.

10. Pleural effusions (see Ch. 55 on malignant pleural effusions). Often respond to chemotherapy.

FURTHER READING

Breast Speciality Group of BASO 1999 British Association of Surgical Oncology Guidelines (BASO). The management of metastatic bone disease in the UK. European Journal of Surgical Oncology 25:3–23

Crown J et al 2002 Chemotherapy for metastatic breast cancer – report of a European expert panel. Lancet Oncology 3:719–726

Royal College of Radiologists' Clinical Oncology Information Network (COIN). Guidelines on the non-surgical management of breast cancer. Available at: www.rcr.ac.uk

Scottish Intercollegiate Guidelines Network (SIGN) guideline No 29. Breast cancer in women. Available at: www.show.scot.nhs.uk

CHAPTER 17

Carcinoid and other neuroendocrine tumours

BACKGROUND INFORMATION

Neuroendocrine tumours (NETs) arise from neuroendocrine cells that are located widely throughout the body. They represent a diverse family of tumours that secrete various tumour products and can arise in almost all tissues. Up to 10% of NETs are associated with multiple endocrine neoplasia (MEN). NETs can be classified according to primary site, histopathology, immunohistochemistry and the type of neuropeptide secreted (Table 17.1). As differentiation between benign and malignant histology is difficult, it is usually the clinical behaviour of the tumour that determines malignant potential. This chapter will focus on carcinoid tumours, which are by far the commonest type of NET. Gastroentero-pancreatic NETs will also be briefly discussed. Phaeochromocytomas are discussed in Chapter 11 on adrenal cancer.

Carcinoid tumours represent over 50% of all NETs but are still uncommon with an incidence rate of approximately 1/100 000 per year in the UK. This is probably an underestimate, as many remain asymptomatic until death, as evidenced by post-mortem studies. They can occur at any age, with a mean of 50–60 years. They are usually classified into foregut, midgut and hindgut carcinoids:

foregut: thymus, lung, stomach, pancreas, duodenum
midgut: jejunum, ileum, proximal colon, appendix
hindgut: colon, rectum.

The gastrointestinal (GI) tract is the commonest site for carcinoids (73%), followed by the bronchopulmonary system (25%). The midgut is the

TABLE 17.1 Neuroendocrine tumours and their products

Neuroendocrine tumour	Tumour product
Carcinoids (mainly gut and bronchopulmonary system)	Serotonin
Gastroenteropancreatic:	
insulinoma	Insulin
glucagonoma	Glucagon
gastrinoma	Gastrin
somatostatinoma	Somatostatin
VIPoma	Vasoactive intestinal polypeptide
PPoma (pancreatic polypeptideoma)	'Non-functioning'
Adrenal: phaeochromocytoma	Catecholamines
Sympathetic nervous system: paraganglionoma	Catecholamines
Thyroid: medullary carcinoma	Calcitonin
Pituitary: pituitary adenomas	e.g. Growth hormone, prolactin, ACTH, follicle-stimulating hormone, luteinising hormone

commonest GI site with most tumours arising in the small bowel and appendix. Rare primary sites include the ovaries, testes, oesophagus, gallbladder and liver. Carcinoid tumours can produce a variety of hormones, including 5-HT (5-hydroxytryptamine – serotonin), ACTH, CRF, ADH, histamine, gastrin, somatostatin, prostaglandins and brady/tachykinins to name but a few. A variety of clinical symptoms can therefore occur in this disease.

Most carcinoid tumours behave in a benign manner and if treated early by surgery, can be cured. They rarely metastasise if they are less than 1 cm in size, but lesions >2 cm commonly metastasise. Traditionally, patients with more malignant behaving carcinoids have a much poorer outlook with 5-year survival of 20% and a median survival of 2 years if liver metastases are present. However, newer treatment modalities have significantly improved the outlook for patients with median survival for advanced disease of 5 years and more.

PRESENTATION

Most GI carcinoids are asymptomatic and discovered incidentally during surgery (or autopsy). However, when these tumours do produce symptoms they can be striking. The carcinoid syndrome is characterised by paroxysmal flushing, diarrhoea, wheezing, abdominal pain and right-sided cardiac failure (due to right-sided cardiac valve fibrosis) and is caused mainly by the midgut carcinoids with liver metastases. These produce brachy/tachykinins (causing the flushing/wheezing) and serotonin and prostaglandins (causing the diarrhoea). Midgut tumours may also present with bowel obstruction. Foregut tumours less commonly present with carcinoid syndrome, but can cause many other clinical symptoms depending on the hormones secreted. Examples include symptoms of Cushing's syndrome, SIADH, and Zollinger–Ellison syndrome (peptic ulcers, gastritis and diarrhoea due to excessive gastrin production). Hindgut tumours tend to be non-functioning and present with GI bleeding, intestinal obstruction and abdominal masses much like colorectal cancer. They tend to be less aggressive than midgut tumours.

DIAGNOSIS

Investigations include full history and examination; routine bloods including FBC, renal and liver function; 24-hour urinary 5-HIAA (5-hydroxyindole acetic acid) levels; serum/plasma chromogranin A levels; and localisation and staging with somatostatin receptor scintigraphy (SRS) with radiolabelled octreotide as the tracer. (This also gives information about somatostatin receptor content in the tumour and this can predict likely response to somatostatin analogue (octreotide) treatment.) CT and MRI scanning aid the staging process. GI and bronchial endoscopy are also useful in localisation and for biopsy of the tumour.

MANAGEMENT

Surgery is the only potentially curative treatment for carcinoid tumours. Cure is possible if the disease is localised to the primary site or to locoregional nodes. Patients with isolated liver metastases also have the possibility of cure. For patients with incurable disease, palliative treatment options include chemotherapy, biotherapy and radiotherapy.

LOCALISED TUMOURS

Appendiceal carcinoids <1.5 cm can be treated adequately with appendi-cectomy with cure rates of essentially 100%. Tumours >2 cm are less common but require more aggressive surgery, especially if the caecum is invaded. This should be a right hemicolectomy with lymph node dissection as performed for colonic cancer.

Small bowel carcinoids <1 cm can be treated by conservative local excision. Tumours >1 cm require more aggressive resection with regional lymph-adenectomy. Multiple primaries are not uncommon in small bowel carcinoid and a careful search should be made.

Carcinoids at other sites are quite rare, but aggressive surgical resection is usually offered.

LOCOREGIONAL DISEASE

If local nodal disease is completely resectable then the chances of long-term survival are good. However, late recurrences at 5–10 years are not uncommon. There is no proven role for adjuvant therapy at present. For unresectable disease, palliative partial resection is often of benefit symptomatically.

METASTATIC DISEASE

Successful management of metastatic disease requires a multi-modality approach. The disease is often indolent with some patients living with metastatic disease for many years, so measures to improve quality of life are paramount.

Surgery

Even if radical curative surgery is not possible, debulking and bypass procedures should be considered at any time during the course of the disease. (Patients with the carcinoid syndrome require special anaesthetic considerations.) Liver metastases can be treated with hepatic artery ligation or more commonly by embolisation with starch powder. Duration of response is 6–12 months (with biochemical response of 50%) and the procedure can be repeated. Embolisation can include the addition of chemotherapy drugs and this is known as chemoembolisation, and although effective, produces more side effects.

Radiotherapy

External beam radiotherapy is only useful for treating bone, skin and brain metastases. However, new tumour targeted radionuclides (radio-immunotherapy) are showing promise. ^{111}In-DTPA-octreotide and ^{90}Y-DOTA-lanreotide can bind to carcinoid tumours that express somatostatin receptors, allowing localised radiation to tumour cells. Results from several worldwide trials are awaited.

Biotherapy

The somatostatin analogues (e.g. octreotide) have been a major breakthrough in the management of malignant carcinoid. They inhibit the release of peptide hormones and also have an anti-proliferative effect on carcinoid tumours. Subjective improvement is seen in 70%, biochemical response in 50%, but tumour shrinkage in only 10%. The drug is given s.c. 2–3 times a day or by monthly depot injection. Side effects include gallstones, steatorrhoea, and slight hyperglycaemia and hypocalcaemia. Interferon alpha can control hormone secretion, clinical symptoms and tumour growth by stimulating natural killer cell activity. Symptomatic response is seen in 60%, with biochemical responses of 50%, and significant tumour reduction in 15%. Median response duration is 32 months. The main side effects are a flu-like syndrome and fatigue.

Chemotherapy

Has limited value and is generally considered not to be a first line treatment. Response rates (RRs) of single agents are around 10%, whilst combinations fare not much better, with RRs of 10–30%. Aggressive, poorly differentiated foregut tumours may respond better, with RRs reported in up to 65% with cisplatin and etoposide.

FUTURE PERSPECTIVES

Current research is focused on combining somatostatin analogues and interferon. Interestingly, interferon is better tolerated when combined with somatostatin analogues. Radio-immunotherapy is also an active area of research.

PROBLEMS IN PATIENTS WITH ADVANCED CARCINOID

See also Chapter 58 on problems in advanced pelvic malignancy.

1. Carcinoid syndrome. Rarely occurs in the absence of liver metastases as vasoactive peptides are efficiently metabolised in the liver. Can usually be effectively treated with octreotide and/or interferon alpha. Surgical measures such as hepatic resection and hepatic artery ligation/embolisation can also be considered. If these are not effective then other measures can be tried: (a) Flushing may be controlled with antihistamines. Prednisolone 20–40 mg daily is useful for flushing, especially from bronchial carcinoids. (b) Bronchospasm responds to bronchodilators. (c) Diarrhoea can be controlled with loperamide 2 mg p.r.n.
2. Carcinoid crisis. This is a life-threatening condition that may occur spontaneously or be precipitated by infection, stress or surgery and

anaesthesia. It most frequently occurs in foregut tumours with high 5-HIAA levels. The patient develops flushing, palpitations, sweating, bronchospasm, headache, hypotension, leading to circulatory collapse, coma and death if untreated. Large doses of octreotide (IV bolus initially, followed by IV infusion) are used in both the treatment and prevention of this condition. IV fluids, steroids, antihistamines and α-adrenergic agents are also used in treatment. β-Adrenergic agents should be avoided as these may promote vasoactive peptide release from the tumour.

3. Carcinoid heart disease and right ventricular failure. Occurs in up to 50% of patients with carcinoid syndrome. Caused by fibrosis of tricuspid and pulmonary valves leading to regurgitation and/or stenosis. The right endocardium can also be involved. This all leads to progressive right heart failure that causes fatigue, dyspnoea, oedema, ascites and cardiac cachexia. Medical therapy is limited to diuretics, which may actually worsen symptoms due to reduced left-sided cardiac output. Cardiac surgery with valvular replacement is the only truly effective treatment, but should be reserved for patients with severe symptoms with an otherwise reasonable long-term outlook.

4. Pellagra. This is a light-sensitive dermatitis that may be accompanied by diarrhoea and dementia. It is caused by nicotinamide deficiency due to conversion of tryptophan to 5-HT. Can be treated with vitamin supplements containing nicotinamide.

GASTROENTEROPANCREATIC NEUROENDOCRINE TUMOURS

INSULINOMAS

These pancreatic tumours are most common in the fifth decade of life. The vast majority are benign. Excess insulin secretion leads to symptoms of hypoglycaemia with headache, sweating, CNS dysfunction, hypotension, weakness and nausea. Patients may appear to be drunk. Hypoglycaemia can generally be managed with dietary modification and oral diazoxide (inhibits insulin secretion). Demonstrating elevated plasma levels of fasting insulin and C-peptide confirms the diagnosis. Most insulinomas are less than 1.5 cm in size and can be missed with CT/MRI. However, endoscopic and/or intraoperative ultrasound are highly sensitive for tumour localisation. Treatment is with surgical enucleation and long-term survival is in excess of 90%. Approximately 7–8% of patients also have multiple endocrine neoplasia (MEN) 1 and a more aggressive resection is required for this group because of the higher rates of recurrence and risk of multiple tumours. In the palliative situation, diazoxide and octreotide may be helpful. Chemotherapy may also be an option.

GLUCAGONOMAS

Glucagonomas are rare pancreatic tumours; 80% are sporadic, 20% are associated with MEN 1. Two-thirds of patients develop a skin condition called necrolytic migratory erythema and this is the commonest mode of presentation. Only 50% have clinically significant hyperglycaemia. Plasma glucagon levels are often very high. Patients with localised disease may undergo a potentially curative resection, but unfortunately the majority have metastatic disease at presentation and the prognosis for these patients is very poor. Cytoreductive surgery may diminish symptoms. Octreotide may also improve symptoms.

VIPomas

These tumours are associated with the Verner–Morrison syndrome of severe diarrhoea, hypokalaemia and achlorhydria. This syndrome is caused by tumour production of vasoactive intestinal polypeptide (VIP). Potentially curative resection is offered to patients with localised disease. Symptomatic patients with metastatic disease respond well to octreotide or cytoreductive surgery.

GASTRINOMAS

The vast majority of gastrinomas occur in the 'gastrinoma triangle', which is an area between the cystic and common bile ducts, pancreas and duodenum. About a quarter of cases are associated with MEN 1. Excessive secretion of gastrin can lead to profound acid secretion and the Zollinger–Ellison syndrome of peptic ulcer disease, diarrhoea and acid reflux. The diagnosis should be suspected if peptic ulcers do not heal or are located in the distal duodenum or jejunum, and if fasting gastrin levels are high. Most tumours are less than 1 cm and therefore difficult to detect with standard imaging techniques. Endoscopic ultrasound may be helpful. Curative surgical resection is possible in over 50% of those with localised disease. Proton pump inhibitors are very effective for controlling symptoms associated with hypersecretion of acid.

FURTHER READING

Oberg K 1998 Carcinoid tumours: Current concepts in diagnosis and treatment. Oncologist 3:339–345
Reed N S 1999 Management of neuroendocrine tumours. Clinical Oncology 11:295–302

CHAPTER 18

Carcinoma of unknown primary site

BACKGROUND INFORMATION

Carcinoma of unknown primary site (CUP) may be defined as metastatic epithelial cancer with no identified primary. It accounts for 3–5% of all malignancies. Historically, the prognosis of CUP has been dismal with median survival of 3–4 months and overall 5-year survival of less than 10%. More recently the treatments and outcomes have improved significantly for some subgroups of patients. Improved immunohistochemical, molecular and cytogenetic techniques have also enabled more tumours to be identified, thus allowing tailoring of more specific treatments. Communication with the pathologist is therefore especially important.

Patients present with symptoms and signs related to the site of metastatic cancer. The commonest sites of metastases are liver, bone, lung, lymph nodes, pleura and brain. The diagnostic work-up including clinical examination, laboratory and radiological investigations fails to identify the primary site. Histological evaluation by light microscopy (after biopsy of the most accessible lesion) allows the tumour to be categorised into one of five groups:

1. Well and moderately differentiated adenocarcinomas (60%)
2. Poorly differentiated carcinomas (30%)
3. Squamous cell carcinomas (<5%)
4. Undifferentiated neoplasms (<5%)
5. Carcinomas with neuroendocrine differentiation (5%).

DIAGNOSIS

Within the above broad categories, more specific groups may be identified by the presence of particular clinical features and/or specialist pathological tests. Patients within these groups, which account for 40% of all CUPs, may benefit from more tumour-specific therapy. The remaining 60% can be offered treatment with empiric therapy where appropriate.

After the initial baseline investigations, immunohistochemistry should be routinely applied in poorly differentiated/undifferentiated cases to exclude potentially curable or chemoresponsive tumours such as lymphomas (CD 45, LCA (leucocyte common antigen)) and germ cell tumours (β-HCG, AFP, PLAP), small cell lung cancer, breast (ER/PR receptors) and ovarian cancer (CA125).

For adenocarcinomas immunostaining for PSA in male patients, and (o)estrogen (ER) and progesterone receptors (PR) for female patients with axillary node metastases, should be undertaken. Thyroglobulin staining is relatively specific for thyroid cancer so may be very useful in some circumstances. TTF1 (thyroid transcription factor 1) is useful for identifying lung cancer. Other less specific stains include CEA, CA19.9, CA125, and the cytokeratins (e.g. CK7/CK20). If a pathological diagnosis can be made, then further investigations such as endoscopy or radiological studies may be appropriate in some cases. Particular examples include: (1) women with axillary nodes should have bilateral mammography (as well as ER/PR status); (2) women with peritoneal carcinomatosis may undergo laparotomy and surgical debulking as they might have ovarian carcinoma; (3) men with bone metastases (especially osteoblastic) should have serum PSA measured. However, in most patients, routine evaluation of organs that are asymptomatic is not very productive.

Most squamous cell carcinomas involve lymph nodes of the neck. Head and neck and lung cancers are the most likely primary sites. Thorough ENT examination including endoscopy/bronchoscopy with biopsy of suspicious areas can be carried out. The presence of inguinal lymph nodes suggests a primary in the anogenital/rectal region, so careful evaluation with proctoscopy and colposcopy may be appropriate.

MANAGEMENT

Around 40% of CUP patients can be defined into a subset where more specific treatment is indicated. The remainder can be classified as undefined CUP.

SPECIFIC PATIENT SUBSETS

Adenocarcinoma

1. Women with axillary nodes should be treated according to guidelines for breast cancer. Mastectomy reveals an occult breast primary in 40–70% of cases even after negative mammography. Prognosis is similar to breast cancer patients with the same stage of disease.
2. Women with peritoneal carcinomatosis should be treated according to guidelines for ovarian cancer. Five-year survival of 15–25% is reported.

3. Men with elevated PSA or osteoblastic bone metastases should be treated according to advanced prostate cancer guidelines.
4. Patient with a single metastatic lesion. Occasionally only one single site of disease can be found, e.g. lymph node, liver, lung, brain, adrenal, bone, etc. An unusual primary should be considered (e.g. a liver metastasis might represent a hepatoma.). Definitive treatment with surgery and/or radiotherapy should be offered. The role of adjuvant chemotherapy is undefined and should be tailored to individual cases.

Squamous cell carcinoma
1. Patients with cervical lymph node involvement should be treated according to guidelines for locally advanced head and neck cancer. Five-year survival of 30–60% is reported.
2. Patients with inguinal node involvement should have lymph node dissection with adjuvant radiotherapy or concurrent chemoradiation in selected cases, in view of anal and cervical cancers being the most likely primaries. Around 25% will enjoy prolonged survival.

Poorly differentiated carcinoma
Young men with mediastinal and retroperitoneal disease or elevated serum HCG/AFP should be treated according to extragonadal germ cell tumour guidelines. This produces cure in 30–40%. Most patients with poorly differentiated tumours do not fit this group, but have traditionally also received germ cell tumour type regimens producing long-term 10-year survival of ~15%.

Neuroendocrine carcinoma
1. Poorly differentiated neuroendocrine carcinomas are usually aggressive but respond well to platinum/etoposide-based chemotherapy. Long-term survival of 15–20% is reported. The addition of paclitaxel may further improve responses.
2. Well-differentiated neuroendocrine carcinomas usually have features of carcinoid tumours and may be treated as such.

UNDEFINED CUP

The majority of patients with CUPs (60%) do not belong to the above subsets. Most of these patients have adenocarcinomas and have traditionally been treated with 5FU-based regimens, commonly used for gastrointestinal cancers. Response rates (20–30%) and median survival (4–7 months) are poor. Platinum regimens are not much better and produce more toxicity, so are inappropriate for many patients.

FUTURE PERSPECTIVES

Current research is focused on new treatments and diagnostic techniques. New imaging modalities such as positron emission tomography and indium-111 pentetreotide scanning need further evaluation. Improvements in immunohistochemistry and molecular genetics will further improve diagnostic accuracy and provide new targets for treatment such as the HER-2/*neu* receptor, which is expressed in ~10% of CUPs. Clinical trials are under way to assess if HER-2/*neu* positive CUPs respond to trastuzumab (Herceptin). Many new chemotherapy agents have already been shown to be effective in phase II trials. The most impressive agents include the taxanes (paclitaxel), gemcitabine, vinorelbine and irinotecan. Further larger phase III studies of these drugs in combination with traditional agents are under way.

FURTHER READING

Hainsworth J D, Greco F A 2000 Management of patients with cancer of unknown primary site. Oncology 14(4):563–574 [A superb overview.]

CHAPTER 19

Cervical cancer

BACKGROUND INFORMATION

There are approximately 3000 new cases of cervical cancer diagnosed each year in the UK, making it the eleventh commonest cancer in women. In 2002, there were 1120 deaths attributable to this disease. The overall incidence seems to be falling, but the incidence of pre-invasive cancer (cervical intra-epithelial neoplasia III – CIN III) has risen dramatically, both of which can partly be explained by screening programmes. Peak incidence is seen in the 45–50 year age group.

The aetiology is complex and there are several risk factors, which include viral infections with the human papilloma viruses (HPV), sexual promiscuity and early age at first intercourse, history of sexually transmitted diseases, smoking and immunosuppression (e.g. HIV, AIDS (HIV is also associated with a higher risk of HPV infection)).

Infection with HPV is found in 90% of squamous carcinomas and these viruses are thought to play a key role in carcinogenesis. There are over 75 different types of HPV, but HPV16 and 18 are the types most commonly associated with invasive disease. At the molecular level, two HPV gene products, proteins E6 and E7, bind to the crucial host cellular p53 and retinoblastoma proteins. This leads to functional loss of these proteins and subsequent resistance to apoptosis, causing uncensored cell growth after DNA damage. This may ultimately result in progression to malignancy.

Pre-invasive disease and squamous cell carcinomas arise in the transformation zone (TZ). Dysplastic changes in the TZ are graded histologically as CIN I, CIN II or CIN III. The higher the grade, the more severe the dysplasia. CIN III (carcinoma in situ) has the potential to develop into invasive cancer but may take many years to do this. Screening programmes are aimed at detecting pre-invasive disease and in the UK cervical screening is recommended for women aged between 25 and 59 years every 3 years, then at 5-yearly intervals until age 64 years. This is now leading to a reduction in mortality from cervical cancer in the UK.

TABLE 19.1 Approximate 5-year survival of cervical carcinoma by stage

	Percentage of patients (%)	Approximate 5-year survival (%)
Stage I	35	80–90
Stage II	34	55
Stage III	26	30
Stage IV	4	7
Overall		50–60

Squamous cell carcinoma accounts for 85–90% of invasive cervical cancer, the other 10% being mainly adenocarcinomas. Rare types include small cell carcinoma, melanoma and lymphoma. Tumours are histologically graded 1, 2 or 3 (i.e. grade 1 well differentiated, 2 moderately differentiated, 3 poorly differentiated).

The overall 5-year survival for cervical cancer is only 50–60% because at least one-third of patients present with stage III and IV disease (Table 19.1). Patients also have lower survival if the primary tumour is greater than 6 cm in size or there is para-aortic lymph node involvement. The commonest sites of distant metastatic disease are the para-aortic and mediastinal nodes, the lungs and the skeleton.

PRESENTATION

Abnormal vaginal bleeding, which may be post-coital, intermenstrual or postmenopausal, is the most common presenting symptom. Vaginal discharge is also common and may have an offensive odour. Pelvic or leg pain are often signs of late disease. Leg oedema, deep vein thrombosis and rectal bleeding are rare presentations. Many patients now present via the screening programme following an abnormal Pap smear.

DIAGNOSIS AND STAGING

Full clinical examination with vaginal, rectal and speculum examinations is required. A cervical smear may be done, but the wait for a result should not delay the referral of the patient with a clinically suspicious cervical lesion.

All patients with suspected invasive cervical cancer should undergo a formal staging procedure, consisting of EUA, cystoscopy and biopsy. If rectal involvement is suspected a proctoscopy should also be performed.

Radiologically, MRI is the investigation of choice, but CT is commonly used. CXR should be obtained to exclude pulmonary metastases. FBC, renal

TABLE 19.2 FIGO staging of cervical cancer

Stage I	Disease confined to cervix (Ia microscopic, Ib macroscopic)
Ia1	Stromal invasion not >3 mm deep and no extension >7 mm
Ia2	Stromal invasion >3 mm, <5 mm and no extension >7 mm
Ib1	Visible lesion ≤4 cm
Ib2	Visible lesion >4 cm
Stage II	Disease beyond cervix but not pelvic wall or lower third of vagina
IIa	Parametrium not involved
IIb	Parametrium involved
Stage III	Extension to pelvic wall or lower third of vagina
IIIa	Extension to lower third of vagina, not pelvic side wall
IIIb	Extension to pelvic side wall or hydronephrosis or non-functioning kidney
Stage IV	Extension beyond true pelvis or involvement of bladder/rectum
IVa	Extension to mucosa of bladder/rectum/or beyond true pelvis
IVb	Distant metastases

and liver function tests are also required. Tumour markers such as CA125, CA19-9 and CEA may be raised but are not used in routine practice.

Staging is by the FIGO system (Table 19.2).

MANAGEMENT

CIN AND MICROINVASIVE (STAGE Ia) DISEASE

CIN I can be managed conservatively with follow-up as most spontaneously regress. CIN II–III is treated by large loop excision of the transformation zone (LLETZ) or cone biopsy which allows the area of abnormal cells to be removed completely together with the transformation zone. Laser, cold coagulation and cryotherapy remove the abnormal cells and allow the normal cells to grow back but are not the treatments of choice. Cure rates are 90–95%. Cone biopsy/loop excision is required if lesions extend into the endocervical canal or if there is microinvasive carcinoma. Wider excision is required for stage Ia2 disease and incompletely resected disease.

GENERAL CONSIDERATIONS IN THE MANAGEMENT OF INVASIVE DISEASE

All patients should be discussed in a multidisciplinary meeting. The main potentially curative treatment options are radical surgery, radical radiotherapy, radical concurrent chemoradiotherapy, or a combination of the above. Advanced incurable disease can be managed with palliative surgery, palliative radiotherapy and chemotherapy.

Radical surgery involves performing a radical hysterectomy and bilateral pelvic lymphadenectomy (Wertheim's procedure). The ovaries may be spared in patients younger than 40–45 years.

Radical primary radiotherapy involves treatment of the pelvis (to include the gross tumour, pelvic nodes and the parametrial tissues) with external beam radiotherapy (e.g. 45–50 Gy over 4–5 weeks) followed by intracavitary brachytherapy to boost the dose to the primary tumour. The role of extending the pelvic field to include the para-aortic nodes is controversial. Intracavitary brachytherapy involves the placement of afterloading applicators into the uterus and vagina (usually one intrauterine tube and two vaginal ovoids), which are then attached to afterloading equipment (see Figs 5.3 and 5.4). This allows remote controlled placement of radioactive sources into the applicators so that a high local dose of radiotherapy is given. This procedure is normally performed under general anaesthetic. The total dose administered depends on the dose rate of the radioactive source and the overall time that it is inserted for. Low dose rate afterloading systems require 3–4 days of hospital admission but only one visit is required. High dose rate systems using radioisotopes such as iridium-192 and cobalt-60 only require a few minutes to give a high dose, but these treatments need to be fractionated (usually 3–5 fractions over 2–4 weeks) to reduce normal tissue toxicity. The brachytherapy dose is prescribed to a reference point called point A. This corresponds to a point 2 cm lateral and 2 cm superior to the cervical os. The optimum total radiation (EBRT + brachytherapy) dose is unknown, but most centres give a total dose of 70–85 Gy to point A.

Radical concurrent chemoradiotherapy has now become the treatment of choice for most patients with stage Ib2–IVa cervical carcinoma. Two important large meta-analyses have recently shown that progression-free survival rates and overall survival are significantly increased in early and advanced disease with concurrent chemoradiotherapy compared to external beam radiotherapy alone. The improvement in absolute survival for chemoradiotherapy versus radiotherapy alone is estimated to be ~10%. The regimen usually involves the administration of weekly cisplatin (the optimum dose is unknown but 40 mg/m^2 is usually recommended) throughout the course of the EBRT. The main disadvantage of chemoradiotherapy is increased acute toxicity (e.g. severe diarrhoea, nausea and vomiting, infection), which requires careful monitoring of patients throughout treatment. Late toxicity data are lacking at present.

During radiotherapy treatment of cervical cancer, it is very important to make sure patients are not anaemic and ideally the haemoglobin level should be maintained at at least 12 g/dl as this has been shown to improve both pelvic control and survival.

STAGES Ib–IIa

The treatment options include radical hysterectomy with lymphadenectomy, radical radiotherapy or chemoradiotherapy. The decision depends on patient age, co-morbidity, suitability for surgery and patient preference. If surgery is performed, adjuvant radiotherapy (e.g. 45–50 Gy over 4–5 weeks) with or without concurrent chemotherapy is recommended for: (1) positive resection margins, (2) close resection margins <3 mm, (3) involvement of pelvic nodes, (4) bulky >4 cm tumours and/or deep stromal invasion >1 cm, (5) lymphovascular space invasion (relative indication only).

STAGES IIb–IVa

External beam radiotherapy to the pelvis (to include important lymph node groups and the parametria), preferably with concurrent chemotherapy followed by intracavitary treatment, is the treatment of choice.

STAGE IVb (METASTATIC DISEASE) AND ALL OTHER STAGES OF DISEASE IN WOMEN NOT FIT ENOUGH FOR RADICAL TREATMENT

Local pelvic control is one of the most important palliative considerations. Palliative radiotherapy to the pelvis to control pain and bleeding is very helpful. It can also be used to treat bulky lymph node disease causing symptoms. Various palliative radiotherapy schedules are used and they may also include intracavitary treatment. Fitter patients may receive high dose palliation, e.g. 40 Gy in 15 fractions of EBRT followed by an intracavitary treatment. Patients of poor performance status may receive lower dose palliation, e.g. single 10 Gy fraction repeated at no more than 4–6-weekly intervals for a maximum of three treatments.

Chemotherapy is also used, but entry into clinical trials should be considered because data on the efficacy of chemotherapy are lacking. Cisplatin dose escalation or combination with other agents may enhance response rates and progression-free survival but these differences are small, or of doubtful clinical significance and have not achieved a statistically significant increase in overall survival. Single agent cisplatin ($50 \, mg/m^2$ every 21 days, $\times 6$) remains the control arm for randomised trials of the GOG (Gynaecological Oncology Group). Response rates are in the order of 20%. Median survival is about 8 months.

RECURRENT DISEASE

Eighty per cent of recurrences occur in the first 2 years following primary treatment. If local recurrence follows surgery, then radiotherapy can offer long-term cure. If local recurrence follows radiotherapy and is a central pelvic recurrence, then surgical pelvic exenteration (complete removal of pelvic contents including bladder and rectum) can offer around 50% 5-year survival. Chemotherapy has a palliative role.

PREGNANCY AND CERVICAL CANCER

This is rare and the treatment depends on both the stage of the pregnancy and the cancer, as well as the wishes of the patient. A multidisciplinary approach including members of the feto-maternal unit is required. In the first and second trimester, surgery or radiotherapy is used depending on the stage of disease. After 20 weeks it may be possible to delay treatment of early disease to allow fetal maturity. In advanced disease, treatment should probably not be delayed and classical caesarean section should be performed followed by the appropriate further management. Vaginal delivery is thought to disseminate the disease. Overall survival is no different from that for non-pregnant women.

FUTURE PERSPECTIVES

Current trials are focused on optimising chemoradiation schedules, e.g. extended field chemoradiation (to include para-aortic nodes) and new chemotherapy agents (paclitaxel). Other trials are assessing the role of cisplatin-based chemotherapy in the neoadjuvant setting and the role of new agents in the metastatic setting, e.g. taxanes, topotecan, liposomal doxorubicin and capecitabine. Another key area of research is the use of HPV vaccines in both the prevention and treatment of cervical cancer.

PROBLEMS IN ADVANCED DISEASE

See Chapter 58 on problems in advanced pelvic malignancy.

1. Massive haemorrhage. Usually occurs with large exophytic lesions. Can be life-threatening and is best treated with vaginal packing and blood transfusions unless it is a terminal event, in which case anxiolytics and analgesics should be used. Urgent external beam or intracavitary treatment usually brings bleeding under control within 24–48 hours, but if radiotherapy has already been used in the prior treatment, then embolisation using angiography or surgical ligation of the anterior division of the iliac artery can be life-saving.

FURTHER READING

Blake P, Lambert H, Crawford R (eds) 1998 Gynaecological oncology. A guide to clinical management. Oxford Medical Publications, Oxford

Lawton F, Friedlander M, Thomas G (eds) 1998 Essentials of gynaecological cancer. Chapman and Hall Medical, London

Colorectal cancer

BACKGROUND INFORMATION

In 2002, colorectal cancer was responsible for 16 220 deaths in the UK, making it the second most common cause of cancer death after lung cancer. There are over 35 000 new cases per year, representing 13% of all new cancer diagnoses. Incidence increases sharply with age, with a rate of over 300/100 000 in those aged 70 and over. The average age at diagnosis is 60–65 years.

Cancer of the colon is approximately twice as common as rectal cancer. The rectum arises below the peritoneal reflection and above the anal canal. It usually extends to 12–15 cm from the anal verge on rigid sigmoidoscopy.

Approximately 75% of patients with colorectal cancer will present at a stage when all gross carcinoma can be resected surgically. Unfortunately, despite this high resectability rate, nearly 50% of all patients die of metastatic disease, primarily because of microscopic disease that is not apparent at the time of surgery. For this reason, adjuvant therapies have evolved in the treatment of this disease.

The aetiology of colorectal cancer is not fully understood, but several factors have been implicated. Western countries have the highest incidence of the disease and people from low risk countries who move to the West have a higher risk if they adopt Western lifestyle, thus implicating environmental factors (especially dietary factors). Two main genetic syndromes, familial adenomatous polyposis (FAP) and hereditary non-polyposis colorectal cancer (HNPCC), are responsible for around 5% of colorectal cancers. In patients with FAP, the risk of colorectal cancer is 100% if untreated (most would develop cancer before the age of 40) and so these patients should be offered a prophylactic total colectomy. The lifetime risk of colorectal cancer in HNPCC is 80% and these patients should be offered regular screening. In addition to these rare syndromes, close relatives of patients with colorectal cancer are also at increased risk themselves. Greater risk is associated with larger numbers of relatives affected, closer family relationship, and younger age of the relative at diagnosis. Patients with pre-existing diseases such as adenomatous polyps and inflammatory bowel disease also have increased risk. Malignant change in polyps is more likely with villous histology and increasing polyp size. Patients with ulcerative colitis have increasing risk with increasing duration of disease, so that after 20 years there is a 30% risk of cancer. Crohn's disease also increases risk, but to a lesser extent.

Many of the above factors have given clues to help unravel the molecular genetic basis of colorectal cancer, which implicates the 'adenoma–carcinoma sequence' model. This model suggests that a number of stepwise genetic events (inactivation of tumour suppressor genes and activation of proto-oncogenes) occur over many years, causing an initial epithelial proliferation, followed by the development of an adenoma and eventually transformation to carcinoma.

Pathologically, 95% of colorectal cancers are adenocarcinomas, many of which are mucin producing. Other primary tumours include lymphomas, carcinoids, GISTs (gastrointestinal stromal tumours) and melanomas. Around 60–70% of colorectal carcinomas are located in the rectum, recto-sigmoid or sigmoid colon and most of these tend to be annular stenosing lesions ('napkin-ring'). Right-sided lesions tend to be polypoid fungating masses. Spread is by direct extension, by the transperitoneal route and via lympho-vascular channels to regional lymph nodes, liver, lungs, bones and brain.

SCREENING

Screening the general population is controversial. The UK government has plans to introduce screening for those aged 50–69 years, but further details are awaited. The two main methods are faecal occult bloods (FOBs) and flexible sigmoidoscopy/colonoscopy. Despite some success, with reduction in mortality, the numbers needed to be screened to save one life are large. High risk groups require follow-up with colonoscopy.

PRESENTATION

Symptoms depend on the site and extent of the tumour. The commonest presenting symptoms are change in bowel habit (diarrhoea, constipation or both) and rectal bleeding. Bleeding may be fresh or altered depending on where the tumour is located. Constricting tumours may cause obstructive symptoms with abdominal pain, distension and vomiting. In right-sided and caecal tumours, weight loss, anorexia and symptoms of anaemia are more commonly seen than obstructive symptoms because the bowel is more distensible and tumours tend not to be constricting. Delay in diagnosis is common due to the non-specific nature of many of the symptoms. Occasionally, patients present with perforation and faecal peritonitis, which carries a significant mortality. Fistulation into other organs such as the bladder, vagina

TABLE 20.1 Staging of colorectal cancer, TNM system (simplified)	
T1	Invades submucosa
T2	Invades muscularis propria
T3	Invades subserosa or non-peritonealised pericolic/perirectal tissues
T4a	Perforates visceral peritoneum
T4b	Invasion of other organs or structures
N1	1-3 regional nodes
N2	4 or more regional nodes
M0	No metastases
M1	Distant metastases
Stage I	T1-2, N0
Stage II	T3-4, N0
Stage III	Any T, N1-2
Stage IV	Any T, any N, M1

and small bowel may cause urinary tract infections, pneumaturia or faecal discharge per vagina/penis. Metastatic disease may produce the presenting features such as abdominal distension and jaundice (ascites/hepatomegaly). Up to 30% of patients will present as surgical emergencies (usually bowel obstruction).

DIAGNOSIS AND STAGING

Investigations include full history and examination including rectal examination (70% of rectal tumours can be detected with this method); routine bloods including liver and renal function, bone profile, FBC and the tumour marker CEA (elevated in 85% of patients with metastatic disease); CXR; colonoscopy (with biopsy) and/or double contrast barium enema and flexible sigmoidoscopy (with biopsy); and CT scan of chest abdomen and pelvis to assess for metastatic disease. Ultrasound is less accurate than CT for detecting liver metastases, but is commonly used because it is cheaper and quicker.

For rectal tumours, the combination of digital rectal examination (DRE) and endoscopic ultrasound has traditionally been the preoperative staging method of choice. This method is likely to be superseded by preoperative high resolution MRI, which provides more accurate information on the local extent of the tumour in relation to the mesorectal fascia. Surgical/pathological studies have confirmed that preoperative MRI is very useful for predicting involvement of the circumferential resection margin (CRM). The improved accuracy of MRI over CT thus allows better patient selection for neoadjuvant treatment (see below).

Current staging uses both the TNM and modified Dukes systems (Tables 20.1 and 20.2).

TABLE 20.2 Modified Dukes system (with associated frequency and survival data)

Modified Dukes system	Frequency (%)	5-year survival (%)
A: Tumour limited to bowel wall	10–20	>90
B1: Tumour penetrates muscularis propria, but not extramural tissue	30–40	60–80
B2: Tumour penetrates muscularis propria and involves extramural tissue		
C1: Regional nodes involved	20–30	30–40
C2: Apical node involved	10–20	10–20
D: Metastatic disease	15–25	<5

MANAGEMENT

Surgery is the mainstay of curative treatment in colorectal cancer. Around 75–80% of patients are operable at presentation. Surgery may also be used with palliative intent. Chemotherapy and radiotherapy are employed in both the adjuvant and palliative settings.

SURGERY

Whenever possible the primary tumour should be resected along with its adjacent mesentery and draining lymph nodes. Even in patients with metastatic disease, the primary tumour may be resected, if technically possible, to improve symptoms and prevent local complications. The surgical mortality rate for elective procedures should be less than 5%.

The type of operation depends on the anatomical site of the tumour. Right- and left-sided colonic tumours may be treated with a right/left hemicolectomy. Sigmoid colectomy or high anterior resections are performed for sigmoid tumours. Extended right or left hemicolectomies are performed for most transverse colonic tumours.

In rectal cancer, surgery is technically more difficult due to the anatomical constraints of the pelvis. In general, tumours of the upper and middle third of the rectum can be treated with an anterior resection, allowing sphincter preservation. Improved surgical techniques, including the staple gun, have led to an increase in lower anterior resections. Construction of colonic pouches can improve functional outcome. An abdomino-perineal (AP) resection with permanent colostomy is usually required for tumours of the lower third of the rectum. Excision of the entire mesorectum as an intact unit reduces the risk of locoregional recurrence to <10% at 2 years. This technique is known as total mesorectal excision (TME) and has been shown to achieve negative circumferential resection margins (CRM) in 93% of resected specimens. A positive CRM is an important risk factor for local recurrence and is associated with a 3-fold higher risk of death compared to CRM-negative patients.

In advanced rectal cancer, the primary tumour may cause intolerable local symptoms. In this situation, good palliation may be achieved with a Hartmann's procedure (anterior resection of tumour with upper end of rectal stump closed and upper bowel formed into descending colostomy). An end colostomy may be fashioned for palliation of unresectable/inoperable rectal cancer.

Surgical excision of resectable liver and lung metastases may offer long-term survival (5-year survival for liver metastases of 20–40% and up to 30% for lung metastases). Good prognostic factors are early stage of primary tumour, fewer than three metastases, negative resection margins and longer disease-free interval between primary resection and metastatic recurrence.

Approximately 30% of colorectal cancers present as surgical emergencies with obstruction or less commonly perforation or bleeding. Surgical morbidity and mortality (up to 20%) is high. Patients are much more likely to have a prolonged hospital stay and require a permanent colostomy. Overall 5-year survival (30%) is also lower compared to patients who have had elective surgery (40%).

RADIOTHERAPY

After 'curative' surgery, patterns of failure differ between colonic and rectal cancers. Locoregional failure in rectal cancer is more commonly seen than in colonic cancer because clear surgical margins are more difficult to obtain due to anatomical constraints. In addition, the risks of radiation injury to adjacent structures such as the small bowel are far greater in colonic than rectal cancer. For these reasons, radiotherapy plays an important role in rectal cancer but not in colonic cancer.

Colonic cancer
Due to the above factors, there is no established role for radiotherapy in the routine management of colonic cancer, except in the palliative setting (e.g. pain relief for bone metastases).

Rectal cancer
Radiotherapy and, more recently, chemoradiotherapy play an important role in improving local control and downstaging inoperable tumours to operable ones. Radiotherapy or chemoradiotherapy may also facilitate sphincter-preserving surgical procedures in patients with low-lying rectal cancers.

In the adjuvant setting, both preoperative and postoperative radiotherapy reduce local recurrence rates and improve disease-free survival. In Europe, short course preoperative radiotherapy (25 Gy in five fractions over 5 days, followed by immediate surgery) for all patients ('blanket approach') with operable rectal cancer is widely used. However, recent improvements in TME surgery have led to local recurrence rates of less than 10%, and the need to offer preoperative short course RT to all patients has thus been questioned. In North America, the preferred adjuvant option is selective postoperative chemotherapy and synchronous chemoradiotherapy for patients with T3/T4 tumours or node-positive disease. In summary, the optimum adjuvant treatment still remains unknown and this problem is therefore the focus of large multicentre clinical trials (e.g. the Dutch TME study and the MRC CR07 trial). Entry into these trials should be encouraged.

For fixed tumours, or tumours predicted to have a positive CRM by MRI assessment, long course preoperative radiotherapy or chemoradiotherapy may be used (e.g. 45 Gy in 25 fractions over 5 weeks, $\pm$ combination with concurrent 5FU $\pm$ folinic acid) to downstage the tumour to increase the chances of successful complete resection (R0 resection). Early results of the chemoradiotherapy option are very encouraging and further trials are ongoing.

RT also plays a useful role in the palliative setting (see section on problems in advanced disease, below).

CHEMOTHERAPY

Chemotherapy is used in the adjuvant and palliative setting for colorectal cancer. For patients with Dukes C carcinomas, 6 months of adjuvant 5-fluorouracil (5FU) and folinic acid (FA) improves absolute 5-year survival by 8–10%. For Dukes B disease, the role of adjuvant chemotherapy is less clear and is still under evaluation (QUASAR study). In metastatic disease, the use of 5FU/FA produces response rates of around 20–30%. The MAYO (bolus 5FU/FA for 5 days every month) and De Grammont (bolus and infusional 5FU/FA for 2 days, every 2 weeks) regimens are the most widely used. Median survival is improved by 6 months and symptom-free survival is improved from 2 months to 10 months. The addition of the newer agents oxaliplatin and irinotecan to 5FU/FA has been shown to improve response rates and survival in the first and second line setting. Outside of clinical trials, the National Institute of Clinical Excellence (NICE) has approved these drugs to be used in the following circumstances:

1. Oxaliplatin in combination with 5FU may be considered for use as first line treatment in patients with metastases confined solely to the liver, with the aim of increasing the chances of resectability by downstaging the disease.
2. Irinotecan monotherapy is recommended as second line treatment following failure of a standard 5FU regimen.

Oral therapy with capecitabine (precursor of 5FU) or tegafur (5FU prodrug) and uracil (in combination with folinic acid) has now also been recommended by NICE as an option for first line treatment of metastatic disease.

FUTURE PERSPECTIVES

Current research is evaluating the new agents oxaliplatin and irinotecan in the palliative and adjuvant settings. The MRC FOCUS trial is assessing the optimum scheduling and sequential use of 5FU, oxaliplatin and irinotecan in the metastatic setting. The optimisation of preoperative and postoperative radiotherapy/chemoradiotherapy is a focus of many clinical trials.

Two particularly exciting developments are: (1) the anti-angiogenesis drug bevacizumab, which has recently been shown to improve survival in combination with chemotherapy in the metastatic setting (phase III trial), and (2) the EGFR receptor inhibitor cetuximab, which has been shown to be effective in patients with metastatic disease refractory to conventional treatment. Both of these drugs are likely to be important additions in the management of colorectal cancer in the near future.

Other studies are addressing the role of intrahepatic and intraperitoneal chemotherapy as well as gene therapy and immunotherapy with vaccines and monoclonal antibodies.

PROBLEMS IN ADVANCED COLORECTAL CANCER

1. Rectal pain, mucous discharge, diarrhoea, tenesmus and bleeding. Pelvic RT may be very useful. If longer-term survival is expected, high dose palliative RT (45–55 Gy over 4–6 weeks) may offer good local control. For patients with poorer outlooks 30 Gy in 10 fractions over 2 weeks or 20 Gy in 5 fractions over 1 week are commonly used schedules. Surgical resection if feasible may be offered.
2. Intestinal obstruction (see Ch. 58 on problems in advanced pelvic malignancy).
3. Liver metastases (see Ch. 51 on liver metastases).
4. Lung metastases. Resection may improve 5-year survival rate to 20–50% if the lung disease is isolated. Chemotherapy offers a small survival benefit for inoperable disease (see also Ch. 59 on pulmonary metastases).
5. Fistula formation (see Ch. 58 on problems in advanced pelvic malignancy).
6. Ascites (see Ch. 52 on malignant ascites).
7. Lymphoedema (see Ch. 58 on problems in advanced pelvic malignancy).

FURTHER READING

Glimelius B, Pahlman L 1999 Perioperative radiotherapy in rectal cancer. Acta Oncologica 38:23–32

Glynne-Jones R, Debus J 2001 Improving chemoradiotherapy in rectal cancer. Oncologist 6(suppl 4):29–34. www.TheOncologist.com

Heald R J 1995 Rectal cancer. The surgical options. European Journal of Cancer 31A:1189–1192

Midgley R, Kerr D 1999 Seminar. Colorectal cancer. Lancet 353:391–399

Seymour M T 1998 Colorectal cancer: treatment of advanced disease. Cancer Treatment Reviews 24:119–131

CHAPTER 21

Endometrial cancer

BACKGROUND INFORMATION

In 2001, there were 5620 new cases of endometrial cancer diagnosed in the UK. The incidence rate is approximately 12 per 100 000 population. It is the fifth most common cancer in women in the UK and most commonly occurs in the two decades after the menopause. About 25% of cases occur in pre-menopausal women, with 5% occurring in women younger than 40 years. The lifetime risk of developing endometrial cancer is 1 in 73. Endometrial cancer results in about 1000 deaths annually in the UK. The overall 5-year survival rate is approximately 70–75%.

The endometrium is a hormone-responsive tissue. Oestrogenic stimulation produces cellular growth and glandular proliferation, which is balanced by the maturational effects of progesterone. Chronic unopposed exposure to oestrogens results in abnormal proliferation and neoplastic transformation of the endometrium. Oestrogen-associated endometrial cancer progresses through a premalignant stage described as atypical adenomatous hyperplasia, characterised by an increase in the number and complexity of endometrial glands, together with cytological atypia. Of these, approximately one-third progress to cancer. Chronic oestrogen exposure includes early menarche and late menopause. Another well-recognised risk factor for endometrial cancer is obesity. Adipocytes convert androstendione to oestrone via the enzyme aromatase. Women with diabetes mellitus and hypertension also have an increased risk which remains independent of other known factors in multivariate analysis.

There is an association between tamoxifen, an oestrogen antagonist and weak agonist, and endometrial cancer but the overall risk is small compared with the risk of recurrent breast cancer. Women who receive tamoxifen should be asked about symptoms of vaginal bleeding and discharge during follow-up and investigated as appropriate.

Progestogens protect against the effects of oestrogen and combined oral contraceptive pill (OCP) preparations actually reduce the risk of endometrial cancer. Smoking reduces risk by inactivating oestrogen and pregnancy reduces risk by interrupting continuous oestrogen stimulation of the endometrium.

Adenocarcinomas (80% endometrioid type) represent 95% of cases. Papillary serous and clear cell carcinomas are uncommon, but have a much poorer prognosis. Uterine sarcomas make up the remainder. Histologically, adeno-carcinomas are graded 1–3, where grade 1 is well differentiated, grade 2 is moderately differentiated and grade 3 is poorly differentiated. Oestrogen and progesterone receptors are found in approximately 70% of tumours. Receptor-negative tumours have a worse prognosis and are more likely to be poorly differentiated. The lung and vagina are the commonest distant metastatic sites.

The 5-year survival rates for stages I, II, III and IV of the disease are 87%, 76%, 63% and 37% respectively. The overall prognosis is excellent because 75% present with stage I disease.

PRESENTATION

The vast majority (75–80%) present with postmenopausal bleeding (PMB). Premenopausal patients may present with heavy and/or irregular periods and post-coital bleeding. Vaginal discharge (which may be due to the tumour or a pyometrium) and pelvic pain indicate advanced disease.

DIAGNOSIS

Full clinical examination with vaginal and rectal examination is required. Transvaginal ultrasound scan (TVS) with measurement of endometrial thickness and assessment of the adnexal structures is required for all patients with PMB. Biopsy with a Pipelle aspiration or at the time of hysteroscopy (curettage) is performed when endometrial thickness exceeds 4 mm. Further investigations should include FBC, renal function, liver function and CXR.

An MRI scan is performed for radiological staging to assess depth of myometrial invasion, presence of occult cervical involvement, and presence of lymphadenopathy.

Staging is by the FIGO system (Table 21.1).

TREATMENT

Surgery and radiotherapy are the major curative treatment modalities in the management of endometrial cancer. Chemotherapy and hormone therapy are used in the palliative setting only. The role of chemotherapy in the adjuvant setting is not clear and further trials are required.

TABLE 21.1 FIGO staging of endometrial cancer

Stage I	Confined to corpus
Ia	Tumour limited to endometrium
Ib	Up to ½ or less than ½ of myometrium
Ic	More than ½ of myometrium invaded
Stage II	Extension to cervix
IIa	Endocervical glandular involvement only
IIb	Invasion of cervical stroma
Stage III	Local and/or regional spread
IIIa	Invasion of serosa/adnexa and/or positive peritoneal cytology
IIIb	Vaginal involvement
IIIc	Regional nodal involvement
Stage IVa	Extension to bladder/bowel
Stage IVb	Distant metastases (includes intra-abdominal nodes and/or inguinal nodes)

STAGE I–IIb

The treatment of choice is total abdominal hysterectomy and bilateral salpingo-oophorectomy (TAHBSO). At operation, peritoneal washings should be taken and a thorough examination of the intra-abdominal structures should be performed. The role of lymphadenectomy is unclear and entry into the surgical randomisation of the MRC ASTEC ('A Study in the Treatment of Endometrial Cancer') trial should be considered.

Following surgery, patients with stage Ia and Ib disease and grade 1 or 2 histology require no further treatment. Patients with stage Ia or Ib, grade 3 disease, and all stage Ic patients should be referred for consideration of adjuvant radiotherapy. The role of adjuvant radiotherapy in this group of patients is uncertain because although local control is improved, no overall survival benefit has been demonstrated with adjuvant radiotherapy (PORTEC study). For this reason entry into the radiotherapy randomisation of the MRC ASTEC trial should be considered. If trial entry is declined, then decisions on adjuvant treatment are made on local policy. In general, because patients <60 years have a low risk of death from endometrial cancer with stage Ia/Ib, grade 3 and stage Ic, grades 1 and 2 disease, it is reasonable to omit adjuvant therapy. Patients over 60 have a higher risk of pelvic relapse (18% risk) and therefore it is reasonable to offer adjuvant radiotherapy in this group and also to patients under 60 with stage Ic, grade 3 disease.

Pelvic radiotherapy reduces the incidence of locoregional recurrences but has no impact on survival. The extent of adjuvant radiotherapy is the subject of ongoing clinical trials (PORTEC 2) comparing the role of pelvic radio-therapy and intravaginal brachytherapy. External radiotherapy to the whole pelvis is given to a dose of 40–45 Gy in 20–25 fractions over 4–5 weeks. This is sometimes given in combination with intravaginal radiotherapy e.g. 12 Gy to 5 mm from the surface applicator in three fractions (high dose rate brachytherapy). Alternatively, intravaginal brachytherapy can be given on its own, e.g. to a dose of 27 Gy at 5 mm from the surface applicator in six fractions (high dose rate brachytherapy).

In medically unfit patients with stage I disease thought to be unsafe to undergo a hysterectomy, intrauterine brachytherapy using Heyman's capsules may be given. This involves packing the endometrial cavity with 5 to 12 capsules that can be connected to an afterloading system to give 30 Gy in five fractions (to the serosa) over 2 days, repeated 3 weeks later to give a total dose of 60 Gy. Crude 5-year survival is 50%. A combination of external beam radiotherapy and Heyman's capsules can be offered to patients with >50% myometrial invasion.

All stage II patients require adjuvant radiotherapy. Those with stage IIa, grade 1–2 disease with less than 50% myometrium invasion can be treated with intracavitary vaginal brachytherapy only. Those with stage IIa, grade 3 disease and IIb with grade 3 and/or >50% myometrial invasion require pelvic RT and intravaginal treatment.

STAGE IIIa–IVb DISEASE

Surgery may be preferred if technically feasible and should be followed by adjuvant radiotherapy including a vaginal intracavitary boost as described above. If residual disease is present, then this requires a higher dose of radiation, which can be achieved with a CT-planned phase II boost to the tumour. If surgery is not possible or likely to be curative, radiotherapy to the whole pelvis followed by a boost to the sites of bulk disease is the treatment of choice (e.g. 45–48 Gy over 5–6 weeks to pelvis, plus 16–18 Gy CT-planned boost to tumour only).

Stage IV disease that is not curable is usually treated with palliative radiotherapy with or without chemotherapy and progesterones. Good performance status patients can receive high dose palliation to pelvic disease (e.g. 40 Gy in 15 fractions over 3 weeks), whereas less well patients should receive lower doses (e.g. 10 Gy single fraction that may be repeated no more than 4–6-weekly to a maximum of three treatments). Chemotherapy drugs commonly used in metastatic endometrial cancer include cisplatin, carboplatin, doxorubicin and paclitaxel. Progression-free survival is only 3–5 months. Further clinical trials are needed to identify the optimum regimen.

Hormone therapy with progesterones (e.g. medroxyprogesterone acetate 200–400 mg daily or megestrol acetate 40–320 mg daily) can be used for patients with progesterone receptor-positive disease, but objective response rates are less than 30% and median duration of response is less than 10 months. Tamoxifen alone or in combination with progesterone may also be of benefit and is thought to work by increasing the progesterone receptor content of the tumour. Luteinising hormone releasing hormone (LHRH) analogues have been used in progesterone refractory tumours, but further research is required.

RECURRENT DISEASE

The vast majority of recurrences occur within 2 years of initial treatment. Local recurrence may be treated with radical radiotherapy (if site not already treated) or radical surgery if technically feasible. Metastatic recurrence may be treated with chemotherapy (response rates of 20–30%) and hormonal treatment.

UTERINE SARCOMAS

This group of tumours represents less than 5% of all endometrial cancers. They can arise from the endometrium or myometrium and usually occur in the 40–60-year age group. Prior pelvic radiotherapy is the only known risk factor.

The main types are carcinosarcoma (malignant mixed mullerian tumour), leiomyosarcoma, endometrial stromal sarcoma and adenosarcoma. Surgery is the mainstay of treatment. Adjuvant radiotherapy reduces pelvic relapse rates by approximately 50%, but this effect is even greater for endometrial stromal sarcomas where pelvic relapse is reduced from 55% to 4%. Early adeno-sarcomas have a good prognosis and adjuvant therapy is not needed.

Chemotherapy and hormone therapy may be helpful in metastatic disease. Endometrial stromal sarcomas with lung metastases have high response rates to progesterones. Overall, uterine sarcomas have a much worse prognosis than adenocarcinomas with overall survival around 15–30%. However, patients with early stage, low grade sarcomas do well.

FUTURE DIRECTIONS

Much of the current research in endometrial cancer is focused on the role of adjuvant radiotherapy and chemotherapy. Concurrent chemoradiotherapy is being studied in the adjuvant and locally advanced disease settings. In the metastatic setting, the role of trastuzumab (Herceptin) and other epidermal growth factor receptor inhibitors is being assessed.

PROBLEMS IN ADVANCED ENDOMETRIAL CANCER

1. * Pelvic pain (see Ch. 58 on problems in advanced pelvic malignancy).
2. * Fistulas (see Ch. 58).
3. * Urinary problems (see Ch. 58).
4. * Leg lymphoedema (see Ch. 58).

5. *Vaginal bleeding and discharge (see Ch. 58).
6. Pulmonary metastases (see Ch. 48 on bone metastases).
7. Ascites (see Ch. 52 on malignant ascites).
8. Bone metastasis (see Ch. 48 on bone metastases).

FURTHER READING

Blake P, Lambert H, Crawford R (eds) 1998 Gynaecological oncology. A guide to clinical management. Oxford Medical Publications, Oxford

Lawton F, Friedlander M, Thomas G (eds) 1998 Essentials of gynaecological cancer. Chapman and Hall Medical, London

Gastric cancer

BACKGROUND INFORMATION

In the UK there were 6360 deaths due to gastric cancer in 2002 (4% of all cancer deaths). There are approximately 10 000 new cases per year but the overall incidence is falling in the UK and many other countries. (The incidence of proximal tumours (gastric cardia) is increasing, but distal tumours are decreasing.) It is very uncommon before the age of 55 years, and most cases are diagnosed in the sixth and seventh decades. Gastric cancer has a dismal prognosis because only 20% of patients have operable tumours at diagnosis and 5-year survival even in this group is 10–20%. Five-year survival in inoperable cases is less than 5%. In Japan, 5-year survival is 60% because of the high number of patients presenting with early gastric cancer detected in screening programmes.

The aetiology of gastric cancer is unknown, but the following factors are associated with increased risk:

1. Environment and diet – high salt and carbohydrate intake and smoked foods increase risk; fruit and vegetables decrease risk. Smoking increases risk. Incidence falls in Japanese who emigrate to the USA. Higher incidence in lower socioeconomic groups.
2. Genetics – more common in patients with blood group A. Also associated with Li–Fraumeni syndrome and hereditary non-polyposis colorectal cancer (HNPCC).
3. Premalignant lesions – gastric adenomatous polyps may become malignant (10–20% risk of transformation, especially if >2 cm).
4. Infection – association with *Helicobacter pylori* infection, which causes chronic atrophic gastritis and production of carcinogenic *N*-nitroso compounds.
5. Miscellaneous – atrophic gastritis, pernicious anaemia, achlorhydria, history of partial gastrectomy.

Pathologically, 95% of gastric cancers are adenocarcinomas. Macroscopically most take the form of an ulcer with a rolled edge that diffusely infiltrates the stomach wall. Some cancers cause a diffuse fibrosis of the whole stomach (linitis plastica –'leather bottle' stomach) and have a particularly bad prognosis. Spread occurs by direct invasion into adjacent organs, via lymphatics, transcoelomically (e.g. to omentum or ovaries (Krukenberg tumours)) and via the bloodstream to liver, lungs and bone. Early gastric cancer is adenocarcinoma that is confined to the mucosa and submucosa (T1 disease) and although it has an excellent prognosis, it accounts for only 10% of all gastric cancer cases in the West, compared to 50% in Japan.

Other tumour types include gastric lymphomas, squamous cell carcinomas, carcinoids and gastrointestinal stromal tumours (GISTs).

PRESENTATION

The commonest symptoms are anorexia, weight loss and upper abdominal pain and discomfort. Dysphagia, nausea and vomiting and haematemesis also occur. An epigastric mass, nodes in the supraclavicular fossa or hepatomegaly may be present and are signs of advanced disease.

DIAGNOSIS AND STAGING

Full history and examination, CXR, FBC, renal and liver function tests are required. Endoscopy with multiple biopsies and cytological washings is the mainstay of diagnosis (95% success rate). Double contrast barium meal may provide further information and is extensively used in Japan as a screening tool. Abdominal CT scan to assess local disease, lymphadenopathy and presence of liver metastases. Endoscopic ultrasound (EUS) provides further information on the T stage and can also detect lymphadenopathy. Staging laparoscopy to rule out peritoneal seedlings and superficial liver metastases can help prevent unnecessary radical surgery in up to a quarter of patients.

Gastric cancer is staged according to the TNM classification (Table 22.1).

MANAGEMENT

SURGERY

Surgery offers the only chance of cure, but should not be offered to patients with multiple liver metastases, distant lymph node spread, peritoneal spread, malignant ascites or extensive invasion into local structures as these are features of incurable disease.

TABLE 22.1 TNM staging for gastric cancer (simplified)

Tis	In situ
T1	Limited to lamina propria or submucosa
T2	Extension to muscularis propria (2a), or subserosa (2b)
T3	Extension through serosa, but not into adjacent structures
T4	Invasion of adjacent structures
N1	1 to 6 nodes involved
N2	7 to 15 nodes involved
N3	>15 nodes involved
M0	No distant metastases
M1	Distant metastases
Stage 0	Tis, N0, M0
Stage Ia	T1, N0, M0
Stage Ib	T1, N1, M0
	T2, N0, M0
Stage II	T1, N2, M0
	T2, N1, M0
	T3, N0, M0
Stage IIIa	T2, N2, M0
	T3, N1, M0
	T4, N0, M0
Stage IIIb	T3, N2, M0
Stage IV	T4, N1–3, M0
	T1–3, N3, M0
	Any T, any N, M1

Early gastric cancer

In the West, standard treatment is with gastrectomy and limited lympha-denectomy. Subtotal gastrectomy is performed if the distal stomach is involved. Five-year survival approaches 90%. In Japan, patients with mucosal lesions less than 1–2 cm are treated with endoscopic mucosal resection as this procedure offers high cure rates and spares the patient from gastrectomy and lymphadenectomy.

Locally advanced gastric cancer

The type of operation depends on the site and stage of the tumour. In general, diffusely infiltrating tumours and tumours of the proximal and middle third of the stomach require total gastrectomy which may include distal oesophagectomy (if the tumour involves the gastric cardia). Subtotal gastrectomy can be performed for more localised tumours that are located towards the distal end of the stomach. An intraoperative frozen section of the proximal resection margin should be carried out and further resection performed if the margin is positive. The extent of lymphadenectomy is one of the most hotly debated topics in gastric cancer surgery. In Japan, it is standard practice to perform extended lymphadenectomies, whereas in the West less extensive lymphadenectomies are generally performed because clinical trials have not shown a clear survival benefit for more extensive procedures. Splenectomy, which may allow easier lymph node dissection, is not performed unless there is direct involvement of the spleen or suspected splenic node involvement. Pancreaticosplenectomy is no longer routinely performed due to increased morbidity and mortality.

RADIOTHERAPY

At present radiotherapy plays a small role in the management of gastric cancer. Postoperative RT (45 Gy in 20 fractions) has shown no survival benefit, although locoregional failures were decreased. Intraoperative RT has shown survival benefits in stage III/IV cancers but is still under investigation. Adjuvant chemoradiotherapy has recently been shown to offer significant survival benefit in a large North American trial (Macdonald et al, 2001) and has become standard practice in the USA. However, this trial has received much criticism and adjuvant chemoradiotherapy is not currently standard practice in Europe.

Palliative RT (e.g. 30 Gy in 10 fractions or a single 8 Gy fraction) with or without chemotherapy is useful for controlling pain, obstructive symptoms (such as dysphagia) and uncontrolled bleeding. RT is generally well tolerated but may cause nausea and vomiting, abdominal pains/cramps and diarrhoea, which are usually short lived. Antiemetics (5-HT$_3$ inhibitors) should be used.

CHEMOTHERAPY

The role of adjuvant and neoadjuvant chemotherapy (5-FU-based regimens) as well as chemoradiation is still under evaluation in clinical trials. A recent meta-analysis has shown a small survival benefit for adjuvant chemotherapy, but this has not been considered sufficient to justify its routine use. Neo-adjuvant chemotherapy has been shown in phase II trials to downstage locally advanced disease, making resection possible, but further evaluation is required. Intraperitoneal chemotherapy has shown no survival benefit to date and toxicity is significant. Early results from the MRC MAGIC trial of perioperative ECF (epirubicin, cisplatin and 5-FU) chemotherapy have shown increased curative resection rates within the chemotherapy arm of the study and longer-term results are eagerly awaited. It is not currently standard practice in the UK to offer any form of adjuvant treatment outside of a clinical trial.

In the palliative setting combination chemotherapy with ECF is the current standard, achieving response rates of 40–50%. There is often useful palliation and prolonged survival (median survival is 9–12 months with chemotherapy versus 3–5 months with best supportive care).

EXPECTED SURVIVAL FOR THE VARIOUS STAGES OF GASTRIC CANCER

Stage I. Total or subtotal gastrectomy with regional lymphadenectomy: 5-year survival ~70%.

Stage II.   Total or subtotal gastrectomy with lymphadenectomy: 5-year
            survival ~30–40%. Superior outcomes are seen in Japan.
Stage III. Even if resection is possible, 5-year survival is only around 15%.
Stage IV.   Five-year survival is less than 5%.

GASTRIC LYMPHOMA

Gastric lymphoma is a rare tumour, but represents the most common extranodal form of non-Hodgkin's lymphoma. The main types are low grade MALT (mucosa associated lymphoid tissue) lymphomas and diffuse large B-cell lymphomas (DLBCL).

Early stage MALT lymphomas respond very well to treatment of *Helicobacter pylori* infection with high complete response rates. Progressive or advanced disease may be treated with single agent chlorambucil or combination chemotherapy. Prognosis is usually very good.

Gastric DLBCL is a high grade lymphoma that has traditionally been treated surgically with gastrectomy ± chemotherapy. However, due to the significant complications of gastrectomy, the non-surgical option of combination chemotherapy alone or with radiotherapy is now being used much more commonly. The optimum management approach remains unknown. The prognosis is similar to other forms of DLBCL. (See Ch. 32 on non-Hodgkin's lymphomas.)

GASTROINTESTINAL STROMAL TUMOURS (GISTs)

GISTs are mesenchymal tumours that express the KIT (CD117) receptor. They can arise anywhere in the GI tract, but 60% arise in the stomach. Surgical resection is the mainstay of treatment, but recurrence rates are high. Chemotherapy and radiotherapy have no role in the adjuvant setting and response rates to combination chemotherapy in the metastatic setting have traditionally been very poor. Recently, the new KIT tyrosine kinase receptor inhibitor imatinib mesylate (Glivec) has achieved response rates of over 65% in patients with metastatic GISTs. Survival data is keenly awaited. This is now the standard treatment in the metastatic setting and may eventually have a role in the adjuvant/neo adjuvant setting.

FUTURE PERSPECTIVES

The role of adjuvant and neo adjuvant therapy including chemotherapy and chemoradiotherapy remains to be defined. Newer agents such as the taxanes, capecitabine and irinotecan continue to be evaluated.

PROBLEMS IN ADVANCED GASTRIC CANCER

1. Pain. Pain is often epigastric, radiating through to the back. RT (30 Gy in 10 fractions) can be useful in some cases but may cause nausea and vomiting. Occasionally a coeliac plexus block may be of help if the pain is not opioid responsive. Dyspepsia can respond to H2 blockers or proton pump inhibitors. Pain may also be due to liver metastases.
2. Obstructive symptoms. Obstructive symptoms usually occur when tumour involves the gastric cardia or pylorus. Nausea and vomiting, which may be projectile, are predominant features. IV fluids and nasogastric suction with high dose steroids (dexamethasone 8 mg o.d.) and prokinetic drugs like metoclopramide (10 mg t.d.s.) may be helpful initially. Endoscopic placement of self-expanding metallic stents can offer useful palliation with minimal risk. Endoscopic laser debulking may also be attempted. Surgical options include venting gastrostomies, gastro-jejunostomy and gastrectomy. Chemotherapy or RT may also have a role.
3. Cachexia (see Ch. 56 on metabolic problems).
4. Ascites (see Ch. 52 on malignant ascites).
5. Steatorrhoea. Invasion into pancreas may cause steatorrhoea. Creon may be helpful.

REFERENCES AND FURTHER READING

Daly J D, Hennessey T P J, Reynolds J V (eds) 1999 Management of upper gastro-intestinal cancer. W B Saunders, Philadelphia

Macdonald J S, Smalley S R, Benedetti J et al 2001 Chemoradiotherapy after surgery compared with surgery alone for adenocarcinoma of the stomach or gastro-oesophageal junction. New England Journal of Medicine 345(10):725–730

Roukos D H 2000 Current status and future perspectives in gastric cancer management. Cancer Treatment Reviews 26:243–255

CHAPTER 23

Head and neck cancer

BACKGROUND INFORMATION

In the UK, 7950 new cases of head and neck cancer were diagnosed in the year 2000, representing 4% of all cancers. In 2002, there were 3000 deaths from head and neck cancers in the UK (2% of all cancer deaths). The sites involved include: larynx, oral cavity, hypopharynx, oropharynx, nasopharynx, salivary glands, paranasal sinuses and nasal cavity.

The main risk factors for head and neck cancers are smoking, high alcohol intake, increasing age (rare before age of 40), male sex, premalignant conditions such as leukoplakia and poor dental hygiene. The Epstein–Barr virus (EBV) and human papilloma virus (especially HPV16) are also thought to have a carcinogenic role. Head and neck cancer is very uncommon in lifelong non-smokers and alcohol abstainers.

There is a high incidence of multiple primary tumours (10%) mainly due to a field change effect caused by chronic exposure to smoking and alcohol. Second malignancies of the lung and oesophagus occur in 18% and 17% of cases, respectively. Many patients also have co-morbidity including heart disease, chronic lung disease and alcohol-related problems such as liver disease and psychosocial problems. These factors are thought to account for up to 30% of deaths among head and neck cancer patients.

The overwhelming majority of head and neck cancers are squamous cell carcinomas (90%) and the most common site of spread is to the lymph nodes in the neck. Distant metastases to other sites are unusual and occur in only about 10% of cases, the lung being the most common site (52% of cases). This means that the majority of patients will die of uncontrolled local-regional disease (a particularly unpleasant mode of death) if treatment fails. Perineural spread is an important mode of spread because it can provide a pathway to the skull base, causing pain (e.g. facial pain and otalgia) and cranial nerve palsies. Its presence is an indicator of poorer prognosis.

GENERAL PRINCIPLES IN THE INVESTIGATION AND DIAGNOSIS OF HEAD AND NECK CANCERS

Full history and thorough clinical examination are needed initially, including dental assessment. Full endoscopic evaluation (oral cavity, pharynx, larynx and oesophagus) is required in most patients because of the significant risk of synchronous tumours. This also allows biopsy of the tumour and any surrounding abnormal mucosa. Imaging of the primary site and lymph nodes is by MRI or CT. Lymph nodes can also be assessed by ultrasound-guided fine needle aspiration (FNA).

A CXR is required in all patients. Abdominal CT or ultrasound of the liver is occasionally required (e.g. in hypopharyngeal cancer or poorly differentiated nasopharyngeal cancer).

Staging is by the 2002 TNM system, which has different T specifications for different primary sites. In general, designations of T1 to T3 indicate increasing size of the primary and T4 indicates involvement of an adjacent structure. The same N (node) specifications are used for all sites (except nasopharynx):

N0: no nodes
N1: single ipsilateral node $\leqslant 3$ cm
N2a: single ipsilateral node >3 cm $\leqslant 6$ cm
N2b: multiple ipsilateral nodes $\leqslant 6$ cm
N2c: bilateral or contralateral nodes $\leqslant 6$ cm
N3: any node >6 cm.

Histologically, tumours are graded using Broder's classification:

grade 1: well differentiated
grade 2: moderately differentiated
grade 3: poorly differentiated
grade 4: undifferentiated.

GENERAL PRINCIPLES IN THE MANAGEMENT OF THE PRIMARY TUMOUR

A multidisciplinary approach is required with the presence of specialists in ENT, maxillofacial surgery, plastics, radiotherapy and chemotherapy.

Specialist nurses, physiotherapists, dieticians, speech therapists, psychologists and dental hygienists are also vital.

About a third of patients will present with confined early stage lesions (T1 and T2). They are usually treated by single modality surgery or radiotherapy (brachytherapy or external beam radiotherapy). Approximately 80% of T1 lesions and 60% of T2 lesions are cured. Failures may be salvaged by surgery or radiotherapy depending on the primary treatment.

Patients with T3 and T4 lesions have a much worse prognosis (cure rates only around 20–40%). Most require combination surgery and radiotherapy. The decision whether to give pre- or postoperative radiotherapy is often difficult. In general, preoperative radiotherapy is used if: (1) the tumour is thought to be unresectable or incompletely resectable; (2) simultaneous primary lesions are present or; (3) if there is dermal invasion.

Sometimes neoadjuvant chemotherapy (e.g. cisplatin and 5FU) is used to shrink down the primary to facilitate surgery or radiotherapy, and can also be used as part of an organ-preserving approach. However, survival benefits of neoadjuvant chemotherapy are debatable.

Concomitant chemoradiotherapy provides better overall and disease free survival in locally advanced, unresectable head and neck cancer, but long-term side effects are considerable. Further studies are ongoing.

The morbidity from surgery and radiation is not to be underestimated, with many patients requiring hospital admission for severe dysphagia, odynophagia (painful swallowing) and problems with deglutition due to surgically related functional loss and radiation mucositis. Other problems include xerostomia (dry mouth), loss of taste and organ loss (e.g. laryngectomy results in voice loss).

Reconstruction surgery has significantly improved the quality of life for many patients with head and neck cancer and there have been significant advances over the last 30 years. Examples include using free tissue flaps from the forearm to reconstruct the tongue following hemiglossectomy with the benefit of improving speech and swallowing, and the use of tracheo-oesophageal voice valves after laryngectomy to allow preservation of good quality speech.

The head and neck is the most technically demanding and complex cancer site for the successful delivery of radiotherapy. Recent improvements in radiation technology with CT conformal radiotherapy and intensity modulated radiotherapy (IMRT) have increased this complexity.

There is great controversy regarding the optimum dose and fractionation schedules that should be used to treat head and neck cancers. For elective neck irradiation (i.e. occult microscopic disease) 50 Gy in 25 fractions over 5 weeks is commonly used. For postoperative irradiation doses of 50–66 Gy in 25–33 fractions over 5 to 7 weeks are used depending on whether there was a positive resection margin or extracapsular nodal spread. Typical schedules for radical radiotherapy vary from 66 Gy in 33 fractions over 6 weeks to 74 Gy in 32 fractions over 7.5 weeks, depending on the size, and site of disease. Some centres use 55 Gy in 20 fractions. The RT is delivered in two to three phases to introduce 'shrinking field' techniques so that only the bulk areas of disease (i.e. the primary site and enlarged nodes) receive the maximum dose, otherwise normal tissue tolerance would be exceeded.

Many groups have investigated the role of altered fractionation with hyperfractionation, accelerated hyperfractionation, and hypofractionation schedules. The most impressive results so far have been seen with the DAHANCA (Danish Head and Neck Study Group) schedule, which accelerated RT by simply increasing the number of fractions from five per week to six per week so that 70 Gy was delivered in 6 weeks instead of 7 weeks. Improvements in local control and disease-specific survival were demonstrated.

The role of concurrent chemoradiotherapy remains under investigation.

GENERAL PRINCIPLES IN THE MANAGEMENT OF NECK NODES

The presence of positive neck nodes has an adverse effect on both survival and locoregional control of disease. A single positive node decreases survival by as much as 50%. If there is nodal extracapsular spread (75% chance if node >3 cm in size), the prognosis is much poorer.

The lymph node groups in the neck are divided into six levels (Fig. 23.1):

level I: submandibular/submental group
levels II, III, IV: upper, middle and lower jugular groups, respectively
level V: posterior triangle group
level VI: pre-/paratracheal group.

Patients with positive nodes in the lower neck (levels IV, V, VI) have a poorer outcome.

SURGICAL CLASSIFICATION OF NECK DISSECTION

Selective
One or more lymph node groups and non-lymphatic structures are preserved. Some are named:

anterior: level VI
lateral: levels II–IV
supraomohyoid: levels I–III
posterolateral: levels II–V.

Comprehensive
Node levels I–V are dissected.

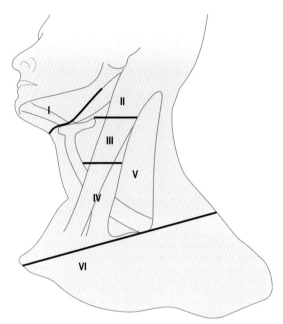

FIGURE 23.1 Anatomical lymph node levels in the neck. I, submandibular/submental group; II, III, IV, upper, middle and lower jugular groups, respectively; V, posterior triangle group; VI, pre-/paratracheal group.

Radical
Reserved for advanced nodal disease. Includes dissection of sternomastoid muscle, internal jugular vein and accessory nerve (XI).

Modified radical
As above, but one or more non-lymphatic structures are preserved and specified.

Extended
Other lymph node groups (e.g. superior mediastinal nodes) or other non-lymphatic structures (e.g. carotid artery, paravertebral muscle) are additionally removed.

MANAGEMENT
Management of the neck is still controversial.

TABLE 23.1 Primary tumour sites and their associated neck node levels for micrometastatic (occult disease) in the clinically negative (N0) neck

	Level I	Level II	Level III	Level IV	Level V	Level VI
Floor of mouth	*					
Anterior tongue	*					
Lower lip	*					
Anterior nasal cavity	*					
Midface structures	*					
Submandibular and sublingual glands	*	*				
Nasopharynx		*	*	*	*	
Oral cavity	*	*	*			
Oropharynx		*	*		*	
Hypopharynx		*	*	*	*	*
Larynx		*	*	*		

Stage N0

Radiotherapy and surgery are equally effective at eradicating subclinical disease. Elective treatment by selective neck dissection or radiotherapy is used for those tumours with an incidence of micrometastasis of more than 20%. The selection of the specific lymph node levels that need treatment is influenced by which primary site is involved (Table 23.1).

Stage N positive

Neck dissection is the usual treatment, although RT may be used if positive nodes are small (<2 cm) and the primary is being treated with RT (e.g. SCC of the tongue). Postoperative RT is recommended if there are: (a) more than two positive nodes involved; (b) nodes at more than one level, (c) nodes greater than 3 cm; and (4) if there is extracapsular spread.

Neck recurrence

The patient should be reinvestigated to exclude a second primary and to restage the disease. If recurrence occurs in a previously untreated neck, then neck dissection is the preferred option with or without postoperative RT. If recurrence follows a previous neck dissection, it is treated with radical radiotherapy. Recurrence following previous RT is treated by salvage neck dissection. Recurrence after combined treatment has a particularly bad prognosis, but may be amenable to further surgery, external beam radiotherapy or brachytherapy. Re-irradiation of previously irradiated tissues is controversial.

Inoperable disease

Radiotherapy is the mainstay of treatment for inoperable disease and can offer cure to a few patients. However, palliation with local control of disease is the main aim of treatment and this requires high dose fractionated radiotherapy. The addition of chemotherapy (e.g. cisplatin and 5FU-based therapy) may bring about further benefit, but the optimum combination of drugs and timing of chemotherapy still requires further research. Occasionally neoadjuvant chemotherapy is employed to try and shrink disease enough to attempt curative surgery or radiotherapy.

POSITIVE CERVICAL NODES WITH UNKNOWN PRIMARY

In a small number of patients with positive cervical nodes, no primary site can be identified, despite a very thorough history and examination including radiological imaging, EUA and surveillance biopsies of the nasopharynx, base of tongue, vallecula, tonsil and hypopharynx.

If the FNA or Trucut biopsy of the cervical node(s) reveals squamous carcinoma, then the patient should be seen by the head and neck team. NB: Open biopsy should be avoided if possible as it is associated with a higher risk of relapse in squamous cancer.

The management of this situation is highly contentious and depending on the clinical scenario, treatment options may vary from a unilateral neck dissection through to bilateral neck dissection and total mucosal irradiation.

Overall 5-year survival is ~50% in this group of patients.

SITE-SPECIFIC CANCERS

LARYNX

The larynx is the commonest site for head and neck cancer. Tumours most commonly occur above (supraglottic) or on the vocal cords (glottic). Subglottic tumours are rare and have a poorer prognosis as they often present at a later stage.

Patients present with a change in voice, hoarseness, airway problems and dysphagia. Supraglottic cancers have a high rate of lymph node metastases with 50% of cases presenting with clinically positive neck nodes and therefore have a poorer prognosis.

Early T1 and T2 glottic tumours are usually treated with radiotherapy with 5-year survival of 60–95%. Endoscopic laser excision or partial laryngectomy are alternatives. The main treatment options for T3 disease (fixed cords) are radiotherapy with the option of salvage surgery later or total laryngectomy (partial laryngectomy may be possible for small tumours) and neck dissection. T4 lesions (invasion into adjacent structures) requires total laryngectomy and neck dissection with postoperative radiotherapy. Five-year survival for glottic T3/T4 disease is 10–50% depending on nodal status.

T1 and T2 lesions of the supraglottis may be treated with radiotherapy including cervical neck nodes or conservation surgery (e.g. partial laryngectomy) with selective neck dissection. Five-year survival is 60–85%. T3/T4 lesions require total laryngectomy and neck dissection with postoperative radiotherapy. Five-year survival is 15–65% depending on nodal status.

Laryngectomy patients may achieve socially useful speech by:

1. Oesophageal speech. Involves the patient pushing air from the oral cavity back into the oesophagus.
2. A neck electrolarynx machine (electrolaryngeal speech). This serves as an outside vibratory source that can be filtered up through the pharynx, nasal and oral cavities, and through the articulators.
3. Tracheo-oesophageal speech. This involves inserting a valve through the stoma and a surgical tracheo-oesophageal fistula. Air is inhaled through the stoma and down the trachea, and transferred through the valve and up through the oesophageal tract to produce voicing.

ORAL CAVITY

The oral cavity includes the buccal mucosa, gingiva, hard palate, tongue and floor of mouth with the latter two being the most frequent sites of cancer. Most patients present with a painless swelling or ulcer, which may have developed in a pre-existing area of dysplasia. In general, early stage disease (T1/T2) may be treated by surgery or radiotherapy (external beam or brachytherapy) depending on the site, anticipated functional deficit, performance status and patient preference. Combined modality treatment is recommended for more advanced disease. Five-year survival is 50–80% for T1/T2, N0 disease, but less than 20% for T4 lesions.

HYPOPHARYNX

Anatomically, the hypopharynx is divided into three sites: pyriform fossa, post-cricoid area, and posterior pharyngeal wall. Patients usually present with a sore throat and worsening dysphagia. Unfortunately, most of these patients have a poor prognosis because lymph node and distant metastases are common at presentation.

In general, T1 and T2 node-negative tumours are usually treated with conservative surgery (if possible) and postoperative RT. Primary RT alone may be an option in some cases (e.g. early post-cricoid tumours). Five-year survival of 50–80% is achievable.

Locally advanced and node-positive disease is best treated with combined radical surgery and postoperative RT, but prognosis is very poor (15–45% 5-year survival). Functional deficit with this approach may be very severe, with loss of speech and normal swallowing. Radiotherapy with or without chemotherapy is an option for patients who refuse surgery or are technically or medically inoperable. Prognosis for these patients is very poor.

OROPHARYNX

The oropharynx includes the base of tongue, tonsillar region, soft palate and posterior pharyngeal wall. Squamous carcinomas of the tonsils and tongue are the commonest tumours in this region and there are high rates of nodal spread. Patients may present with dysphagia, dysarthria and aspiration of liquids.

In general, surgery and radiotherapy have similar local control and 5-year survival rates in early tumours and the choice of therapy will depend on the likely functional outcome and the medical condition of the patient.

For T1/T2 (<4 cm) tonsillar cancers, RT is the treatment of choice with 5-year survival of 50–70% and local control rates of 88–100%. For more advanced lesions combined surgery and radiotherapy are used. T4 tonsillar lesions have a dismal 5-year survival of 14%.

For T1/T2 base of tongue cancers, surgical resection or radiotherapy including neck nodes gives 50–60% 5-year survival. T3/T4 lesions have 5-year survival rates of around 20%.

For recurrent disease, salvage surgery is used if possible with the option of postoperative radiotherapy if not given previously. Cures are sometimes achieved, but overall prognosis is poor.

NASOPHARYNX

The nasopharynx extends from the base of skull to the superior part of the soft palate. Cancer of the nasopharynx is very rare in the UK with an incidence of 0.1/100 000 compared to 10–20/100 000 in Hong Kong. It may present with ear pain and discharge, nasal blockage, cranial nerve palsies or most commonly a lump in the neck. Over 70% have clinically palpable nodes at presentation and 25% have base of skull involvement, radiologically.

Concurrent chemoradiotherapy is the treatment of choice. Large radiation fields are required and acute and late toxicity is common. Long-term problems include xerostomia, trismus (due to fibrosis of masseter muscles and temporomandibular joint), hearing loss, hypothyroidism and hypopituitarism. Overall 5-year survival rates are around 40–65% depending on the histological type.

PARANASAL SINUSES AND NASAL CAVITY

The nasal sinuses include the maxillary, ethmoid, sphenoid and frontal sinuses. Most cancers (two-thirds) arise in the maxillary antrum and may present with nasal stuffiness, dental pain, cheek swelling and ophthalmoplegias. Eighty per cent are squamous carcinomas, others being minor salivary gland tumours (10–15%), lymphomas (5%), melanomas (1%), and sarcomas. Lymph node involvement occurs in only a quarter of cases.

Treatment involves surgery with postoperative RT for all stages except stage I disease, when postoperative RT is only required for histologically unfavourable tumours. Neck dissection is only required for patients with positive nodes. Topical 5FU may be applied to the cavity.

Overall 5-year survival is around 30–40%. Many of these patients now manage to have fairly normal appearances despite extensive resections, due to advances in prosthetics (obturators and dentures) and surgical reconstruction.

SALIVARY GLANDS

The salivary glands comprise the major and minor glands. The major glands are the parotid, submandibular and sublingual glands. The minor glands are located throughout the upper aerodigestive tract. There are a wide variety of histological types of tumour. Most parotid tumours are benign (pleomorphic adenomas), whereas most minor gland tumours are malignant. Malignant histological types are grouped into low, intermediate and high grade malignancy. The commonest types are adenocarcinoma, mucoepidermoid, adenoid cystic, acinic cell, squamous and mixed malignant.

For all tumours, treatment is by surgical excision if possible, followed by postoperative RT if the tumour is high grade or surgical margins are close or involved. If the parotid gland is involved, the surgeon should attempt to spare the facial nerve if possible.

Overall prognosis varies according to histological grade and stage, but overall 5-year survival is around 70%. Recurrent cancer has a dismal prognosis regardless of histological type but salvage may be attempted by surgery and/or radiotherapy depending on previous treatment. Chemotherapy (cisplatin, 5FU, doxorubicin, cyclophosphamide) is still under evaluation.

FUTURE PERSPECTIVES

Much of the current research interest is focused on the use of altered fractionation schedules and the role of chemotherapy especially when given concurrently with radiotherapy. Biological therapies such as epidermal growth factor receptor inhibitors (e.g. gefitinib) are also being studied in combination with radiotherapy.

Intensity modulated radiotherapy (IMRT) is a particularly exciting development in the treatment of head and neck cancers as it potentially offers the chance of dose escalation due to greater sparing of normal tissues. However, further studies are needed to confirm its benefits and the technical and time demands on radiotherapy departments using this technology are high.

In the locally advanced and metastatic setting newer chemotherapy drugs such as the taxanes, capecitabine and gemcitabine are under evaluation. There are also clinical trials assessing the role of biological therapies such as epidermal growth factor receptor inhibitors (e.g. gefitinib), angiogenesis inhibitors (e.g. anti-VEGF antibodies such as bevacizumab) and gene therapy.

PROBLEMS RELATED TO ADVANCED HEAD AND NECK CANCER AND TOXICITIES OF TREATMENT

1. Dysphagia and aspiration. Usually caused by tumour mass, but may be secondary to or exacerbated by nerve infiltration or previous RT and surgery. Simple measures such as analgesia and lubrication with artificial saliva or water may improve swallowing. If there is complete dysphagia or danger from aspiration then nasogastric (for short term) or PEG (for long-term) feeding should be commenced. High dose steroids can occasionally help.
2. Stridor. Often terrifying for the patient. Depending on the severity it may be treated with high dose steroids initially, but a tracheostomy may be required (sometimes as an emergency procedure). Nebulised adrenaline (epinephrine; 10 ml of 1:10 000 solution up to six times daily) and heliox (21% oxygen in helium which allows greater laminar flow, therefore easing breathing) can also be tried. Some centres may offer palliative endoscopic laser resection or stenting for lesions below the cricoid. Patients with particularly poor prognoses should be heavily sedated and kept comfortable.
3. Pain. Pain is very common in head and neck cancer and is particularly important to control, because this region is so vital for communication, nutrition and social functioning. Direct infiltration of tumour into adjacent structures including nerves and bone is the main cause of pain, but other factors include post-surgical neural damage, radiation mucositis, lymphoedema and psychological problems. Pain should be treated according to the WHO analgesic ladder, but may also respond to palliative chemotherapy and/or RT. Neuropathic pain is a particular problem and can be treated pharmacologically or by nerve blocks to the stellate ganglion, trigeminal nerve, glossopharyngeal nerve, and cervical plexus. TENS machines, acupuncture and psychological interventions are also sometimes helpful.
4. Trismus. This is difficulty in opening the mouth (<35 mm interincisal distance) due to fibrosis of the muscles of mastication and may be caused by direct tumour infiltration and/or surgical/radiation damage. This causes problems with eating, speech and oral hygiene and should be aggressively treated with regular exercises for jaw stretching (e.g. using stacks of wooden tongue depressors between the teeth, gradually increasing their numbers over a period of weeks).

5. Infection. This is common and may be a cause of severe pain and odour. Gram-negative organisms are commonly involved and can be treated with systemic and topical antibiotics (e.g. metronidazole). Candidiasis should be treated with antifungals (nystatin 1 ml q.d.s. or fluconazole 50 mg o.d.).

6. Base of skull involvement. Can cause pain and cranial nerve palsies and may respond to palliative RT and/or high dose steroids.

7. Fistulae. Can result in leakage of saliva and oral contents to the skin surface (e.g. orocutaneous fistula) or into the lung (tracheo-oesophageal fistula). Treatment options include stenting over the fistula, plugging the fistula with moulded occlusive dressings, using absorbent dressings, avoiding oral feeding, and using a wound drainage bag to collect the leakage.

8. Disfigurement. Has complex psychosocial and psychosexual implications. Can be helped with maxillofacial prosthetics, cosmetic camouflage and counselling.

9. Haemorrhage. Light bleeding from fragile tumour capillaries is common and may be treated with non-adherent dressings. Ligation and cautery can be used for heavier bleeds. Tranexamic acid is also used (e.g. 500 mg b.d.). Erosion of the carotid artery may lead to a carotid 'blow out', where exsanguination causes death within 2–3 minutes. It is more likely in patients who have had both RT and surgery. It is often preceded by a herald or sentinel bleed and in the terminally ill patient should be managed with someone staying with the patient, heavy sedation (e.g. midazolam 10 mg IV/IM or diamorphine) and using green towels to minimise visual impact.

10. Xerostomia. Dry mouth is most often caused by RT, which may cause permanent loss of salivary function. Exacerbated by drugs (e.g. antidepressants, diuretics, opioids etc.) and dehydration. It affects eating, taste, speech and sleeping, and increases the risk of oral infection and dental caries.

11. Osteoradionecrosis. Severe necrosis of bone may occur following radical RT if there is a portal of entry for infection and therefore patients with poor dentition are most at risk. It is notoriously difficult to treat but can respond to debridement and hyperbaric oxygen therapy. If these fail then further surgical excision may be required.

12. Lymphoedema. The main causes are neck dissection, RT and tumour infiltration of lymphatics. It may cause disfigurement and pain as well as functional deficits of speech and swallowing, airway problems and visual disturbance. Can be helped with manual lymphatic drainage (massage), exercises (e.g. facial muscle contractions), skin moisturising and aggressive treatment of cellulitis.

13. Loss of special sensory functions. Vision, smell, taste, hearing and balance can all be affected by direct involvement of tumour, nerve infiltration or as complications of treatment (e.g. deafness caused by cisplatinum).

Palliative RT and steroids may be of benefit in some situations, e.g. orbital infiltration.

14. Communication and speech problems. Caused and/or exacerbated by tumour infiltration, nerve involvement, xerostomia, lymphoedema, RT and surgery. Patients should be referred to a speech therapist and any treatable causes corrected, e.g. ensuring adequate lubrication with artificial saliva.

FURTHER READING

Feber T (ed) 2000 Head and neck oncology nursing. Whurr, London

Million R R, Cassisi N J 1994 Management of head and neck cancer. A multidisciplinary approach, 2nd edn. JB Lippincott, Philadelphia

Shah J 2001 Atlas of clinical oncology. Cancer of the head and neck. BC Decker, Hamilton, Ontario

Vokes E E, Weichselbaum R R, Lippman S M, Hong W K 1993 Head and neck cancer (review). New England Journal of Medicine 328(3):184–194

CHAPTER 24

Hepatobiliary cancer

BACKGROUND INFORMATION

Hepatobiliary cancers include cancers of the liver, bile ducts and gallbladder. In 1999, there were just under 3000 new cases of hepatobiliary cancer in the UK. The death rate is similar to the incidence rate, emphasising the poor prognosis of this group of cancers. Approximately 65% of these tumours are hepatocellular carcinomas (HCC), 20% are gallbladder cancer and the remainder are bile duct cancers.

Hepatocellular carcinoma (HCC) is by far the commonest primary malignant tumour of the liver. Other primary malignant tumours of the liver include intrahepatic cholangiocarcinoma, angiosarcoma (extremely rare, associated with polyvinyl chloride exposure, very poor prognosis) and hepatoblastoma (very rare, occurs mainly in children <3 years old). Although worldwide HCC is common and accounts for between 300 000 and one million deaths a year, in the UK (and the West) it is relatively uncommon, with an incidence of 4.7/100 000 in men and 3/100 000 in women. Chronic liver damage and cirrhosis are major factors in the development of liver cancer. About 80% of HCCs worldwide are associated with hepatitis B (HBV) infection. In Europe, HCC is most commonly related to hepatitis C infection (HCV) (60–80%). Other risk factors include aflatoxin B1 (found in peanuts and corn), alcohol (co-carcinogenic with HCV), smoking, haemochromatosis, autoimmune hepatitis and Budd–Chiari syndrome. Pathologically, HCC is macroscopically a single mass (30%), multiple nodules (60%), or diffusely infiltrating (10%). Approximately 70% of HCCs produce alpha-fetoprotein (AFP). Fibrolamellar carcinoma is a rare variant of HCC that does not produce AFP. It occurs in younger patients with non-cirrhotic livers and has a better prognosis (60% 5-year survival). Overall survival in HCC is less than 10%.

Bile duct cancers are uncommon. They are classified as:

1. Intrahepatic (20–25%)
2. Perihilar (50–60%) – includes Klatskin tumours which occur at the hilum of the ducts
3. Distal (20–25%).

Histologically, 95% are adenocarcinomas, otherwise known as cholangio-carcinomas. Other histological types include squamous cell carcinoma, and small cell carcinoma. Risk factors include primary sclerosing cholangitis (PSC), choledochal cysts, environmental agents (nitrosamines, radon, radionuclides), chronic inflammation and biliary stasis. Most patients are inoperable at presentation, so overall 5-year survival is poor.

Gallbladder cancer is most frequently seen in patients aged between 70 and 75 years and is commoner in women than men by a factor of 2.4:1. Pathologically 85% are adenocarcinomas, the remainder being squamous and mixed types. Cholelithiasis is an associated factor, but only 1% of patients with this condition develop cancer. Other associations are inflammatory bowel disease, gallbladder polyps, gallbladder calcification ('porcelain' gallbladder) chronic typhoid infection and carcinogens (e.g. nitrosamines). Unfortunately, although the disease is highly curable in the early stages, the vast majority present with advanced disease, so overall 5-year survival is only around 5%.

PRESENTATION

HCC

Most patients present with late stage disease. The commonest symptoms are of right upper quadrant pain, sometimes referred to the shoulder, and non-specific symptoms such as weight loss and anorexia. Fever due to tumour necrosis is sometimes experienced. Around 10% of patients present with gastrointestinal (GI) bleeding (half caused by oesophageal varices) and 2–5% with an acute abdomen secondary to tumour rupture. Paraneoplastic syndromes are not uncommon and include hypoglycaemia, hypercalcaemia and erythrocytosis. Hepatic decompensation leads to jaundice, ascites and encephalopathy. A vascular bruit is present in 25%.

BILE DUCT CANCER

Intrahepatic bile duct cancer presents in a similar manner to HCC. Perihilar and distal tumours present with obstructive jaundice, pruritus, abdominal pain, weight loss and anorexia. Right upper quadrant pain, fever and rigors suggest cholangitis.

GALLBLADDER CANCER

Symptoms are often vague and non-specific. Pain in the right upper quadrant is common (60–95% of patients) and may be identical in nature to biliary colic. Jaundice is present in 25–50% and anorexia and weight loss are also typical. Patients may have a palpable gallbladder mass, hepatomegaly and ascites.

About 20% of gallbladder cancers are discovered incidentally during cholecystectomies for benign disease.

DIAGNOSIS AND STAGING

Investigations used in the diagnosis of hepatobiliary cancer include: history and clinical examination; FBC, liver and renal function; clotting studies; calcium; CXR; ultrasound abdomen; CT/MRI of the abdomen; hepatitis B and C serology (for HCC); tumour markers – AFP (for HCC) and CA19.9, CEA, CA125 (for cholangiocarcinomas only if diagnosis is in doubt).

For cholangiocarcinomas, invasive cholangiography with ERCP (endoscopic retrograde cholangiopancreaticography) and PTC (percutaneous transhepatic cholangiography) can yield a tissue diagnosis, help assess resectability, and allow palliative stent insertion. MRCP (magnetic resonance cholangio-pancreatography) is non-invasive and can determine the extent of duct and liver involvement.

A liver mass and AFP >500 ng/dl is virtually diagnostic of HCC. In non-surgical candidates, an image-guided FNA or core biopsy confirms the diagnosis. FNA should not be undertaken in patients who are going to have potentially curative treatment as biopsy can be taken at laparotomy, thus avoiding the risk of tumour seeding along needle tracks. Gallbladder cancer has a particularly high propensity to spread along needle tracks, and so the above principles are applied regarding FNA.

Staging is by the 2002 TNM classification (Table 24.1).

MANAGEMENT

HEPATOCELLULAR CARCINOMA

Surgery with hepatic resection, either partial or total (orthotopic liver transplant) offers the only chance of cure. Palliative options include ablative therapies, radiotherapy, systemic therapy (immunotherapy, chemotherapy, hormones) and supportive care.

Surgery
Only 10–20% of patients are thought to be operable prior to surgery and a significant number of these will be found inoperable at laparotomy. In patients without cirrhosis, partial hepatectomy of up to two-thirds of the liver can be tolerated. Patients with cirrhotic livers have a much higher risk of morbidity and mortality and should have liver function assessed according to the Pugh–Child scoring system, before curative resection is attempted. Despite resection, recurrence is a major problem and 5-year survival is only

TABLE 24.1 TNM staging for liver, gallbladder and bile duct cancers

Liver (summary)

TI	Solitary lesion without vascular invasion
T2	Solitary lesion with vascular invasion or multiple lesions ≤5 cm
T3	Multiple >5 cm or invasion of major branch of portal/hepatic vein
T4	Invades adjacent organs other than gallbladder or perforates visceral peritoneum
NI	Regional nodes
Stage I	TI, N0
Stage II	T2, N0
Stage IIIA	T3, N0
Stage IIIB	T4, N0
Stage IIIC	Any T, NI
Stage IV	Any T, any N, MI

Gallbladder (summary)

TI	Gallbladder wall (Ia lamina propria, Ib muscle)
T2	Perimuscular connective tissue
T3	Serosa, one organ and/or liver
T4	Portal vein, hepatic artery, or 2 or more extrahepatic organs
NI	Regional nodes
Stage IA	TI, N0
Stage IB	T2, N0
Stage IIA	T3, N0
Stage IIB	TI–3, NI
Stage III	T4, any N
Stage IV	Any T, any N, MI

Extrahepatic bile ducts (summary)

TI	Ductal wall
T2	Beyond ductal wall
T3	Liver, gallbladder, pancreas, or unilateral vessels
T4	Other adjacent organs, or main or bilateral vessels
NI	Regional
Stage IA	TI, N0
Stage IB	T2, N0
Stage IIA	T3, N0
Stage IIB	TI–3, NI
Stage III	T4, any N
Stage IV	Any T, any N, MI

30%. Patients with multiple lesions may be offered resection if all the lesions are confined to one lobe (24–28% 5-year survival). Although controversial, orthotopic liver transplantation (OLT) is an option for some patients (tumour <5 cm, up to three tumours <3 cm in size, cirrhotic liver, no portal vein or hepatic vein involvement, no extrahepatic spread), but obviously limited due to the shortage of donor livers and high cost. Five-year survival is 20–45%. There is no role for adjuvant therapy outside the setting of a clinical trial.

Ablative therapy

Numerous methods of ablative therapy have been used and are still under evaluation for patients with unresectable disease. Ablative therapies may eradicate tumour and minimise loss of functioning normal liver.

1. Percutaneous ethanol injections (PEI) for small tumours (<5 cm) have achieved 5-year survival rates of 33% in selected cases.
2. Transcatheter arterial chemo-embolisation (TACE) utilises the fact that the majority of the blood supply to HCCs comes from the hepatic artery and not the portal vein, which is the main supply of the normal liver. A variety of embolic (oils and coils) and chemotherapeutic agents have produced response rates of 60–80% with 5-year survival of 10%.
3. Cryosurgery with liquid nitrogen probes requires laparotomy and is limited to the research setting.
4. Radiofrequency ablation (RFA) involves inserting needle electrodes (percutaneous or laparotomy) into tumours and applying a high frequency alternating current across them, which causes thermal injury (>60°C) to surrounding tissues. It is suitable for tumours <5–6 cm, but is still investigational.

Radiotherapy

Conformal external beam radiotherapy may offer useful palliation, but whole liver irradiation has no convincing role. Intrahepatic arterial administration of radioisotopes such as yttrium-90 and iodine-131 is experimental.

Systemic treatments

1. Chemotherapy has traditionally been very disappointing in HCC with response rates of single agent and combination regimens of 10–25%, with no clear survival benefit convincingly demonstrated. This may partly be due to the presence of the multidrug resistance (MDR) gene product, p-glycoprotein, which has been found in over 65% of HCC patients. Active agents include doxorubicin, cisplatinum, 5FU, methotrexate, capecitabine and etoposide. More recent phase II studies with new combinations of these drugs have shown some promise, but need further evaluation. Hepatic arterial infusion (HAI) chemotherapy has shown better response rates (up to 50%), but randomised trials are needed.
2. Biotherapy with interferon alpha has shown some activity in HCC, especially when combined with chemotherapy; e.g. PIAF regimen (platinum, interferon, adriamycin, 5FU) gave a 26% response rate.
3. Hormone treatment with tamoxifen has been advocated because a third of HCCs express oestrogen receptors. Unfortunately, results have been very disappointing with no benefit shown for tamoxifen alone.

As there is no proven benefit to systemic therapies, patients with metastatic disease should only be offered treatment in a clinical trial setting. Patients not entered into trials receive supportive care only.

CHOLANGIOCARCINOMA

Any chance of long-term survival depends on complete surgical resection.

Intrahepatic cholangiocarcinomas

These are treated surgically in a similar manner to HCC, but very few patients present with operable disease. Median survival after surgery is 1–2 years. Patients with inoperable disease have a median survival of 3–6 months. The role of chemotherapy and radiotherapy in both the adjuvant and palliative settings remains undefined, so participation in clinical trials should be encouraged. Ablative therapy can be useful for those with unresectable disease.

Extrahepatic cholangiocarcinomas

If operable, the type of curative surgery depends on location of the tumour. Proximal/hilar tumours require major liver resection with biliary and vascular resection and reconstruction. Mortality of surgery is ~10%. Five-year survival is 30% with median survival of 2 years. Inoperable disease is fatal within 6–12 months.

Distal tumours are more often resected (up to 70% of cases in some centres). Whipple's procedure is often the operation of choice, offering 5-year survival of 20–40%. There is currently no established role for adjuvant chemotherapy or radiotherapy, but some centres do give concurrent chemoradiotherapy if there are positive resection margins.

Patients found to be unresectable at laparotomy may undergo palliative biliary-enteric bypass. Palliative biliary drainage with PTC stenting can be performed for inoperable tumours. Two or three stents may be required for proximal/hilar tumours. Radiotherapy and 5FU-based chemotherapy have been used in the palliative setting but results are poor.

GALLBLADDER CANCER

Unfortunately, very few patients present with operable disease. Patients with ascites, peritoneal metastases, hepatoduodenal ligament involvement, invasion/encasement of major vessels or distant metastases are unresectable. Median survival in this group is dire at 2–4 months with <5% surviving 1 year.

Operable disease

Incidental gallbladder cancer   If the cancer is discovered incidentally during a 'routine' cholecystectomy for benign disease, then a radical cholecystectomy should be performed if the disease is operable. This involves removal of gallbladder and at least 2 cm of the gallbladder bed, and regional lymphadenectomy ± partial liver resection.

If the diagnosis was made incidentally postoperatively, then further surgical exploration is required for T2 tumours and above if radiological staging (CT/MRI) excludes the presence of metastatic disease. Radical surgery should be performed if disease is resectable. Patients with T1 tumours require no further surgery and can be observed, as 5-year survival is 85–100%.

Clinically diagnosed gallbladder cancer Most have advanced locoregional or metastatic disease and are inoperable. Those with organ-confined disease may be treated with radical surgery, although 5-year survival is only around 30% as most have T3/T4 disease.

Adjuvant therapy
The role of adjuvant radiotherapy and chemotherapy requires further evaluation and these are not offered routinely.

Advanced unresectable and metastatic disease
Those with obstructive jaundice may be palliated with surgical biliary enteric bypass or endoscopic/percutaneous (PTC) stenting. Palliative radiotherapy to the primary tumour mass may be useful for pain relief. Palliative chemotherapy has been used with limited success, but requires further evaluation. Active agents include 5FU, mitomycin C, cisplatin and gemcitabine.

FUTURE PERSPECTIVES

In HCC, current research is focused on prevention and screening, the use of multimodality therapy with biological and chemotherapeutic agents, regional intrahepatic therapies, radiofrequency ablation, octreotide and gene therapies involving replacement of the absent tumour suppressor gene p53 using viral vectors. For bile duct and gallbladder cancer, the main focus is on new chemotherapy and chemoradiation schedules, as well as evaluation of radiosensitisers such as hyperthermia or drugs.

PROBLEMS IN ADVANCED DISEASE

1. Abdominal pain. Caused by stretching of liver capsule. May also get pressure symptoms on other organs. In addition to the WHO pain ladder, phenytoin 100 mg nocte, carbamazepine 100 mg b.d. or amitriptyline 10 mg nocte may be helpful. Steroids may be very helpful because they reduce

oedema and inflammation, thereby decreasing stretching of liver capsule (e.g. dexamethasone 8–16 mg o.d.). Referred pain to lower thoracic or upper abdomen may respond to a coeliac axis block.

2. Obstructive jaundice. More commonly seen in the bile duct cancers than in HCC. (See above and Ch. 36 on pancreatic cancer.)

3. Ascites (see also Ch. 52 on malignant ascites). Common in liver cancer. Pressure effects may cause diaphragmatic splinting and respiratory compromise as well as gaseous GI disturbance and early satiety due to gastric compression. Abdominal paracentesis offers good palliation, but is often short-lived due to reaccumulation. Peritoneal infection is a potential serious complication. Spironolactone 100 mg escalating to 600 mg daily may also offer good palliation, but may cause electrolyte and renal problems. Peritoneovenous shunting may be considered for resistant cases, but may be hazardous in patients with poor clotting and low platelets.

4. GI bleeding. Usually a terminal or pre-terminal event, with a median survival of 21 days after bleeding. Often due to varices caused by portal hypertension, but can also be due to peptic ulceration. Patients with a good pre-morbid condition may undergo emergency endoscopic sclerotherapy.

5. Spontaneous rupture of liver. This is a rare complication seen in 2.7% of cases of HCC in England. Most patients present with an acute abdomen. Those who are haemodynamically unstable, but previously fit, should have a laparotomy and alcohol injection of the bleeding point. This controls bleeding in >50%. Those who continue bleeding may undergo hepatic artery ligation, and failing this hepatic resection may be attempted, but this has a high mortality rate. Stable patients may have an ultrasound and angiogram to identify the bleeding point. Selective angiographic embolisation can then be employed.

6. Paraneoplastic syndromes (HCC). (a) Hypoglycaemia. Type A is seen in end-stage disease when there is rapid tumour growth and cachexia. It is usually mild and responds well to glucose administration. Type B is rare in the West and is usually seen early in the disease. Severe symptomatic hypoglycaemia occurs, which may lead to convulsions, coma and death. It is difficult to control with glucose, glucagon and steroids. Tumour production of insulin-like growth factor II (IGF-II) and similar peptides is thought to be responsible. Growth hormone is thus a useful holding measure, whilst patients await more definitive treatment (i.e. resection, ablation, etc.). (b) Erythrocytosis (haemoglobin >16 mg/dl, haematocrit >48%) is seen in 10% of HCC patients. Ectopic production of erythropoietin is the suggested cause. Symptomatic patients can be venesected.

7. Hepatic encephalopathy. An end-stage event. It may occur gradually or be acutely precipitated by an adverse event such as infection or bleeding. Management is aimed at (i) removing or treating precipitating factors, (ii) minimising nitrogenous intake by decreasing intake, evacuating the bowel, and using antibiotics (neomycin) to kill gut flora.

FURTHER READING

Hepatocellular carcinoma. Seminars in Oncology 2001;28(5) [Whole issue dedicated to hepatocellular carcinoma]

Hussain S A, Ferry D R, El-Gazzaz G et al 2001 Review: Hepatocellular carcinoma. Annals of Oncology 12:161–172

Khan S A, Davidson B R, Goldin R et al 2002 Guidelines for the diagnosis and management of cholangiocarcinoma: Consensus document. Gut 51(Suppl VI):vi1–vi19

Misra S, Chaturverdi A, Misra N C, Sharma I D 2003 Carcinoma of the gallbladder. Review. Lancet Oncology 4:167–176

Ryder S D 2003 Guidelines for the diagnosis and treatment of hepatocellular carcinoma (HCC) in adults. Gut 52(suppl III):iii1–iii8

CHAPTER 25

Hodgkin's lymphoma

BACKGROUND INFORMATION

Thomas Hodgkin first described this disease in 1832 and it is one of the great success stories in oncology, with current 5-year survival rates of 80%+. There are approximately 1400 new cases of Hodgkin's disease (HD) in the UK per year and in 2001 there were only 264 deaths. This illustrates the high cure rates that are now achievable with combination chemotherapy and/or radiotherapy. The disease is more common in males (M : F 3 : 2) and Caucasians. There is a bimodal age distribution, peaking in 15–34-year-olds and over 60s.

The aetiology is unknown, but the Epstein–Barr virus (EBV) may be involved in the pathogenesis, as tumour cells are EBV-positive in up to 50% of patients with HD. Patients with HIV infection have a higher incidence of HD and almost 100% of HIV-associated HD cases are EBV-positive. However, HD is still not considered an AIDS-defining neoplasm. Genetic predisposition may play a role as approximately 1% of patients with HD have a family history of the disease, and siblings of an affected individual have 3–7 times the risk compared to the normal population. This risk is higher in monozygotic twins.

Histologically, the picture is unique, with 1–2% of neoplastic cells (Reed–Sternberg (RS) cells) in a background of a variety of reactive mixed inflammatory cells consisting of lymphocytes, plasma cells, neutrophils, eosinophils and histiocytes. HD is classified by the WHO into classical HD, of which there are four subtypes, and lymphocyte predominant nodular HD.

Classical (95%)
1. Nodular sclerosing (NSHD) (70%). This is usually seen in young adults and most commonly involves the mediastinum and supradiaphragmatic nodes. Prognosis is excellent.
2. Mixed cellularity (MCHD) (15–30%). Often more advanced disease at diagnosis and tends to affect infradiaphragmatic nodes and spleen. Prognosis is good.

3. Lymphocyte depleted (LDHD) (1%). This is more commonly seen in older patients and HIV-positive patients, and is often advanced at presentation. May be mistaken for large-cell anaplastic non-Hodgkin's lymphoma (NHL). The prognosis is less good.
4. Lymphocyte-rich (LRHD) (5%). Excellent prognosis. Relapse is rare following complete remission.

Lymphocyte predominant nodular HD (LPNHD) (5%)

Typical RS cells are rarely seen and instead atypical 'popcorn' RS cells are abundant. It is typically seen in young males who present with lymphadenopathy in the neck or axilla. B symptoms and mediastinal disease are rare. The prognosis is good, but late relapses and transformation into aggressive NHL (2–10% of cases) may occur.

PRESENTATION

Most patients present with an enlarged, painless lymph node in the neck (70%), axilla (25%) or inguinal region (10%). Constitutional symptoms (B symptoms) such as fever, drenching night sweats and weight loss occur in up to 40%. Generalised pruritus occurs in 5–10% at presentation, but this is more of a problem in advanced disease. The classic Pel–Ebstein fever (cyclical fever in which periods of fever lasting from 3 to 10 days are separated by an afebrile period of about the same length) is unusual and not specific to HD. Patients with mediastinal disease may complain of chest pain and dyspnoea, but haemoptysis is rare. Alcohol-induced pain at sites of nodal disease is specific for HD, but is uncommon and usually associated with mediastinal disease. Bone marrow involvement is rare at presentation (~2% of cases), but may cause bony aches and pains and is usually associated with systemic symptoms. Abdominal pain may be due to hepatosplenomegaly or bulky abdominal nodal disease.

Clinical signs may include palpable rubbery lymphadenopathy, hepatomegaly, splenomegaly, and skin excoriations due to pruritus. SVCO due to mediastinal lymphadenopathy is occasionally seen. CNS disturbances are very rare, but if present, may be due to direct tumour involvement (usually spinal rather than cerebral) or paraneoplastic syndromes including cerebellar degeneration, neuropathy, Guillain–Barré syndrome, or multifocal leukoencephalopathy.

The disease tends to spread predictably to lymph node groups in a contiguous manner. Splenic, liver and bone marrow involvement usually occur late in the natural history of the disease.

TABLE 25.1   Ann Arbor staging of lymphoma

Stage I	Single lymph node area (I) or single extranodal site (IE)
Stage II	2 or more lymph node areas on the same side of the diaphragm (II) or localised single extralymphatic organ or site and its regional node(s) (IIE)
Stage III	Lymph nodes involved on both sides of the diaphragm
Stage IV	Disseminated or multiple involvement of extranodal organs (e.g. liver, bone marrow, lung, skin)
The designation of A or B is also applied:	
A	No constitutional symptoms
B	Presence of 1 or more of the following: (1) unexplained fevers (temperature >38°C), (2) drenching night sweats, and (3) unexplained weight loss of more than 10% in the preceding 6 months

DIAGNOSIS AND STAGING

Investigations include full history and examination; full blood count (usually normal in early disease); ESR; renal and liver function tests; LDH; β2 microglobulin; CXR; CT scan of the neck, chest, abdomen and pelvis. Bone marrow aspiration and trephine (~2% will have bone marrow involvement at presentation). Biopsy of an accessible node should be by excision biopsy and needle and core biopsies should only be used in cases where excision biopsy would be a hazard to the patient. Staging laparotomy is no longer necessary.

The Ann Arbor staging classification is used (Table 25.1).

MANAGEMENT

Combination chemotherapy has revolutionised the treatment of HD and this has led to the dramatic shift in the use of wide field radiotherapy to more localised 'involved field' techniques in many centres. The gold standard chemotherapy regimen is ABVD (doxorubicin, bleomycin, vinblastine, dacarbazine) as it has a low risk of impairing fertility and is not associated with an increased risk of secondary leukaemia. Other regimens used include Stanford V, MOPP and BEACOPP.

Identification of unfavourable prognostic factors has allowed the design of risk-adapted therapy in HD. Three main categories are recognised:

1. Limited stage. Clinical stage I and II without risk factors.
2. Intermediate stage. Clinical stage I and II and at least one of the following poor prognostic factors:
   - bulky mediastinal disease (defined as a mass >7.5 cm or a mediastinal mass ratio >0.35)
   - high ESR (≥30 mm/h for B stages, >50 mm/h for A stages)
   - massive splenic disease
   - multiple lymph node sites (≥3 lymph node areas)
   - extranodal disease.
3. Advanced stage. Clinical stage III or IV.

Entry into clinical trials should be encouraged as standard treatments for HD remain to be elucidated. Outside of trials, the following treatment options are acceptable.

Stage I/IIA lymphocyte predominant nodular HD (LPNHD)
Involved field RT alone is appropriate (e.g. 30–36 Gy over 4 weeks).

Limited stage
Chemotherapy (e.g. two to four cycles of ABVD) followed by involved-field RT (e.g. 30 Gy). This achieves >90% cure rate.

Intermediate stage
Chemotherapy (e.g. four cycles of ABVD) followed by involved-field RT (e.g. 30 Gy). This achieves ~80% cure rate.

Advanced stage
Chemotherapy (e.g. eight cycles of ABVD). Involved-field RT (e.g. 30 Gy) is only required if there is residual disease or if the original tumour was bulky. This achieves ~60–70% cure rate.

Relapsed or resistant disease
Patients who relapse after radiotherapy alone (~25%) can be salvaged with chemotherapy. At least 60% of these patients will be cured.

Some patients (~15%) do not achieve a complete response (CR) after initial ABVD chemotherapy or relapse within a couple of months and this predicts a poor outlook. The treatment of choice for this group of patients is high-dose chemotherapy (HDCT) with an autologous stem cell transplant (ASCT), which offers a 5-year survival rate of ~30%. A commonly used regimen is ifosfamide and mitoxantrone (four cycles) followed by a stem cell harvest, which is then followed by high-dose BEAM (BCNU, etoposide, ara-C, melphalan) and the stem cell autograft. Patients who relapse between 2 and 12 months after initial chemotherapy should also be offered HDCT with ASCT.

Patients who relapse with localised disease over 12 months following chemotherapy may be treated with further conventional chemotherapy and RT, but HDCT and ASCT may offer a greater chance of survival. All other forms of late relapse are best treated with HDCT and ASCT, which offers cure rates between 30 and 70%.

Those who relapse following HDCT and ASCT pose a very difficult problem and entry into experimental phase I and II clinical trials should be considered if appropriate.

FUTURE PERSPECTIVES

Although current treatment is often very successful, this comes at a price for some patients cured of their disease, with secondary malignancies (leukaemia, lung cancer and breast cancer) and coronary artery disease resulting in a premature death. For these reasons many clinical trials are seeking to obtain the same excellent cure rates for patients with early favourable prognosis disease, whilst trying to minimise late toxicity. The identification of prognostic factors in early stage and late stage HD is helping in the design of risk adapted therapy. Treatment of refractory and relapsed disease also remains a great challenge and several new therapies are being evaluated. These include non-myeloablative allogeneic stem cell transplants, immune therapies such as EBV-specific autologous cytotoxic T-lymphocytes, anti-CD30 immunotoxin, and single-agent chemotherapy drugs such as gemcitabine, vinorelbine, paclitaxel and fludarabine.

PROBLEMS IN ADVANCED DISEASE

1. Bone marrow suppression. Heavy bone marrow involvement causes pancytopenia, resulting in transfusion dependent anaemia, thrombocytopenia and bleeding complications, and neutropenia and lymphopenia causing increased risk of bacterial and viral infections. Blood and platelets should be transfused and infections treated as appropriate.
2. Painful bulky lymph nodes. These may ulcerate if large and are best treated with chemotherapy and radiotherapy if possible. Previously irradiated sites may be re-irradiated to within normal tissue tolerances.
3. Ascites and effusions (see Chs 52, 54 and 55 on malignant ascites, pleural/pericardial effusions).
4. Dyspnoea. May result from pleural/pericardial effusions, massive mediastinal disease, SVCO or treatment related pneumonitis (e.g. RT, bleomycin).
5. Obstructive jaundice. Can occur due to bulky nodes at the porta hepatis. Local RT or placement of stent may help.

6. Constitutional symptoms. May respond to dexamethasone.
7. Tumour lysis syndrome (see Ch. 56 on metabolic problems in cancer).

FURTHER READING

Hancock B W, Selby P J, Maclennan K A, Armitage J O (eds) 2000 Malignant lymphoma. Edward Arnold, London

Horwitz S M, Horning S J 2000 Advances in the treatment of Hodgkin's lymphoma. Current Opinion in Hematology 7(4):235–240

CHAPTER 26

Leukaemias – acute

Andrew John Ashcroft

BACKGROUND INFORMATION

Acute leukaemias arise from proliferation of immature malignant clones of haematopoietic progenitors in the bone marrow or lymphatic system. Bone marrow infiltration can then lead to pancytopenia and the clinical manifestations of weakness, fatigue, recurrent infections, and bleeding.

In adults, approximately 80–85% of acute leukaemias are myeloid leukaemias (AML) and the remainder are acute lymphoblastic leukaemias (ALL). ALL conversely is the most common childhood cancer with most cases reported in the 2–10-year age group. The annual incidence of acute leukaemias is 4–7 cases/100 000 population. Over 90% of patients with AML are over 15, and the incidence increases with age (median 60 years). In adult ALL, the incidence is slightly higher in the young (15–24 years) and peaks again in those over 80 years of age.

The aetiology is unknown, but factors associated with the development of some acute leukaemias include exposure to ionising radiation (peak incidence after 6–7 years, e.g. in Chernobyl survivors), exposure to chemical agents such as benzene and chemotherapy drugs (alkylating agents), viruses, and congenital disorders such as Down's syndrome (20-fold increased incidence), Klinefelter's syndrome, Fanconi's anaemia, Bloom's syndrome, ataxia telangiectasia and neurofibromatosis.

AML and ALL are diagnosed by examination of peripheral blood and bone marrow. The classifications of ALL and AML were until recently based on the French-American-British (FAB) classification, which divided ALL into L1, L2, and L3 subtypes, depending on primarily morphological features and AML into M0–M7, depending on the degree of cellular maturation and the degree of myeloid, monocytoid, erythroid or megakaryocytic differentiation. This system has been replaced by the WHO classification. WHO divides ALL into

B and T precursor lymphoblastic leukaemia/lymphomas and blastic NK (T cell) lymphomas whilst AML is divided into:

AML with recurrent genetic abnormalities t(8,21) (FAB M2), inv(16), t(16,16) (FAB M4Eo), t(15,17) (FAB M3) or 11q23 abnormalities
AML with multilineage dysplasia
AML and myelodysplastic syndromes, therapy related
AML not otherwise categorised (which consists of FAB classification M0–2 and M4–7, acute basophilic leukaemia, acute panmyelosis with myelofibrosis and myeloid sarcoma).

Hence, rather than the previous morphological classifications, immunophenotyping and cytogenetic analysis to identify prognostic factors (e.g. various chromosomal abnormalities such as translocations) are now considered essential for the accurate identification and appropriate treatment of different leukaemias (e.g. ATRA in the treatment of AML with t(15,17). Many texts still however refer to the FAB classification.

Significant progress has been made in the treatment of adults with acute leukaemia. However, the outlook for children is still far better. In adults with ALL, complete remission (CR) rates of 75–90% can be achieved with modern treatment regimens. However, most will relapse and 5-year survival of 10–40% can now be expected. In AML, CR rates are in the order of 70% and the overall 5-year survival is 35–50%. The mainstay of treatment for acute leukaemia is chemotherapy. Patients should be entered in Medical Research Council (MRC) clinical trials if possible.

PRESENTATION

AML

Patients often present with malaise, fever, sweats, anaemic symptoms, bleeding (gums, nosebleeds and menorrhagia), bruising, chest infections, and occasionally skin/mucosal infections. Hyperleucocytosis (white cells > 100×10^9) can lead to symptoms of leucostasis (sludging of the blood) such as dyspnoea associated with diffuse pulmonary shadowing, CNS and visual disturbance.

On examination there may be gum hypertrophy, which is classically associated with M4 and M5 (FAB classification), occasionally solid tumour lesions (chloroma) and skin lesions due to infiltration. AML M3 is particularly associated with bleeding due to disseminated intravascular coagulopathy (DIC).

ALL

Presenting symptoms can be similar to AML with weakness, malaise, sweats, bleeding, bruising, and symptoms relating to infections being the most common clinical manifestations. Hyperleucocytosis can occur but is much less common than in myeloid leukaemias. CNS involvement, which is seen in 6% of patients at presentation, can cause meningism, visual disturbances and cranial nerve palsies.

On examination, there may be lymphadenopathy (55%), splenomegaly (50%), hepatomegaly (45%), CNS signs (6%) or skin infiltration (6%). Superior vena caval obstruction is occasionally present due to mediastinal nodes, and testicular involvement can also occur.

DIAGNOSIS

Full history and examination may reveal a number of the findings outlined above.

Full blood count (FBC) and a differential count from a Wright–Giemsa-stained smear will often give the diagnosis to an experienced morphologist. AML can be diagnosed if Auer rods (rod-like cytoplasmic inclusions) are present. The white cell count is usually raised with circulating blasts, but can be low. Very high white counts due to the presence of leukaemic blast cells are more common in ALL than AML but occur in either condition. Anaemia, thrombocytopenia and neutropenia are usually evident.

The bone marrow aspirate and trephine usually reveal a heavy blast cell infiltration. Normal haemopoietic cells are often absent or reduced with normal fat spaces being replaced by infiltrating blasts.

Cytochemistry, immunophenotyping and cytogenetic analysis give further information to confirm the diagnosis, aid classification and provide prognostic information.

Immunophenotyping
AML: Allows the differentiation of myeloid, monocyte, erythroid and megakaryocyte components, blast cell percentages and maturation status of cells.
ALL: Distinguishes early or null cell ALL from pre-B or common ALL and T ALL (T ALL <10% of total).

Cytogenetics
AML: Chromosomal abnormalities, t(15,17) in M3, t(8,21) in M2 and inv(16) in M4Eo (M4 with eosinophilia), are all good prognostic markers. Monosomy 7 and multiple deletions/breakages are usually associated with AML arising from a previous myelodysplastic syndrome (MDS) and are poor prognostic markers.
ALL: Presence of the Philadelphia chromosome t(9,22) is a very poor prognostic marker and occurs in 10–20% of adult ALL; t(4,11) is also a poor prognostic marker.

Other investigations

Lumbar puncture (LP) for examination of the CSF is routinely performed in ALL patients. LP is only necessary in AML if clinically indicated. Other investigations should include blood group, antibody screen, coagulation screen, renal and liver function tests, LDH, urate, calcium, glucose, virology, HLA typing, immunoglobulins, autoantibody screen, midstream specimen of urine, blood and stool cultures if the patient is septic, CXR and ECG.

MANAGEMENT

Many patients present acutely unwell, and some of the initial complications of the disease such as septic shock, metabolic disturbances and bleeding may require emergency treatment. Alongside more immediate measures to resuscitate and stabilise the patient, prophylactic and supportive measures to prevent and manage other complications of the disease and its treatment should also be instigated. These include:

1. Adequate IV fluid intake and electrolyte replacement to improve urine output, reduce risk of urate crystal formation, and decrease risk of tumour lysis syndrome.
2. Allopurinol to decrease risk of gout and urate uropathy.
3. Antifungal prophylaxis with fluconazole or itraconazole decreases risk of candida and aspergillosis infection and is utilised depending on specific circumstances. Aciclovir may be used as prophylaxis if there is a previous history of HSV infection. In the bone marrow transplant (BMT) setting, co-trimoxazole reduces risk of *Pneumocystis carinii* (PCP) infections.
4. Early treatment of febrile neutropenia is essential. Antibiotics as per local protocols should be used.
5. Platelet transfusions are indicated if the platelet count is less than 10×10^9 and there is no active bleeding, or if less than 20 and the patient is septic (these levels may vary depending on local/national guidelines). Blood transfusions should be used to treat symptomatic anaemia.

TREATMENT OF ACUTE LEUKAEMIA – GENERAL PRINCIPLES

The aim of therapy is to achieve a complete remission and cure. Remission, when described by morphology alone, was traditionally defined as normal marrow cellularity, less than 5% leukaemic blast cells with recovery of peripheral blood counts. However, cytogenetics detecting residual chromosomal abnormalities in remaining malignant cells, polymerase chain reaction (PCR) techniques and flow cytometry are now often used in the assessment of minimal residual disease not visible by morphological examination. CR also requires the CSF to be clear of blast cells.

Patients should be offered entry into the various MRC trials (AML 14/15, UKALL XII) or other high quality leukaemia trials. The exact course of treatment is based on selection criteria, which include age, type of leukaemia, various prognostic factors, previous therapies and response to therapy within the trial.

SPECIFIC THERAPY

AML

Treatment of AML is conventionally divided into two phases: Remission induction and post-remission consolidation. In addition, patients with AML M3 (acute promyelocytic leukaemia) should receive retinoid therapy with all-*trans*-retinoic acid (ATRA), which produces maturation of the leukaemic clone in this group of patients and also helps to resolve DIC if present. The use of this agent should be combined with chemotherapy.

Remission induction

The drugs most commonly used in the remission induction phase are daunorubicin, ara-C and etoposide given over 8–10 days depending on the trial protocol, or the FLAG IDA regimen (fludarabine combined with ara-C, G-CSF and idarubicin). The role of the monoclonal antibody (Myelotarg) is also being assessed in current trials. This intensive treatment causes periods of profound myelosuppression.

Post-remission consolidation

Following induction therapy a majority of patients will enter CR. The trial options for young patients who achieve CR are: (1) further chemotherapy with additional drugs including mitoxantrone, etoposide and idarubicin (alongside retinoids (ATRA) if AML M3), or (2) allogeneic mini stem cell transplantation (or possibly conventional allogenic transplant for younger patients) if standard or poor risk.

Traditionally, allogeneic transplants have the lowest rate of relapse (15%), probably due to the graft-versus-leukaemia effect, but have the disadvantage of treatment-related morbidity/mortality. Chemotherapy has higher relapse rates, but lower early morbidity/mortality. Patients over 60 tend to have adverse cytogenetics and a worse prognosis. Current trials are studying the role of high versus low dose treatment for this group who traditionally have only a 10–15% chance of cure.

Relapse

Most relapses occur in the first 2–3 years. About 50% will re-enter remission, and ~15% of these will survive over the next 3–5 years.

ALL

The treatment of adult ALL has been based upon protocols used in childhood ALL. The definitive therapy of adult ALL is at present considered in three to four parts: remission induction, intensification/consolidation, CNS prophylaxis and maintenance therapy or high dose procedure. For Ph$^+$ adults (and children) allogenic transplant offers the only realistic possibility of cure.

Remission induction

Two induction phases of multi-agent chemotherapy including daunorubicin, vincristine, prednisolone and L-asparaginase followed by cyclophosphamide, ara-C, 6-mercaptopurine and intrathecal methotrexate are given to induce a CR, which is possible in about 80% of cases. (There are significant periods of cytopenia during induction, and prophylaxis for both *Aspergillus* and PCP are utilised.)

Intensification and consolidation

High dose methotrexate and L-asparaginase are given and autologous bone marrow harvest performed prior to either auto- or allograft, or further chemotherapy (four cycles of consolidation) and maintenance treatment.

CNS prophylaxis

Without CNS prophylaxis, 30% of patients will have a CNS relapse. Intrathecal methotrexate, ara-C and craniospinal radiotherapy (for those not undergoing transplant) are currently the methods used.

Maintenance

Lasts for 18 months post consolidation and consists of outpatient 6-mercaptopurine, methotrexate, vincristine, prednisolone and intrathecal ara-C.

Relapse

The best cure rates approach 90% and are achieved in young girls <10 years of age with a low presenting white cell count and no CNS disease. Overall childhood cure rates approach 70%. The picture in adults is much worse, with only up to 40% of the best prognostic groups achieving cure after allogenic BMT. In the adult group as a whole cure rates are <20%.

In total over 60% of adults in first remission will relapse. Bone marrow transplantation offers the only realistic chance of cure in these patients and can be offered to patients who achieve a second complete remission following combination chemotherapy. CNS relapse requires systemic and intrathecal treatment.

FUTURE PERSPECTIVES IN TREATMENT

Treatment outcomes have gradually improved over recent years. These improvements in both mortality and morbidity are undoubtedly due to both greater knowledge and utilisation of effective chemotherapy regimens and as importantly, significant improvements in general patient care. The most exciting progress in the foreseeable future is likely to come from novel agents, such as monoclonal antibodies and cellular proteosome inhibitors.

FURTHER READING

Catovsky D, Hoffbrand A V 1998 Acute leukaemia. In: Hoffbrand A V, Mitchell Lewis S, Tuddenham E G D (eds) Postgraduate haematology, 4th edn. Butterworth Heinemann, Oxford

Hoelzer D, Burnett A K 2002 Acute leukaemias in adults. In: Souhami R L, Tannock I, Hohenberger P, Horiot J-C (eds) Oxford textbook of oncology, 2nd edn, volume 2. OUP, Oxford, pp 2191–2215

Lowenberg B, Downing J R, Burnett A 1999 Acute myeloid leukaemia. New England Journal of Medicine 341(14):1051–1062

CHAPTER 27

Leukaemias – chronic

Andrew John Ashcroft

BACKGROUND INFORMATION

Chronic myeloid leukaemia (CML) and chronic lymphocytic leukaemia (CLL) are the more commonly occurring chronic leukaemias. Other disease entities including chronic myelomonocytic leukaemia (CMML), which can be classed amongst the myelodysplastic syndromes, conditions such as hairy cell leukaemia, which is a chronic curable lymphoproliferative disease, and more aggressive conditions such as T-prolymphocytic leukaemia are beyond the scope of this discussion.

CML

CML is a malignant clonal myeloproliferative disorder of a pluripotent haemopoietic stem cell and accounts for ~15% of adult leukaemias. The incidence is 1–1.5/100 000 population with a peak in the 40–60 years age group; the male to female ratio is 1.4:1. CML is characterised by the presence of the Philadelphia chromosome (created by a balanced translocation between the long arms of chromosomes 9 and 22). The t(9,22) results in fusion of two genes that produce a hybrid (chimeric) *bcr-abl* gene. This gene encodes a tyrosine kinase, which plays a central role in the pathogenesis of CML. Irradiation is the only known aetiological risk factor.

CML typically has a biphasic course. The initial chronic phase lasts for a mean period of 4.5 years (range 3 months–22 years) before spontaneously transforming to an accelerated phase which is usually associated with the acquisition of additional chromosomal abnormalities and terminates in a blast crisis (which is myeloid in 80% and lymphoid in 20% of cases). Once transformed, survival is in the order of 6–9 months.

The disease is potentially curable with either sibling or matched unrelated donor (MUD) allogeneic stem cell transplantation. These procedures offer

5-year survival rates of between 45–60%. Unfortunately, very few patients have the opportunity of transplantation due to either their clinical state or lack of a suitable donor. Overall median survival at present is 5–7 years.

Previous mainstays of treatment have been hydroxyurea and interferon; however, the biological agent imatinib mesylate (Glivec), which is a protein-tyrosine kinase inhibitor, has become the treatment of choice outside the transplant setting, and is now used in both chronic and accelerated phase disease. Many patients who would previously have been transplanted or died due to accelerated phase disease have obtained molecular remissions with this drug. Longer-term follow-up is, however, not yet available to assess how overall survival will be affected or if a proportion of patients are in fact cured with this treatment.

CLL

CLL is produced by proliferation of a monoclonal population of B-lymphocytes. B- and T-cell chronic leukaemias other than B-CLL are relatively rare. CLL is the commonest adult leukaemia, accounting for 30–40% of all leukaemia cases seen in clinical practice. The annual incidence of CLL is 2.5/100 000 and it is primarily a disease of older age groups with 70% over the age of 70 at diagnosis; the male to female ratio is 2:1. The aetiology of CLL is unknown, but some cases are familial (~2%), suggesting a genetic link. CLL is generally characterised by the gradual accumulation of small mature lymphocytes in the bone marrow and peripheral blood; lymphadenopathy and splenomegaly are often present. The disease can run an indolent course and patients can, probably due to the age of presentation, die of unrelated causes. The median overall survival is 10 years; however,

Table 27.1   Rai and Binet staging systems for CLL

Stage	Clinical features	Risk level	Median survival
Rai system for CLL			
0	Lymphocytosis alone	Low	>10 years
I	Lymphocytosis + lymphadenopathy	Intermediate	7 years
II	Lymphocytosis, spleen ± liver		
III	Lymphocytosis + anaemia (<11 g/dl)	High	1.5 years
IV	Lymphocytosis + thrombocytopenia (platelets < 100 × 10⁹)		
Binet system for CLL			
A	Lymphoid involvement in <3 sites		14 years
B	Lymphoid involvement in 3 or more sites		5 years
C	Myelosuppression (Hb < 10 g/dl or platelets < 100 × 10⁹)		2.5 years

this varies considerably from patient to patient and cannot usefully be used as a guide at diagnosis for any individual case. Probably the most clinically relevant staging systems to assess prognosis are those of Rai and Binet (Table 27.1).

Other features of CLL include the development of autoimmune haemolytic anaemia and thrombocytopenia (Evans' syndrome) and hypogamma-globulinaemia. A proportion of patients (<5%) can undergo Richter's transformation to a diffuse large B-cell lymphoma in one or more lymph nodes or can develop increasing numbers of prolymphocytes (>10%) becoming CLL/PLL.

PRESENTATION AND CLINICAL FEATURES

CML

The majority of patients present in the chronic phase of disease, many with symptoms related to hypermetabolism such as fatigue, weight loss, sweating or pallor, dyspnoea and tachycardia due to anaemia. Other features include abdominal discomfort from splenic enlargement or infarction, infections, bleeding, bruising and gout due to hyperuricaemia. Rare presenting problems include those due to leucostasis leading to visual disturbance, hyperviscosity and priapism. In 10–30% of patients, there are no symptoms as the diagnosis is made incidentally on routine blood testing.

The main examination finding is usually palpable splenomegaly, which is present in 75% of cases and is occasionally massive. Patients in the advanced phase have more frequent and severe symptoms; infectious complications are a particular problem.

CLL

Symptoms tend to be related to lymphocyte mass. Early CLL is usually asymptomatic and diagnosed incidentally on a routine blood count when there is lymphocytosis of $>5 \times 10^9$/litre. It is, however, recognised that CLL cells are present in a proportion of the population at levels much lower than this. As the disease progresses the patient often develops anaemia, which can be due to either bone marrow infiltration or autoimmune haemolysis. Infections become common due to neutropenia, abnormal lymphocyte function and disordered innate immunity including in some cases a para-protein. Organ involvement leads to splenomegaly, hepatomegaly and painless lymphadenopathy. Constitutional symptoms such as fever, night sweats, lethargy and weight loss are usually late features.

DIAGNOSIS

CML

FBC and blood film shows a leucocytosis (neutrophils and myeloid precursors), basophilia and eosinophilia. Raised platelets with clumping may also be seen. The neutrophil alkaline phosphatase (NAP) score is low. The bone marrow is hypercellular and cytogenetic studies showing the presence of the Philadelphia chromosome confirm the diagnosis. In a proportion of cases, molecular analysis with the polymerase chain reaction (PCR) to detect the bcr-abl product may be necessary if cytogenetic studies are inconclusive. In advanced disease, there is a rise in the blast cell population, an increase in the NAP score and loss of disease control despite treatment.

CLL

Blood count and film classically show a lymphocytosis of at least $5 \times 10^9/l$ with characteristic morphology. In some cases the lymphocytosis may be $>300 \times 10^9/l$. A bone marrow examination reveals $\geqslant 30\%$ lymphocytes with characteristic immunophenotypic markers. Cytogenetics may reveal a loss of one p53 or deletion of 11q23 (poor prognosis) or single deletion of 13q (good prognosis). Additional tests should include serum electrophoresis and immunoglobulins, Coombs' test and reticulocyte count to exclude haemolytic anaemia, and either CT or ultrasound scanning to assess disease bulk.

MANAGEMENT

Entry into high quality clinical trials should be encouraged.

CML

Chronic phase

Allogeneic stem cell transplantation (allo-SCT) at present offers the only known chance of cure and may be offered to selected patients who are biologically fit for the procedure with a suitable HLA-matched donor and should be received within a year of diagnosis. Cure depends on a poorly defined 'graft versus leukaemia' effect. The overall 5-year leukaemia-free survival is 55–60%, but may approach 70–80% if the patient is young (<40 years old), cytomegalovirus (CMV) seronegative, is transplanted within 1 year of diagnosis, and has a young male donor. There is a significant risk of morbidity and mortality with this procedure and the decision to offer allo-SCT has been made more complex with the success of imatinib mesylate (Glivec).

Other treatment options include the use of hydroxyurea, interferon-α ± ara-C and imatinib mesylate (Glivec).

1. Interferon-α induces haematological remission in 70–80%; however, it produces major or complete cytogenetic response (Philadelphia negative) in a much lower percentage of patients. Those who achieve major or complete cytogenetic response survive significantly longer than those who do not. Five-year survival is better with interferon-α (57%) than with chemotherapy (42%), but toxicity with interferon may be significant and the optimum doses and duration of treatment are unclear. The addition of cytosine arabinoside has been shown to further improve cytogenetic response and survival.

2. Hydroxyurea is very useful for controlling leucocytosis and improving symptoms and if possible is combined with interferon-α.

3. Imatinib mesylate (Glivec) is an extremely promising agent. It is a tyrosine kinase inhibitor of the *bcr-abl* tyrosine kinase. In a recent international trial, the complete cytogenetic response rate was 63% for imatinib versus 7% for interferon-α + ara-C, but overall survival data are still awaited. It also produces high response rates in interferon-α resistant disease. Current NICE guidelines indicate imatinib should be the first treatment considered in newly diagnosed CML. Imatinib is also recommended as an option in those patients presenting in accelerated phase or blast crisis or in those patients who progress to accelerated phase without previous imatinib treatment. It has low toxicity, is easy to administer (given orally) and has rapidly become the drug of choice in the haematologist's therapeutic armoury. Imatinib resistance does, however, occur and similar molecules with potentially little cross-resistance are in development.

4. Leucophoresis using a cell separator can lower WBC counts rapidly and safely in patients with leucostasis and tends to be used as an emergency measure.

Accelerated and blast phase

There is still a chance of cure for the few patients eligible for transplantation, with leukaemia-free survival rates of 30–50%. Imatinib is effective in the accelerated phase, producing complete haematological response in 53%, with 19% returning to chronic phase disease. Median survival at 1 year is 78%, but longer-term survival data are awaited.

In the blast crisis, imatinib produces median survival of 7 months, with 1-year survival of 32%. Hydroxyurea is still helpful in this setting for both leucocytosis and splenomegaly. Interferon-α has no place in blastic transformation, but combination chemotherapy similar to that used in the acute leukaemias can be offered with limited success. Around 20% with myeloid transformation and 50% with lymphoid transformation will achieve a second chronic phase.

CLL

Apart from the occasional patient treated with allogenic transplant, CLL is to date an incurable disease. As the natural history of the disease is often very long, patients with Binet stage A and B disease may be kept under review without treatment. However, if the patient is symptomatic, has progressive anaemia, thrombocytopenia, lymphocytosis, autoimmune disease or repeated infections, then systemic therapy should be initiated. Therapeutic options include:

1. Chlorambucil. Is still considered to be a standard therapy in many situations, produces response rates of 50% with reduction in symptoms and improvement in blood counts, but CR is rare (3%). Treatment is stopped when a normal lymphocyte count is achieved or continued for up to 6–12 months if the disease continues to respond. Overall survival is not improved.
2. Purine analogues. Fludarabine produces higher overall response rates and CR than chlorambucil and this translates into better disease-free survival (33 versus 17 months). However, there is no evidence for an overall survival benefit. It is currently recommended as a second line agent by NICE. The MRC CLL IV trial is comparing chlorambucil versus fludarabine versus fludarabine/cyclophosphamide as first line treatments.
3. Steroids. Are useful in reducing lymphocytosis in patients with neutropenia and thrombocytopenia, where chemotherapy could carry a high risk. Steroids are also used in patients with autoimmune manifestations of CLL.
4. Combination chemotherapy (e.g. CHOP) produces better response rates than chlorambucil, but is more toxic and has no overall survival benefit. It has now been superseded by the purine analogues for second line treatment.
5. Monoclonal antibodies (alemtuzumab) either as single agent or in combination with purine analogues can produce dramatic responses in relapsed disease but is associated with significant atypical infection risk (e.g. CMV/*Aspergillus*).
6. Transplantation. Autologous SCT and allogeneic BMT have had some success in young patients but remain investigational; the MRC CLL V trial is studying the role of transplant in CLL.

FUTURE PERSPECTIVES

In CML, there is much interest in assessing imatinib in combination with interferon ± ara-C (e.g. the SPIRIT trial). Other areas of interest in CML include the use of non-myeloablative stem cell transplants (NMSCT) – 'mini-allos'. This procedure involves a less aggressive conditioning regimen and relies on the 'graft versus leukaemia' effect of donor lymphocyte infusions (DLI). There is also renewed interest in the role of autografting as imatinib offers the opportunity of in vivo purging, potentially providing a Ph chromosome-negative stem cell harvest.

FURTHER READING

Besa E C. Chronic myelogenous leukaemia. Available at: www.emedicine.com
Chronic lymphocytic leukaemia. Still an incurable disease. Drugs and Therapy Perspectives 2000; 16(10):4–9
Goldman J H 2002 Treatment of chronic myeloid leukaemia. Lessons and challenges. International Journal of Haematology 76(Suppl 2)
Guidelines Working Group of the UK CLL Forum 2004 Management of chronic lymphocytic leukaemia. British Journal of Haematology 125(3):294–317. Available at: www.bcshguidelines.com
Perry M. Chronic lymphocytic leukaemia. Available at: www.emedicine.com
Souhami R L, Tannock I, Hohenberger P, Horiot J-C (eds) 2002 Chronic myeloid leukaemia and chronic lymphocytic leukaemia and other chronic lymphoid leukaemias. In: Oxford textbook of oncology, 2nd edn. OUP, Oxford

Lung cancer

BACKGROUND INFORMATION

Lung cancer is the second commonest cancer in the UK, with 38 410 new cases registered in 2000. It is the third commonest cause of death in the UK, with 33 600 deaths in 2002, representing nearly a quarter of all cancer deaths. Approximately 80% of patients die within a year of diagnosis and only 5.5% survive 5 years (UK figures). This appalling statistic is due not only to the aggressive nature of lung cancer, but also to the fact that it mainly affects older people (median age 72 years), many of whom have co-morbid medical conditions related to smoking. More encouragingly, male death rates from lung cancer in the UK continue to fall. However, female death rates are slowly climbing as the number of young female smokers continues to increase.

Lung cancer is a global health problem. Worldwide, the annual number of new cases is around one million per annum and this is predicted to rise to 25 million by 2025 due to increased consumption of tobacco in the developing world. Lung cancer is a preventable disease that requires a strong government health policy to reduce tobacco consumption. Currently around 14 million people smoke in the UK.

There is no doubt that the main cause of lung cancer is smoking. The risk of smokers developing lung cancer is 10–20 times that of non-smokers and about 85–90% of lung cancer patients are smokers. However, since less than 20% of smokers develop lung cancer in their lifetime, an inherited predisposition may be an important factor. At least 50 carcinogens have been identified in tobacco smoke. Poly-aromatic hydrocarbons (PAHs) and nitrosamines are the most important carcinogens. Other causative agents are radon gas, asbestos, nickel, arsenic, cadmium and chromates. Asbestos exposure increases risk of lung cancer by 5 times in non-smokers but this risk increases to 50–90 times in smokers.

The molecular events that lead to lung cancer involve a multistage process that includes overexpression of growth factors and their receptors, loss of control of the cell cycle and apoptosis, loss of DNA repair mechanisms and development of immune escape mechanisms. New strategies for treatment of lung cancer are being aimed at these processes.

Pathologically, lung tumours are classified by the WHO schema. The main histological types are: squamous cell (30–35%), adenocarcinoma (25–35%), large cell carcinoma (10%) (non-small cell lung cancer) and small cell carcinoma (20–25%). Mixed tumours are relatively common (10–20%). The majority of lung cancers arise in the large and medium-sized bronchi. Distant spread to brain, bone, adrenals and liver is common.

In terms of clinical management, lung cancer is simply classified as non-small cell lung cancer (NSCLC) and small cell lung cancer (SCLC).

At present, screening with CXR and sputum cytology has not been shown to be an effective strategy and further data are awaited regarding spiral CT screening.

PRESENTATION

Unfortunately, most lung cancers are clinically silent for the majority of the time, so most patients present with advanced disease. Incidental finding on CXR in an asymptomatic patient occurs in 5–10% of cases. Cough is the most common symptom, occurring in 45–75%. Dyspnoea, haemoptysis, bronchorrhoea, anorexia and chest pain are also common. Other local symptoms include wheeze, stridor, hoarseness and dysphagia. Bone pain, right upper quadrant pain, headache and neurological symptoms suggest distant metastases (bone, liver, brain). Superior sulcus tumours (Pancoast) may cause Horner's syndrome. Paraneoplastic effects are more common in lung cancer than in any other tumour and their clinical manifestations are mediated by ectopic production of biologically active peptides, cytokines and antibodies. A few examples include hypercalcaemia, SIADH, ectopic ACTH (Cushing's syndrome), Lambert–Eaton myasthenia, clubbing, HPOA (hypertrophic pulmonary osteoarthropathy) and dermatomyositis. Clinical examination may reveal signs of cachexia, clubbing, cervical lymphadenopathy, SVCO, pleural effusion/lung collapse, hepatomegaly and neurological impairment.

DIAGNOSIS AND STAGING

History and examination, CXR and sputum cytology are required. Baseline blood tests should include renal and liver function tests, calcium and LDH levels.

Spiral CT of the chest/abdomen including liver and adrenals is an essential tool for staging purposes and surgical evaluation of the primary tumour. MRI may offer additional information for superior sulcus tumours and for tumours abutting the chest wall/vertebrae. Positron emission tomography (PET) is very useful for assessing mediastinal nodes as well as distant dissemination of disease. PET can indicate presence of metastatic disease in normal-sized mediastinal lymph nodes, which may save the patient from an unnecessary thoracotomy. Unfortunately, PET is only available in a few UK centres at present.

Bronchoscopy may provide a histological diagnosis with biopsies, brushings and washings. In addition, bronchoscopy can offer very important information regarding tumour resectability and assessment of optimum lung resection volume.

Percutaneous CT-guided biopsy may be used for peripheral lesions and achieves a tissue diagnosis of 80–90%.

Histological confirmation and further staging information may be obtained by cervical mediastinoscopy or anterior mediastinotomy (Chamberlain procedure with the incision through second intercostal space). Video-assisted thoracoscopic surgery (VATS) may be used to sample small indeterminate peripheral nodules, lymph nodes and pleural disease. NSCLC patients fit for surgery but with mediastinal nodes >1 cm on CT scan should undergo biopsy by staging mediastinoscopy prior to any definitive procedure. The mediastinoscopy and, if appropriate, definitive lung resection, can be performed either as a staged procedure, or under a single anaesthetic if a suitable frozen section service is available.

Diagnostic imaging of bones and the brain is only required if there is clinical suspicion of metastatic disease of these sites.

The TNM staging system is used (Table 28.1), but is not so useful for small cell cancer as the disease is often occultly disseminated at diagnosis and therefore only weakly correlated with outcome. Therefore, the VALG (Veterans Administration Lung Group) staging system is more widely used for small cell lung cancer (Table 28.2).

MANAGEMENT

The management of NSCLC and SCLC are very different and every effort should be made to obtain a histological diagnosis.

NON-SMALL CELL LUNG CANCER

Surgery offers the greatest chance of cure for patients with NSCLC. Unfortunately only around 20% have operable disease at presentation. Radical radiotherapy may offer a chance of cure to patients who are medically unfit for surgery. Inoperable patients can be palliated with radiotherapy and/or chemotherapy.

TABLE 28.1 Lung cancer

(a) 2002 TNM staging

TX	Positive cytology, but tumour not apparent on bronchoscopy or imaging
T0	No evidence of primary tumour
Tis	Carcinoma in situ
T1	Tumour ≤3 cm, surrounded by lung or visceral pleura
T2	Tumour >3 cm, or any size invading visceral pleura or associated partial atelectasis/obstructive pneumonitis extending to hilum. Tumour must be within a lobar bronchus or ≥2 cm from carina
T3	Tumour of any size invading chest wall, diaphragm, pericardium, mediastinal pleura, main bronchus <2 cm from carina but not involving carina, total atelectasis
T4	Tumour of any size involving mediastinum, heart, great vessels, carina, trachea, oesophagus, vertebra; separate nodules in same lobe, malignant pleural effusion
N1	Ipsilateral peribronchial nodes and/or ipsilateral hilar and intrapulmonary nodes
N2	Ipsilateral mediastinal node(s) and/or subcarinal node(s)
N3	Contralateral mediastinal or hilar node(s), scalene or supraclavicular node(s)
M0	No distant metastases
M1	Distant metastases present. Includes nodule(s) in different lobes

(b) TNM staging and 5-year survival

Stage	TNM group	5-year survival (approx) (%)
Stage IA	T1, N0, M0	60
Stage IB	T2, N0, M0	35–40
Stage IIA	T1, N1, M0	30–35
Stage IIB	T2, N1, M0	25
	T3, N0, M0	20
Stage IIIA	T1–3, N2, M0	10–15
	T3, N1, M0	10
Stage IIIB	T1–3, N3, M0; T4, N0–3, M0	0–7
Stage IV	Any T, any N, M1	0–1

TABLE 28.2 The VALG (Veterans Administration Lung Group) staging system for small cell lung cancer

Limited disease (LD)	Disease confined to one hemithorax, including involvement of ipsi- and/or contralateral hilar, mediastinal or supraclavicular nodes. Patients with ipsilateral pleural effusion are included in this group[a]
Extensive disease (ED)	Includes all patients with disease beyond the confines of limited disease

[a]Some clinicians suggest that limited disease should be defined as disease encompassable within a single tolerable radiation portal.

Surgery in NSCLC

All patients being considered for surgery require thorough preoperative assessment of fitness for surgery. Age, pulmonary function, cardiovascular fitness,

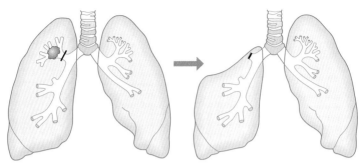

FIGURE 28.1 Right upper lobectomy.

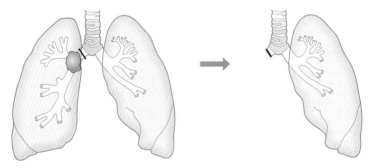

FIGURE 28.2 Right pneumonectomy.

weight loss, performance status, nutrition and multiple other risk factors are taken into account as per the British Thoracic Society (BTS) guidelines, 2001.

Surgical resection of lung cancer may be performed with a wide variety of surgical techniques. Standard major pulmonary resections (i.e. lobectomies and pneumonectomies) require thoracotomy. Lobectomy (Fig. 28.1) is by far the commonest procedure. Mortality from this operation is 2–4%. Pneumonectomy (Fig. 28.2) is the preferred operation when lobectomy would be unable to remove all locoregional disease. Mortality is ~6–8%. Extended radical resections are occasionally warranted in selected patients with involvement of structures such as the chest wall, vertebral body, pericardium, diaphragm and major vessels (e.g. superior vena cava). Bronchoplastic or 'sleeve' resections (Fig. 28.3) may be performed when a tumour would normally lie at the resection margin; e.g. a sleeve lobectomy may be performed instead of a pneumonectomy for cancer of a proximal bronchus with suitable anatomy. These procedures allow sparing of lung parenchyma in patients with impaired pulmonary reserve, but are technically demanding.

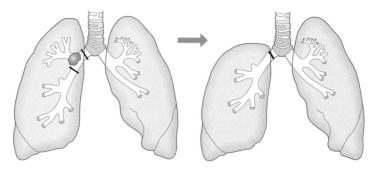

FIGURE 28.3 Sleeve lobectomy of right upper lobe.

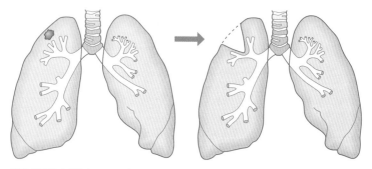

FIGURE 28.4 Wedge resection.

Wedge resection (Fig. 28.4) and segmentectomy (sublobar resections) can be performed for peripheral lesions in patients with poor lung function, although local recurrence rates are higher than with lobectomy. VATS lobectomy is a newer technique, which is rarely performed at present (<2% of UK practice), but is minimally invasive and causes less postoperative pain than open surgery. Early results are comparable to open lobectomy, but further evaluation is required.

The therapeutic value of radical lymph node dissection is unclear, but systematic node dissection is essential for accurate staging of the disease.

Potential surgical candidates are all patients with stage I and II disease. Five-year survival is 40–60% for stage I and 25–35% for stage II. Patients with stage IIIA (T3, N1; or T1–3, N2) and selected IIIB disease (T4N0, T4N1) have poor 5-year survival (5–30%) with surgery alone and so they should be offered surgery in the context of a clinical trial incorporating adjuvant chemotherapy. In general, stage III tumours with mediastinal nodal (N2) involvement and stage IV disease should be considered inoperable.

Radiotherapy in NSCLC

Radiotherapy is commonly used in the management of NSCLC. For medically inoperable stage I and II patients, primary radical conformal RT (55–65 Gy in 4–6 weeks) offers a chance of cure. Two-year survival is around 40% and 5-year survival 10–15%. Selected patients with stage IIIA and IIIB disease may also receive radical RT, which improves local control and survival (~20% 2-year survival). Recently, CHART (continuous hyperfractionated accelerated radiotherapy – 54 Gy in 36 fractions over 12 days) has been shown to improve 2-year survival in patients with all stages of disease (except stage IV) by 9% from 20% to 29% compared to conventional radiotherapy (60 Gy in 30 fractions). The survival benefit has been maintained at 5 years (7% versus 12%). CHART has therefore been suggested as the standard of care, but unfortunately this has resource implications (due to patients needing three treatments a day including weekends), so most centres in the UK still offer 60 Gy in 30 fractions over 6 weeks or 55 Gy in 20 fractions over 4 weeks. The role of concurrent chemoradiotherapy remains to be defined in the UK, but this has become the standard of care for locally advanced disease in the USA.

The role of postoperative radiotherapy (PORT) is controversial. A recent large meta-analysis (PORT Meta-analysis Trialists Group) showed that radiotherapy was detrimental in terms of overall survival in patients with completely resected early stage disease (T1–3, N0), but in N2 disease there was reduced locoregional recurrence and a strong trend to improved survival. (This meta-analysis has been much criticised because the trials included used older radiotherapy techniques and not the gold standard of CT-planned conformal RT with mega-voltage equipment.) Currently, postoperative RT is not offered following complete resection, but it may be given to patients with N2 disease and/or positive resection margins.

The majority of radiotherapy is given with palliative intent. Approximately 70% of patients obtain symptomatic benefit. In locally advanced disease higher palliative doses (39 Gy in 13 fractions) modestly improve survival in good performance status patients. In those with a poor prognosis and chest symptoms, a single 10 Gy fraction, or 17 Gy in two fractions 1 week apart, can improve symptoms such as dyspnoea, haemoptysis, chest pain and cough.

Endobronchial brachytherapy (which involves bronchoscopic insertion of ^{192}Ir bronchial catheters to deliver 10–15 Gy in less than 20 minutes) can be very effective for relieving bronchial obstruction in patients already treated with external beam RT.

Chemotherapy in NSCLC

Despite the considerable use of chemotherapy in the management of NSCLC, its value in improving survival is still unclear. A recent meta-analysis of over 9000 patients in 52 trials assessed the value of chemotherapy within four primary treatment groups: surgery, surgery plus radiotherapy, radical radiotherapy and supportive care. It showed that modern cisplatin-based chemotherapy might improve absolute survival by about 5% in the first three groups and prolong median survival in the supportive care group by 2 months.

Evidence is not currently strong enough to recommend the routine use of neoadjuvant (preoperative) or adjuvant (postoperative) chemotherapy. However, there is now good evidence from a very large international trial (International Adjuvant Lung Trial – IALT) that adjuvant chemotherapy offers an absolute 5-year survival benefit of 4–5% and it may be an option for selected patients with good performance status.

Patients receiving concurrent chemoradiotherapy have not shown a consistent increase in survival but have shown an increase in morbidity and further trials are ongoing.

In advanced (stage IV) NSCLC, combination chemotherapy with platinum-based regimens compared to best supportive care improves survival at 1 year by 10% with an increase in median survival of 2 months. Symptomatic benefit is also seen, especially in patients with better performance status. Previously, commonly used regimens included MIC (mitomycin C, ifosfamide, cisplatin), MVP (mitomycin C, vinblastine, cisplatin). These are now being superseded by 'doublets' such as (i) vinorelbine, cisplatin – VP, (ii) gemcitabine and carboplatin/cisplatin, (iii) paclitaxel and carboplatin, or (iv) docetaxel and cisplatin. These combinations produce 1-year survival rates of 35–40% and tend to be better tolerated than MIC or MVP.

The new epidermal growth factor receptor tyrosine kinase inhibitor (EGFR-TKI), gefitinib (Iressa), has recently shown response rates of ~20% in patients pretreated with chemotherapy. It is currently unlicensed in the UK, but is being offered to some patients on a compassionate basis.

Superior sulcus (Pancoast) tumours

Around 2–4% of NSCLC patients have a Pancoast tumour, which arises in the apex of the lung and involves the structures of the apical chest wall. This may result in the Pancoast syndrome if the nerve roots of C-8, T-1, T-2 and lower brachial plexus, cervical sympathetic chain and stellate ganglion are involved. Spinal cord compression may result from invasion of the vertebral body.

Unfortunately, the optimum management of these tumours is unknown due to their rarity. Traditionally, treatment by 2 weeks of RT followed by radical surgery (Paulson regime) produces 5-year survival of up to 30% in patients with node-negative and completely resectable disease. Radical treatment with RT and surgery is possible for selected patients with T3–4, N0–1 disease. Patients with positive mediastinal nodes (N2) should be considered inoperable due to very poor survival after resection. Improved resectability rates and overall survival have recently been reported with neoadjuvant concurrent chemoradiation followed by surgery.

High dose palliative radiotherapy should be offered to inoperable patients to gain local control in the hope of avoiding severe symptomatic brachial plexus or spinal cord involvement.

SMALL CELL LUNG CANCER

SCLC is highly chemosensitive and therefore chemotherapy forms the mainstay of treatment for SCLC. Prior to the use of effective chemotherapy, the median survival for untreated patients with limited disease (LD) was 12 weeks and with extensive disease (ED) only 6 weeks. With current therapy, median survival is 12–15 months for LD and 8–10 months with ED. Around 5–10% of patients achieve long-term survival and almost all of these patients have LD at presentation. Unfortunately only 30% present with LD.

Patients can be stratified into prognostic groups using scoring systems based on various prognostic factors. This helps in selecting patients for the most appropriate treatment strategy. The Manchester system is commonly used and based on the following prognostic factors: LDH, stage, sodium, performance status and alkaline phosphatase (Table 28.3). 'Good' prognosis patients usually receive combination chemotherapy with consolidation/concurrent radiotherapy to the chest and prophylactic cranial irradiation (PCI). 'Poor' prognosis patients usually receive less aggressive chemotherapy regimens, palliative RT or supportive care only.

Surgery is rarely an option, as most patients have disseminated disease at presentation.

Chemotherapy in SCLC

Combination chemotherapy gives response rates of 85–95% (CR 50%) in limited disease and 65–85% (CR 25%) in extensive disease. Frequently used regimens in 'good' prognosis patients are PE (cisplatin, etoposide), CAV (cyclophosphamide, doxorubicin, vincristine), ACE (doxorubicin, cyclo-phosphamide, etoposide) and ICE (ifosfamide, carboplatin, etoposide). Four to six cycles of treatment are normally given and some of these regimens can be alternated, e.g. CAV/EP. In limited disease, 4–6 cycles of PE is generally considered the standard of care. High dose chemotherapy with autologous bone marrow transplantation has not been promising in phase I/II trials

---

TABLE 28.3 Manchester prognostic scoring system for small cell lung cancer

LDH: >normal – 1 point
Stage: extensive disease – 1 point
Sodium: less than normal – 1 point
WHO performance status: 2 or worse – 1 point
Alkaline phosphatase: >1.5 times normal – 1 point

Score	Prognosis	2-year survival (%)
0–1	Good	15
2–3	Intermediate	8
4–5	Poor (6-month survival 40%)	2

so far. Patients should be offered entry into clinical trials assessing new therapies where possible. Very encouraging results from phase III trials using the combination of cisplatin and irinotecan have recently been reported in Japan.

Poor prognosis and elderly patients cannot tolerate the more intensive regimens, but may respond well (up to 60–70% response rates) to less toxic schedules such as low dose CAV, carboplatin and etoposide, VE (vindesine and etoposide) or single agent carboplatin. Prophylactic antibiotics are often given to these patients due to their increased risk of sepsis.

Radiotherapy in SCLC

SCLC is a radiosensitive disease. Thoracic consolidation radiotherapy (e.g. 40–50 Gy in 3–5 weeks) improves local control and survival in patients with LD who achieve a complete response to chemotherapy (3-year survival is increased from 10% to 15% in LD). There is now compelling evidence that radiotherapy given concurrently with chemotherapy improves locoregional control and survival, and this is now standard therapy in the USA and some UK centres for good prognosis patients with limited stage disease. The optimum dosing and scheduling is currently unknown and subject to ongoing clinical trials.

Prophylactic cranial irradiation (PCI) (e.g. 30 Gy in 10 fractions to the whole brain) in complete responders following chemotherapy reduces the incidence of brain metastases from 58.6% to 33.3% at 3 years and increases 3-year survival from 15% to 21%. The main side effect of PCI is somnolence syndrome, which occurs a few weeks after treatment but is usually self-limiting. It is characterised by excessive tiredness, anorexia and poor concentration.

Palliative radiotherapy may be offered to patients unfit for chemotherapy at presentation or to patients with relapsed disease not suitable for more chemotherapy.

Surgery in SCLC

Some studies report long-term survival following surgery for highly selected patients with very early disease, but there are no randomised studies that show an advantage over chemotherapy and radiotherapy. Surgery is therefore not routinely recommended. A few patients are diagnosed with SCLC as a consequence of excision biopsy of a solitary peripheral lung lesion and these patients should be referred on for adjuvant chemotherapy (e.g. three cycles of PE).

Relapsed SCLC

For patients who initially had a CR or PR lasting for more than 3 months, 25–75% will respond to further chemotherapy (same or different regimen) but the duration of response is much shorter (median 2–4 months). The decision to offer further treatment to those who relapse quickly (<3 months – refractory), or do not respond at all, is difficult and these patients may be offered entry into clinical trials. Palliative radiotherapy may be an option if not already given.

FUTURE PERSPECTIVES IN NSCLC AND SCLC

NSCLC

The role of chemotherapy is still under investigation in all stages of disease, although further improvements are likely to be minimal. The optimum sequencing of chemotherapy with surgery and radiotherapy remains to be determined. Newer chemotherapy agents (taxanes, gemcitabine, vinorelbine and irinotecan) and biological therapies (trastuzumab (Herceptin), gefitinib (Iressa), gene therapy, tumour vaccines, and angiogenesis inhibition (thalidomide)) continue to be evaluated.

Radiotherapy research is focused on concurrent chemoradiotherapy, CHART/hyperfractionation, radiosensitisers (tirapazamine), the role of PCI, and dose escalation with 3D conformal techniques.

The role of PET scanning continues to be evaluated with potential benefits in diagnosis, staging, assessment of response to treatment and radiotherapy planning.

SCLC

The optimum scheduling, dosing and sequencing of chemoradiation is a key question in the management of SCLC and this is the focus of several trials. New combination chemotherapy regimens with agents such as taxanes, irinotecan, gemcitabine, vinorelbine and thalidomide are being evaluated. High dose chemotherapy with stem cell transplantation remains investigational.

PROBLEMS IN ADVANCED DISEASE

1. Breathlessness. Numerous causes including airway obstruction by tumour (extrinsic/intrinsic), lung infiltration, lymphangitis, pleural/pericardial effusions, atelectasis/lobar collapse, infection, pulmonary embolism, anaemia, SVCO, radiation pneumonitis, generalised weakness of respiratory muscles (cachexia, myasthenia), anxiety, chest pain and co-morbid medical condition (e.g. chronic obstructive pulmonary disease, left ventricular failure). Treatment should include simple measures such

as relaxation techniques, chest physiotherapy, facial cooling (fans) and oxygen therapy. Bronchodilators (inhalers or nebulisers) are helpful in the presence of reversible airflow obstruction. Medical conditions should be treated appropriately including antibiotics for chest infections. Pleural effusions may be drained and pleurodesed (see Ch. 55 on malignant pleural effusions). For patients with tumours obstructing large airways, palliative EBRT (17 Gy in two fractions, 10 Gy single fraction) may provide excellent symptom relief. Endobronchial brachytherapy is also effective. Other useful endobronchial treatments include Nd:YAG laser treatment, electrocautery, cryotherapy, stent placement and photodynamic therapy (PDT). Corticosteroids (e.g. prednisolone 40–60 mg o.d.) are helpful if there is bronchial inflammation, oedema, reversible small airway airflow obstruction, lymphangitis or radiation pneumonitis (usually occurs 6–12 weeks following RT and responds to 3–4 weeks of high dose steroids which should then be tailed off). Opioids, benzodiazepines and nebulised local anaesthetics can decrease the sensation of breathlessness and reduce anxiety (e.g. morphine 5–10 mg 4-hourly p.o., s.c., nebulised), lorazepam 0.5–2 mg 6-hourly sublingually, 2% lidocaine (lignocaine) 5 ml nebulised 4-hourly). In the terminal situation, IV/IM/s.c. midazolam 2.5–5 mg (or 20–60 mg via 24-hour s.c. syringe driver) and diamorphine 5 mg (or 20–30 mg via 24-hour s.c. syringe driver) can be used.

2. Cough. This is a very common and distressing symptom in lung cancer, which can lead to insomnia, exhaustion, vomiting, rib fracture and syncope. It may be caused by the local effect of the tumour, infection, radiation/chemotherapy-induced pneumonitis, COPD, asthma and gastro-oesophageal reflux. The underlying cause should be addressed first. Further measures include the use of antitussive linctuses, e.g. morphine (5–10 mg 4-hourly), codeine (30 mg 6–8-hourly), methadone (1–2 mg nocte), and nebulised local anaesthetics, e.g. 2% lidocaine 5 ml 4-hourly, 0.5% bupivacaine 5 ml 4-hourly. Nebulised saline/steam inhalations and physiotherapy may loosen tenacious secretions. Steroids may also be helpful if there is an inflammatory cause of the cough.

3. Haemoptysis. Most haemoptysis in lung cancer is scanty and settles spontaneously. Persistent or massive haemoptysis (arbitrarily defined as >500 ml per 24 hours or life-threatening intrabronchial bleeding) is quite rare. Minor bleeding may settle with tranexamic acid 1–1.5 g t.d.s. Palliative radiotherapy is also effective. Other measures include nebulised adrenaline (epinephrine; 1 mg/1 ml) diluted in 5 ml of saline, and endobronchial treatment (brachytherapy, laser, cryotherapy, electrocautery), although careful patient selection is required. Massive fatal haemoptysis requires heavy sedation with IV/IM opioids (e.g. diamorphine 5–10 mg) and benzodiazepines (e.g. midazolam 2–5 mg) with repeated 5 mg increments after 2 minutes.

4. Pain. Direct tumour invasion is the commonest cause of pain, e.g. bone destruction, nerve compression/infiltration, pleural/mediastinal

invasion. Non-specific vague chest pain is often visceral and unrelated to local invasion. Post-thoracotomy pain is common and may persist for many years following surgery. Radiotherapy can also cause chest pains. Obvious treatable causes should be tackled, e.g. RT to bone metastases. Tricyclic antidepressants and anticonvulsants may be used for neuropathic pain. Early referral to a pain specialist should be considered for particularly refractory cases. Psychological assessment and treatment may also be of benefit.

5. Stridor. This is due to narrowing of the glottis, trachea or major bronchi. Initial treatment is with oxygen (or heliox – 21% oxygen in helium), high dose steroids (dexamethasone 16 mg) and nebulised adrenaline (10 ml of 1 : 10 000 up to 4-hourly). In fitter patients with external compression, endotracheal/endobronchial stenting may be helpful. Laser therapy may be considered for intraluminal tumour. EBRT may be helpful if not pretreated or outside previous radiation portal. Chemotherapy may benefit patients with untreated SCLC. Patients with particularly poor prognoses should be heavily sedated and kept comfortable.

6. Dysphagia. Usually caused by extrinsic compression by tumour mass. Therapeutic options include using steroids, stenting (especially if there is an oesophagotracheal fistula) and palliative RT. Occasionally PEG feeding is required. Dysphagia is also caused by oral thrush (treat with antifungal, e.g. nystatin or fluconazole) and is a side effect of mediastinal radiotherapy (treat with mucaine liquid, 10 ml t.d.s. p.o.).

7. Hoarseness. Usually caused by left recurrent laryngeal nerve palsy due to compression or invasion by tumour. A Teflon injection performed by an ENT surgeon can improve voice quality and volume.

8. SVCO (see Ch. 61 on SVCO).

9. Lymphangitic carcinomatosis (see also Ch. 59 on pulmonary metastases). Caused by spread of tumour from mediastinal nodes peripherally along lymphatics. Usually due to adenocarcinoma. Results in severe breathlessness and hypoxaemia. Symptomatic relief anecdotal with oxygen, steroids, diuretics and nebulised salbutamol.

10. Malignant pleural effusion (see also Ch. 55 on malignant pleural effusions). In NSCLC, effusions often reaccumulate after aspiration, and so early pleurodesis should be performed, preferably with the surgical VATS talc technique, which is 90% effective. An intercostal drain may be inserted, followed by talc or bleomycin pleurodesis if the surgical expertise is not easily available. In previously untreated SCLC, pleural effusions usually resolve if chemotherapy is successful.

11. Bone metastases (see Ch. 48 on bone metastases). If painful, may be treated by EBRT (single 8 Gy fractions) to good effect.

12. Brain metastases (see Ch. 49 on brain metastases). In patients with NSCLC, 5-year survival rates of 10% have been reported for patients with a solitary brain metastasis and an operable primary tumour (T1–2, N0–1). A radical approach with neurosurgery, postoperative whole brain

radiotherapy (WBRT) and resection of the primary tumour should be considered in these cases. In SCLC, chemotherapy followed by WBRT or WBRT alone are the main options.

13. Spinal cord compression (see chapter on spinal cord compression). Oncological emergency that requires urgent radiotherapy (e.g. 20 Gy in five fractions). Surgical decompression is not usually indicated, as most patients with stage IV lung cancer are unwell and have a very poor prognosis.

14. Paraneoplastic syndromes (see also Ch. 57 on paraneoplastic syndromes). Seen in 10–20% of lung cancer patients. The course of the paraneoplastic syndrome usually follows the clinical course of the underlying lung cancer. Hypercalcaemia is the commonest syndrome and can be treated with IV hydration and pamidronate. SIADH may be treated with fluid restriction and demeclocycline. Ectopic ACTH (Cushing's syndrome) may be suppressed by ketoconazole (300–400 mg b.d.). Lambert–Eaton myasthenic syndrome may be treated by 3,4 diamino-pyridine. HPOA (hypertrophic pulmonary osteoarthropathy) is a painful condition usually affecting ankles, wrists and knees for which there is no effective treatment other than analgesics and treating the primary tumour.

FURTHER READING

BTS 2001 Guidelines on the selection of patients with lung cancer for surgery. Thorax 56:89–108

COIN Guidelines on the non-surgical management of lung cancer. February 1999. Available via www.rcr.ac.uk

Hansen H (ed) 2000 Textbook of lung cancer. Martin Dunitz, London

START European oncology guidelines. SCLC and NSCLC. Available at: www.startoncology.net

CHAPTER 29

Malignant mesothelioma

BACKGROUND INFORMATION

Over the next 20 years, the UK incidence of mesothelioma is expected to increase from the present total of 1300 to more than 3000 cases per year. Half of all cases occur in those aged 70 and over and 80% occur in men. A history of occupational exposure to asbestos can be obtained in about 90% of cases. All types of asbestos may cause mesothelioma, but crocidolite (blue) and amosite (brown) asbestos are the most potent. The average latent period between exposure and disease is very long (30–40 years). The fact that peak imports of asbestos into the UK occurred in the late 1970s probably explains the current increasing incidence.

Pathologically, the main histological types are epithelioid, sarcomatoid and biphasic (mixed epithelioid and sarcomatoid). Epithelioid is the most common type and has a more favourable prognosis. However, it is easily confused with adenocarcinoma and numerous immunohistochemical stains are required to aid diagnosis.

The disease tends to spread by local extension rather than haematogenous spread and encasement of an entire hemithorax is common. Primary involvement of the peritoneum is also seen but this is rare.

Overall prognosis is poor with median survival of 8–14 months. There are now over 1800 deaths per year in the UK. Poor prognostic features are older age, extensive disease and sarcomatoid or biphasic histology. Patients with epithelioid histology have a better than average outlook and a few may enjoy longer-term survival.

PRESENTATION

Most patients present with chest pain or dyspnoea. The pain often has neuropathic elements due to involvement of nerves (e.g. brachial plexus, intercostal nerves). Dyspnoea in early stage disease may be due to a pleural effusion, but in later stages may be due to restrictive pleural thickening. Less common presenting features include a chest wall mass, weight loss, abdominal pain, ascites and profuse sweating.

Clinical examination may reveal clubbing, and signs consistent with pleural thickening/effusions. Cervical lymphadenopathy, haemoptysis and symptoms relating to metastatic disease are unusual presenting features since the disease initially progresses locally. Occasionally the diagnosis is suspected following a routine CXR, which may show pleural thickening, effusions, a mass or pleural plaques (associated with asbestosis).

DIAGNOSIS

Investigations should include: history (including a detailed occupational history) and examination; baseline FBC, renal and liver function tests; CXR; CT of the chest, which may include CT-guided biopsy. MRI may offer further information with tumours that are invading the chest wall, diaphragm, pericardium and spine.

TABLE 29.1 IMIG staging of mesothelioma	
Primary (T)	
T1a	Tumour limited to ipsilateral pleura (may include mediastinal and diaphragmatic pleura)
T1b	As above, but also scattered foci of tumour involving visceral pleura
T2	Tumour involves ipsilateral pleura and at least one of: extension into diaphragmatic muscle/pulmonary parenchyma, or confluent visceral pleural tumour
T3	Tumour involves ipsilateral pleura and at least one of: extension into endothoracic fascia, mediastinal fat, soft tissue of chest wall, pericardium
T4	Tumour involves ipsilateral pleura and at least one of: diffuse multifocal mass tumour in chest wall, rib/vertebral destruction, peritoneal extension, contralateral disease, mediastinal organ involvement
Lymph nodes (N)	
N1	Ipsilateral bronchopulmonary or hilar nodes
N2	Subcarinal or ipsilateral mediastinal nodes
N3	Contralateral mediastinal, ipsi/contralateral supraclavicular nodes
Staging	
Stage Ia	T1a, N0, M0
Stage Ib	T1b, N0, M0
Stage II	T2, N0, M0
Stage III	T1–3, N1–2; T3, N0
Stage IV	T4, any N; any T, N3; any T, any N, M1

Thoracoscopic biopsy is the best way to obtain a histological diagnosis (90% success rate) and also affords the opportunity to perform an effective pleurodesis. Aspiration cytology of pleural effusions has only 32% specificity and blind pleural biopsy with an Abrams needle is diagnostic in less than 50% of cases.

The staging was traditionally based on the Buchart system, but a more detailed system based on the TNM classification has recently been proposed by the International Mesothelioma Interest Group (IMIG) (Table 29.1).

MANAGEMENT

Standard treatment for all but localised mesothelioma is generally not curative.

SURGERY

It is estimated that only 1–5% of all patients with mesothelioma are suitable for surgery. The role of radical surgery even in early stage disease is controversial as there are no randomised controlled trials. Extrapleural pneumonectomy (EPP) in carefully selected early stage disease may improve recurrence-free survival, but its impact on overall survival is unknown. (Operative mortality is 6–30%.) Five-year survival of ~10–15% has been reported following EPP. Pleurectomy and decortication can provide palliative relief of symptomatic effusions, discomfort caused by tumour burden and pain caused by invasive tumour.

More recently, multimodality therapy with radical surgery followed by postoperative radiotherapy and chemotherapy has shown some promising results (Sugarbaker et al, 1998), but overall very few patients are eligible for this approach.

RADIOTHERAPY

There is no evidence to support the use of radical radiotherapy as a primary single modality treatment. The addition of postoperative RT has not demonstrated a survival advantage. Palliative radiotherapy provides pain relief in at least 50% of patients. Prophylactic RT (21 Gy in three fractions) should be given within one month of any invasive procedures as it reduces the risk of seeding and chest wall implantation from 40% to 0%.

CHEMOTHERAPY

There are no published randomised trials of chemotherapy showing improvement of survival or quality of life compared with best supportive care. The best single agent chemotherapies have response rates of 10–20% (doxorubicin, epirubicin, platinum, mitomycin, ifosfamide). Combination chemotherapy has not been shown to be consistently better than single agents.

A large study of combination chemotherapy versus single agent chemotherapy versus best supportive care is currently under way (MESO 1). A recent North American phase III trial has shown a significant survival advantage for the combination therapy of pemetrexed and cisplatin versus cisplatin alone (median survival 12 months versus 9 months). There was also greater symptom relief and improvement in lung function in the pemetrexed arm of the study.

FUTURE PERSPECTIVES

Newer chemotherapy agents such as capecitabine, gemcitabine, raltitrexed and oxaliplatin, and anti-angiogenesis agents such as thalidomide and bevacizumab are being evaluated. The role of pemetrexed will need to be defined. Gene therapy and immunotherapy have no established role at present.

PROBLEMS IN ADVANCED DISEASE

1. Pain. Chest pain due to pleural disease is very common. Early referral to pain specialists is required for poorly controlled pain, which may respond to TENS machines, intervertebral/paravertebral nerve blocks, interpleural, epidural or intrathecal analgesia. Occasionally a percutaneous cervical cordotomy is performed. Radiotherapy may be useful for localised pain secondary to chest wall invasion (e.g. 20 Gy in five fractions).
2. Breathlessness (see Ch. 28 on lung cancer).
3. Cough (see Ch. 28 on lung cancer).
4. Anorexia, fever, weight loss and fatigue. Common and difficult to treat. May respond to steroids (e.g. dexamethasone 2–4 mg o.d.) and megestrol acetate. Dietary advice.

REFERENCES AND FURTHER READING

British Thoracic Society Standards of Care Committee 2001 Statement on malignant mesothelioma in the UK (BTS Statement). Thorax 56:250–265
Parker C, Neville E 2003 Management of malignant mesothelioma. Thorax 58:809–813
Sugarbaker D J, Norberto J J 1998 Multimodality management of malignant pleural mesothelioma. Chest 113:61S–65
Treasure T, Waller D, Swift S, Peto J 2004 Radical surgery for mesothelioma. BMJ 328:237–238
Van Ruth S, Baas P, Zoetmulder N 2003 Surgical treatment of malignant pleural mesothelioma. Chest 123(2):551–561

CHAPTER 30

Melanoma

BACKGROUND INFORMATION

Malignant melanoma accounts for only 5% of all skin cancers, but causes three-quarters of all skin cancer deaths. In 2002, there were 1640 deaths from melanoma in the UK compared to less than 400 for non-melanoma skin cancer. It occurs most frequently in patients between 40 and 70 years. The incidence of melanoma has been increasing rapidly worldwide in the white population over the last several decades. There was a 50% increase in the number of new cases in England and Wales between 1991 and 2000 and the current incidence is now approximately 8/100 000 per year with nearly 7000 new cases per year. The highest rates are seen in Australia and New Zealand where the incidence rate reaches 42/100 000 per year. Fortunately death rates seem to be stabilising due to earlier detection and removal of lesions.

The major risk factors for melanoma are: white race (especially blue eyes, fair/red hair, light complexion, freckling), history of sunburn, family history of melanoma and dysplastic naevi, history of prior melanoma, presence of dysplastic naevi, immunosuppression and higher socioeconomic status. Exposure to ultraviolet B radiation is a major exogenous cause. Preventative measures such as reducing sun exposure and using sun screens should be encouraged. Familial melanoma accounts for 5–10% of cases and a genetic abnormality has been located in the tumour suppressor gene p21 on chromosome 9.

Melanoma is a malignant tumour of melanocytes that are derived from neural crest tissue. Most melanomas arise in the skin but some can occur in extradermal sites where neural crest tissue has migrated. Examples include mucosal surfaces and the uveal tract of the eye. Most melanomas arise in a previously normal area of skin in a sun-exposed area, but around one-third develop in a pre-existing lesion (usually a dysplastic naevus, congenital naevus or lentigo maligna). Worrying signs in a lesion are increasing size, change in colour/pigmentation, irregularity and elevation, itching, presence of satellite lesions, bleeding and ulceration. In women, most lesions are located in the extremities, whereas in men most are found in the trunk and head and neck regions. In blacks and Asians, melanomas usually occur on the palms and soles (acral areas) and mucosal sites. Malignant melanoma occasionally spontaneously regresses, but this occurs in less than 1% of cases.

Early melanomas are highly curable, but metastatic disease has a dismal prognosis and is highly resistant to treatment. Public awareness campaigns to increase knowledge of the symptoms and signs of skin melanomas are an important way to increase the number of melanomas diagnosed at an earlier, more treatable stage.

PRESENTATION

There are four main types of melanoma:

1. Superficial spreading malignant melanoma is the commonest type (70%) and usually has a prolonged period of superficial (radial) growth (1–7 years). The prognosis is usually good at this stage. However, it may enter a vertical growth phase and invade deeply, increasing metastatic potential.
2. Nodular melanomas (15%) usually arise from normal skin. They appear as a nodule or papule in the vertical growth phase. They have a rapid onset developing over months. Unlike other melanoma types, most have uni-form borders and colour. Around 5% are amelanotic. They have a worse prognosis due to vertical growth pattern and invasion.
3. Acral lentiginous melanomas (5–10%) arise on the palms, soles and beneath the nail plate (subungual). They usually have a radial growth pat-tern over long periods and often go undiagnosed because of their location. Vertical growth may be seen as a papule or nodule and ulceration may occur. Delays in diagnosis are common.
4. Lentigo maligna melanoma (5–15%). Usually occurs on sun-exposed skin in elderly patients, especially the head and neck regions. The precursor lesion is lentigo maligna, but few (<5%) of these lesions become cancerous.

DIAGNOSIS AND STAGING

Full history and clinical examination are required, including complete skin examination with special attention to tumour satellites (tumour nests or nodules <2 cm from the primary tumour), in-transit metastases (skin/subcutaneous metastases >2 cm from primary tumour but not beyond regional lymph nodes), regional lymph node groups and distant metastases. Skin surface microscopy (dermoscopy) improves diagnostic accuracy. CXR, ultrasound of the abdomen or CT of the chest/abdomen, full blood count, LDH, liver and renal function tests are recommended for patients with stage IIB disease and above.

The ABCDE concept is useful for early recognition and is widely used:

A: Asymmetry
B: Border irregularity
C: Colour change
D: Diameter >6 mm
E: Enlargement or Elevation.

Total full-thickness excisional biopsy is the standard option as this allows accurate measurement of tumour depth (microstaging), which is prognostically important. Incisional biopsies (full-thickness) are sometimes used when excisional biopsy is not possible (e.g. with large tumours or when excision would be mutilating).

Pathological staging (microstaging) uses two systems: Breslow and Clark's. The Breslow system involves accurate measurement of the actual tumour thickness and is more reliable prognostically than Clark's level, which measures the depth of infiltration into the skin. Both of these systems have been included in the new TNM 2002 staging system (Tables 30.1, 30.2 and 30.3).

TABLE 30.1 Clark's levels of invasion

Level I	Melanoma in situ
Level II	Melanoma in the papillary dermis
Level III	Melanoma filling the papillary dermis
Level IV	Melanoma in the reticular dermis
Level V	Melanoma in the subcutis

TABLE 30.2 TNM 2002 melanoma staging

T1a	Breslow ≤1 mm thick, Clark's level II or III, no ulceration
T1b	Breslow ≤1 mm thick, Clark's level IV or V, or ulceration
T2a	Breslow >1 mm ≤2 mm thick, no ulceration
T2b	Breslow >1 mm ≤2 mm thick, ulceration
T3a	Breslow >2 mm ≤4 mm thick, no ulceration
T3b	Breslow >2 mm ≤4 mm thick, ulceration
T4a	Breslow >4 mm thick, no ulceration
T4b	Breslow >4 mm thick, ulceration
N1	One node
N1a	Microscopic
N1b	Macroscopic
N2	2–3 nodes or satellites/in-transit lesions without nodes
N2a	2–3 nodes microscopic
N2b	2–3 nodes macroscopic
N2c	Satellites or in-transit without nodes
N3	≥4 nodes; matted; satellites or in-transit with nodes
M1a	Distant skin, subcutaneous, or lymph node metastases with normal LDH
M1b	Lung metastases with normal LDH
M1c	LDH elevated and/or non-pulmonary visceral metastases

TABLE 30.3 UICC TNM 2002 staging and 10-year survival

Stage	TNM	10-year survival (%)
Stage IA	T1a, N0, M0	88
Stage IB	T1b/2a, N0, M0	79–83
Stage IIA	T2b/T3a, N0, M0	64
Stage IIB	T3b/4a, N0, M0	51–54
Stage IIC	T4b, N0, M0	32
Stage IIIA	Any Ta, N1a/N2a, M0	57–63
Stage IIIB	Any Tb, N1a/N2a, M0	36–48
Stage IIIC	Any Tb, N1b/N2b, M0	15–25
	Any T, N3, M0	18.5
Stage IV	Any T, any N, M1a	16
	Any T, any N, M1b	2.5
	Any T, any N, M1c	6.0

MANAGEMENT

TREATMENT FOR LOCALISED DISEASE

Surgery is the mainstay of treatment for localised primary melanoma. Wide excision with a margin of 1 cm is required for tumours <1 mm thick. For lesions 1–2 mm thick, 2 cm margins may be more appropriate, although there is no survival benefit over 1 cm margins. For lesions more than 2 mm thick, a 2 cm wide excision margin is mandatory. For lesions on the fingers, toes or ears, surgical compromise on the width of these margins may be required for preservation of function. Larger lesions may require skin grafting. Elective regional lymph node dissection (ERLND) or irradiation is not recommended as no survival benefit has clearly been shown. Recently, the use of sentinel node biopsy techniques has revealed the presence of occult micrometastases in 20% of melanomas thicker than 1 mm. This technique is still investigational, but has been shown to have prognostic importance and is a promising step towards the clinical detection and early treatment of occult lymph node metastases. There is no established role for adjuvant immunotherapy and it therefore remains investigational at present. Ten-year survival in this group is ~70% overall.

LOCOREGIONAL DISEASE

Surgical excision of the primary site with full therapeutic lymph node dissection is the standard treatment. If the primary tumour is very close to the lymph node station then the lymph node dissection should include (en-bloc) the biopsy scar of the primary melanoma. Post-surgical adjuvant therapy with chemotherapy and immunotherapy remains investigational because although there is improvement in disease-free survival, there is no clearly proven overall survival benefit. Postoperative radiotherapy may be considered for residual disease, extranodal spread or head and neck melanoma, which is thought to be a separate entity with different biological behaviour. Isolated regional perfusion with chemo-immunotherapy (e.g. melphalan and tumour necrosis factor (TNF)) may be considered for patients with in-transit metastases or inoperable primary tumours. Ten-year survival in patients with locoregional disease is ~30% overall.

DISTANT METASTATIC DISEASE

Patients with distant metastases have an extremely poor outlook with a median survival of 2 to 6 months, as melanoma is notoriously resistant to conventional therapies. Radiotherapy can be used to palliate bone pain, brain metastases, skin lesions and bleeding/ulcerated lesions. Systemic chemotherapy has very little activity, with the most effective drugs having single agent response rates of 10–20% (e.g. DTIC (dacarbazine), nitrosoureas). Responses are usually short-lived, ranging from 3 to 6 months. Combination chemotherapy is slightly better in terms of response rate, but there is no improvement in median survival over single agents. Immunotherapy with interferon alpha has response rates of 12–18% and interleukin-2 (IL-2) 15–25%, but toxicity is often a problem. Combinations of chemotherapy and immunotherapy may achieve higher responses but no survival improvements have been demonstrated over single agent dacarbazine.

Potentially curative surgical resection of isolated visceral metastases of the brain, liver or lung may be possible for highly selected patients with good performance status.

FUTURE PERSPECTIVES

Much current research has focused on the role of lymph node mapping and sentinel lymph node biopsy, which may aid early detection and treatment of nodal disease. The role of adjuvant therapy with high dose interferon alpha is still under investigation. Chemo-immunotherapy for advanced disease is an active area of research and some promising results have been seen with the combination of cisplatin, vinblastine, temozolomide (CVT) with IL-2 and interferon alpha. Vaccine therapies have demonstrated some responses in advanced disease and there is potential for use in the adjuvant setting. Gene therapy and anti-angiogenesis agents are also being studied.

PROBLEMS IN ADVANCED DISEASE

1. Brain metastases (see Ch. 49 on brain metastases). Poor prognosis with median survival of 2–5 months. Palliation of multiple metastases can be

achieved with whole brain radiotherapy. Surgical resection of solitary lesions may be offered with postoperative radiotherapy.

2. Bone metastases and spinal cord compression (see Chs 48 and 60 on bone metastases and spinal cord compression, respectively). Good palliation can be achieved with RT.

3. Lymph node metastases. Can cause significant pain, nerve compression and lymphoedema. Ulceration, bleeding and infection may also occur. If possible, nodes should be surgically resected, but inoperable symptomatic nodes can still be treated with palliative radiotherapy, e.g. 20 Gy in five fractions.

4. Skin metastases. May become painful, ulcerated and start bleeding. Palliative radiotherapy may be very helpful, e.g. single 8–10 Gy fraction, which may be repeated if necessary.

5. Liver and lung metastases (see Chs 51 and 59 on liver and pulmonary metastases, respectively). Removal of solitary lesions may be curative.

FURTHER READING

Hall P N, Javaid M 1998 Cutaneous melanoma: diagnosis and at risk patients. Hospital Medicine 59(11):866–871

START oncology group. Melanoma. Available at: www.startoncology.net

CHAPTER 31

Multiple myeloma

BACKGROUND INFORMATION

Multiple myeloma (MM) is a malignant disease of plasma cells. The annual UK incidence is 5–6 cases per 100 000 population, with 3730 new cases registered in 2000. There are 10 000–15 000 patients with the condition in the UK at any one time. The median age at diagnosis is 60–65 years with less than 2% of cases occurring in patients under 40 years of age. It is more common in males (M : F 1.5 : 1), and Afro-Caribbean ethnic groups.

MM is characterised by the production of monoclonal immunoglobulin (Ig) detectable in the serum in 80% of cases (usually IgG or IgA). Free light chains may pass into the urine as Bence Jones protein (BJP) and this may cause renal tubular damage. Malignant plasma cells interact with bone marrow stromal cells via a complex process involving cell-to-cell contact and cytokine production. These interactions lead to stimulation of myeloma cell growth, new vessel formation, activation of osteoclasts, inhibition of osteoblasts and effects on the stroma itself. Activation of osteoclasts leads to bone resorption and the development of osteolytic bone lesions, a key feature of MM.

Most cases of MM arise de novo, but a minority evolve from a condition called monoclonal gammopathy of undetermined significance (MGUS). In a patient with MGUS there will be a detectable serum paraprotein, but no other features to suggest myeloma (i.e. no lytic bone lesions, normal haemoglobin, bone marrow plasma cells <10%, normal calcium and normal renal function). The annual risk of transforming to MM is ~1%. Indolent or smouldering myeloma are terms used to describe patients where the diagnostic criteria of MM are met, but in whom the disease is asymptomatic and stable over a long period of observation. MM may also develop from a solitary plasmacytoma of bone, where the risk of developing MM is approximately 50% over a 15-year period. Extramedullary plasmacytomas rarely progress to MM.

Median survival for patients with MM is approximately 4 years, but is highly variable depending on prognostic factors described later in this chapter and the therapy received. Despite advances in treatment with responses in approximately two-thirds of patients, MM remains incurable, as it eventually becomes refractory to treatment. In the UK, there were 2600 deaths attributable to MM in 2002.

CLINICAL PRESENTATION

The clinical presentation of MM is highly variable. However, common presentations include bone pain (60%), recurrent or persistent infections, anaemia, renal impairment or a combination of these factors. The number of asymptomatic patients diagnosed with the disease is increasing mainly due to the incidental findings of a raised ESR or abnormal protein electrophoresis.

The spine and ribs are the most common sites of pain, and vertebral collapse may lead to kyphosis and loss of height. Osteoporosis, pathological fractures, spinal cord compression and hypercalcaemia also occur. Renal impairment is present in 25–30% and severe in ~5% of patients. This is mainly due to damage to renal tubules by BJP ('myeloma kidney'), but other predisposing factors include hypercalcaemia, infection, dehydration, hyper-uricaemia, amyloid, and the use of non-steroidal anti inflammatory drugs in the treatment of bone pain associated with the disease. Anaemia is very common, but severe pancytopenia is rare at presentation. Impairment of both humoral and cell-mediated immunity is common and leads to increased susceptibility to viral and bacterial infections.

Other less common problems include primary amyloidosis (which may cause renal problems, peripheral neuropathy, and congestive cardiac failure) and hyperviscosity syndrome due to high paraprotein levels. Occasionally, patients can present with circulating plasma cells detectable on a blood film; this group have a particularly poor prognosis.

DIAGNOSIS AND INVESTIGATIONS

A full history and examination is essential. Laboratory investigations should include as a minimum: FBC, renal and liver function, albumin, uric acid, calcium, β2 microglobulin, LDH, CRP, plasma viscosity, serum electrophoresis and paraprotein estimation, and a bone marrow aspiration and trephine. Other diagnostic tests should include 24-hour urinary BJP and skeletal X-ray survey.

Classically the diagnosis is confirmed by demonstration of >10% plasma cells in bone marrow, a paraprotein in the serum/urine with immunoparesis and/or lytic lesions on X-ray.

The most powerful predictors of a poor prognosis are high β2 microglobulin levels, and complete or partial deletion of chromosome 13.

Other adverse factors are anaemia, hypercalcaemia, renal impairment, advanced lytic bone lesions, low albumin, raised LDH and raised CRP.

A new staging system and clinical classification of MGUS and myeloma is currently in preparation.

MANAGEMENT

Before embarking on any specific therapies, general supportive measures should be a key part of management (see section on problems in advanced disease).

Chemotherapy is the mainstay of management for patients with symptomatic myeloma, but is not indicated for MGUS or for those with indolent or smouldering myeloma. Patients without symptoms and a normal haemoglobin, calcium, renal function and no bone lesions remain stable for long periods without treatment, and early intervention has no proven benefit. Patients who are asymptomatic but have radiological evidence of bone lesions are at high risk of progression.

There are two main chemotherapy pathways available to patients with MM:

1. VAD (vincristine, doxorubicin and high dose dexamethasone) and similar regimens, which include high dose dexamethasone but not alkylating agents. These are usually followed by high dose therapy (HDT) with stem cell rescue.
2. Single agent melphalan or cyclophosphamide with or without prednisolone, or combination chemotherapy regimens (with alkylating agents). The aim is to achieve a stable response or 'plateau'.

The choice of initial therapy depends on factors such as age, performance status, and whether stem cell harvesting and high dose therapy are planned.

OUTLINE OF THERAPY REGIMENS

VAD and related regimens

A VAD-type regimen should be offered to patients being considered for HDT as it will not damage stem cells. It is also suitable for patients with severe renal failure or in whom a rapid response is required.

High dose therapy (HDT)

High dose therapy (melphalan) with autologous stem cell transplant (ASCT) should be considered as part of the primary treatment strategy in newly diagnosed patients who are deemed medically fit for the procedure. It is normally given after establishing initial responsiveness to VAD-based regimens and offers complete remission rates of 24–75% and median survival of 4–5 years. Patients aged 60–70 may also be considered, but there is no current evidence for a survival benefit in this group. The role of allogeneic stem cell transplantation is controversial due to high transplant-related mortality, but it may be offered to patients less than 50 years. Up to one-third of these patients remain in persistent molecular remission with a low rate of relapse. Those patients who do relapse post allogeneic BMT may respond to donor lymphocyte infusions (DLI), as may those with persisting disease, suggesting a significant graft versus myeloma effect can occur. The role of mini-allogeneic transplantation is under study in the MRC myeloma IX trial.

Melphalan with or without prednisolone
This is suitable for most patients in whom HDT is not planned and produces around 50% partial response (PR) rates (defined as >50% decrease in paraprotein levels). Complete response (CR) is rare, but most reach a stable plateau phase (defined as stable paraprotein level for at least 3 months and transfusion independent with minimal symptoms), which usually lasts 18–24 months. Median survival is 2–4 years. Continuing chemotherapy during the plateau phase does not prolong remission. (Note: the evidence for the benefit of steroids is controversial.)

Cyclophosphamide with or without prednisolone
This produces very similar results to melphalan. Weekly cyclophosphamide is less myelotoxic than melphalan and is preferred in patients with bone marrow suppression.

Alkylator combination regimens
These consist of cyclophosphamide (C) and melphalan (M) with other drugs such as vincristine (V), adriamycin (A), prednisolone (P) and BCNU (B). There is no clear survival benefit over single alkylating agents. ABCM is a commonly used regimen.

High dose dexamethasone alone (HDD)
HDD can induce responses in over 40% of patients with few serious side effects. It is recommended as initial treatment when cytotoxic chemotherapy is contraindicated (e.g. severe pancytopenia or patients requiring extensive local radiotherapy) or severe renal failure is present.

Interferon
IFN-α does have a role in MM, but only small survival benefits have been demonstrated. It is mainly used as maintenance therapy in the plateau phase, but side effects can be significant.

Thalidomide
This drug has enjoyed a return to favour in recent years and it has been shown to be an effective treatment for myeloma, often producing responses

in otherwise chemotherapy resistant disease. The effectiveness of thalidomide is being assessed in a formal trial setting in MRC myeloma IX.

Bisphosphonates

Long-term therapy with bisphosphonates (e.g. clodronate orally or pamidronate IV) reduces skeletal morbidity, improves quality of life and reduces the need for surgery and radiotherapy. Bisphosphonates are therefore recommended to all patients requiring treatment, whether or not bone lesions are evident. Newer bisphosphonates such as zoledronic acid are becoming available and have been shown to be at least as effective as present treatment options. The efficacy of zoledronic acid versus clodronate is being assessed in the current MRC myeloma IX trial.

REFRACTORY AND RELAPSED DISEASE

Patients with refractory disease initially treated with alkylating agents may be offered VAD-type regimens, and young patients failing with VAD may still be offered high dose melphalan.

Almost all patients will relapse and management should still be aimed at disease control, symptom relief, improving quality of life (QoL) and prolonging survival. Early relapse predicts a poor response to further chemotherapy, but most patients who had a long plateau phase will respond to further treatment. The options for further management are numerous and should be determined on an individual basis depending on age, timing of relapse, performance status, prior therapy and other clinical circumstances.

FUTURE PERSPECTIVES

There is much current research interest in the role of 'mini' allogeneic (non-myeloablative) transplants and early reports demonstrate lower rates of transplant-related mortality. A wide range of agents are being evaluated in clinical trials and these include conventional chemotherapy (e.g. taxanes, vinorelbine and topotecan), thalidomide, cytokines (e.g. interleukins 2 and 12), proteasome inhibitors (e.g. bortezomib), VEGF inhibitors (e.g. bevacizumab), and donor lymphocyte infusions. Gene therapy and vaccine strategies are also being investigated.

In the management of bone disease, new bisphosphonates such as zoledronic acid are already standard therapies, but their role continues to be evaluated. Encouraging results have also been reported with the new technique of vertebroplasty. This involves injection of methylmethacrylate cement into collapsed vertebral bodies in order to recover bone strength and structure, thereby reducing kyphosis and height loss.

PROBLEMS IN ADVANCED DISEASE

1. Bone disease (see Ch. 48 on bone metastases). Adequate analgesia should be ensured with simple analgesics, opiates and NSAIDs (avoid NSAIDs in renal impairment). The use of bisphosphonates is essential to maintain skeletal integrity and local RT can be used to treat specific lesions and pain, which may also require orthopaedic intervention.

2. Renal impairment. A degree of renal impairment can occur in up to 50% of patients with MM at some stage during their illness. It is important to maintain adequate hydration (3 litres of fluid per day), avoid nephrotoxic drugs and treat infections vigorously. Occasionally dialysis is required for patients with severe renal failure.

3. Hypercalcaemia (see Ch. 56 on metabolic problems).

4. Spinal cord compression (see Ch. 60 on spinal cord compression). RT is usually the treatment of choice because spinal surgery in myeloma patients may be difficult due to bone disease. Surgery may, however, be indicated for spinal instability.

5. Anaemia. This is a common problem at presentation and during treatment and becomes more so as the disease progresses. Any contributing factors should be addressed. Packed red cell transfusion in patients with high paraprotein levels must be given with caution due to the risk of exacerbating hyperviscosity. Erythropoietin (EPO) therapy is a useful alternative to blood transfusion and there is a growing body of evidence to support its use. Over 80% of patients show an increase in haemoglobin of 1 g/dl after 4 weeks of EPO and QOL is also improved. EPO is especially useful in patients with associated chronic renal impairment.

6. Hyperviscosity. Symptomatic patients require urgent plasma exchange or isovolaemic venesection if plasma exchange not available. If blood transfusion is required then exchange transfusion should be performed. Treatment with chemotherapy should start promptly.

7. Infection. Prophylactic influenza, pneumococcal and *Haemophilus* vaccinations can be offered. Urgent admission for systemic antibiotics is required for severe infections. Prophylactic immunoglobulin infusions may offer some protection against serious infections and reduce the risk of recurrent infection, but do not improve overall survival.

FURTHER READING

UK Myeloma Forum on behalf of the British Committee for Standards in Haematology. Guidelines on the diagnosis and management of multiple myeloma. Updated March 2002. Available at: http://www.ukmf.org.uk/guidelines.shtml

CHAPTER 32

Non-Hodgkin's lymphomas

BACKGROUND INFORMATION

Non-Hodgkin's lymphomas (NHLs) are a heterogeneous group of lympho-proliferative malignancies with differing patterns of behaviour and responses to treatment. In 2000, there were over 9190 new cases diagnosed in the UK representing 3% of all new cancer diagnoses. In 2002 there were 4750 deaths attributable to NHL (3% of all cancer deaths).

NHL represents a progressive clonal expansion of B-cells or T-cells and/or natural killer (NK) cells. The vast majority (85%) are of B-cell origin, with only 15% originating from T-cells/natural killer (NK) cells. The World Health Organisation (WHO) has recently proposed a new classification of these tumours based on the Revised European-American Lymphoma (REAL) classification (Table 32.1).

The potential for cure is highly variable and depends on the histological subtype of NHL, the stage at presentation and patient response to initial therapy. In general, low grade lymphomas are indolent tumours associated with a predicted median survival time of 5–10 years, but are usually incurable. They have a characteristic relapsing and remitting course, with response rates to treatment and length of remissions decreasing over time. Intermediate grade and high grade lymphomas are more aggressive but are more responsive to chemotherapy and potentially curable. The predicted median survival time is 2–5 years for intermediate grade NHL and less than 2 years for high grade NHL.

Low grade NHL (~25%): Follicular lymphoma (70%) represents the vast majority of this group. Most patients are over 50 and usually present with disseminated disease at diagnosis (bone marrow involved in 50%). Transformation into a high grade lymphoma occurs in 10% and this is associated with a poor outcome. Other types include lymphoplasmacytic lymphoma, small lymphocytic lymphoma and marginal zone lymphoma.

TABLE 32.1 REAL-WHO classification of NHL

B-cell neoplasms
Precursor B-cell
B-cell lymphoblastic leukaemia/lymphoma

Peripheral (mature) B-cell
Chronic lymphocytic leukaemia/prolymphocytic leukaemia/small lymphocytic lymphoma
Lymphoplasmacytic lymphoma
Mantle cell lymphoma
Follicular lymphomas (three grades)
Marginal zone lymphoma (extranodal form/nodal form)
Splenic marginal zone lymphoma
Hairy cell leukaemia
Plasmacytoma/plasma cell myeloma
Diffuse large cell lymphoma (five subtypes)
Primary mediastinal lymphoma
Burkitt's lymphoma/leukaemia
Effusion lymphoma

T-cell/natural killer neoplasms
Precursor T-cell
T-cell lymphoblastic leukaemia/lymphoma

Peripheral (mature)
T-cell/NK
T-cell prolymphocytic leukaemia
T-cell chronic lymphocytic leukaemia
T-cell large granular lymphocyte leukaemia
Aggressive NK leukaemia
Adult T-cell leukaemia/lymphoma (HTLV-1 positive)
Extranodal T/NK cell lymphoma (nasal-type)
Enteropathy-type T-cell lymphoma
Hepatosplenic T-cell lymphoma
Subcutaneous panniculitic-like T-cell lymphoma
Mycosis fungoides/Sézary syndrome
Anaplastic large cell lymphoma, T/null cell types/primary cutaneous type
Peripheral T-cell lymphomas, not otherwise characterised
Angioimmunoblastic T-cell lymphoma
Anaplastic large cell lymphoma, T/null cell types/primary systemic type

Aggressive NHL (intermediate and high grade NHL) (~75%): Diffuse large B-cell lymphoma is the most common type of NHL and usually presents with rapidly enlarging nodes and B symptoms. Others include immunoblastic, anaplastic large cell, lymphoblastic, Burkitt's and Burkitt-like lymphomas. Mantle cell lymphomas also behave aggressively and are somewhat resistant to treatment.

The aetiology of NHL is complex and not fully understood. Chromosomal translocations and molecular rearrangements play an important role in many lymphomas. Viruses have been implicated in some lymphomas (e.g. Epstein–Barr virus (EBV) and Burkitt's lymphoma, human T-cell leukaemia virus type

1 (HTLV-1) and adult T-cell leukaemia/lymphoma, hepatitis C and lymphoplasmacytic lymphoma, and Kaposi's sarcoma associated virus and body cavity-based lymphomas). Other factors include immunosuppression, congenital conditions (severe combined immunodeficiency disease (SCID), Wiskott–Aldrich syndrome), autoimmune disorders, environmental factors (e.g. chemical pesticides, chemotherapy and radiotherapy) and *Helicobacter pylori* infection (causes marginal zone lymphoma (MALToma) of stomach).

PRESENTATION

There is an enormous spectrum of clinical behaviour with NHL. In general, indolent (low grade lymphomas) tend to present with slow-growing painless adenopathy. Weakness, fatigue and B symptoms may also be present, especially if the disease is advanced at presentation. Primary extranodal involvement is not common. Examination findings include adenopathy and splenomegaly. In aggressive NHL, most present with adenopathy (which may be rapidly growing) and over a third will have extranodal site involvement. B symptoms are present in over 30%. The commonest extranodal sites are the gastrointestinal (GI) tract, Waldeyer's ring, skin, bone marrow, sinuses, thyroid and CNS, but any site can be affected. Clinical symptoms and signs will depend on which sites are involved.

DIAGNOSIS AND STAGING

The following are required: full history and examination including all lymph node groups; full blood count (usually normal in early disease); ESR; renal and liver function tests; LDH; β2 microglobulin; protein electrophoresis; marker studies on peripheral blood if involvement suspected; CXR; CT scan of the chest, abdomen and pelvis; bone marrow aspiration and trephine. Biopsy of an accessible node should be by excision biopsy and needle and core biopsies should only be used in cases where excision biopsy would be a hazard to the patient. Additional investigations depending on the clinical scenario include MRI of the craniospinal axis, bone scans, lumbar puncture, GI endoscopy and testicular ultrasound.

The Ann Arbor staging classification is used (Table 32.2). Data from the investigation and staging of patients are used to calculate the International Prognostic Index (IPI) (Table 32.3). This was initially designed for use in diffuse large B-cell lymphoma, but has also been shown to be a valid guide to outcome for many types of lymphoma. It is particularly helpful in selecting patients for clinical trial entry.

TABLE 32.2 Ann Arbor staging of NHL

Stage I	Single lymph node area (I) or single extranodal site (IE)
Stage II	2 or more lymph node areas on the same side of the diaphragm (II) or localised single extralymphatic organ or site and its regional node(s) (IIE)
Stage III	Lymph nodes involved on both sides of the diaphragm
Stage IV	Disseminated or multiple involvement of extranodal organs
The designation of A or B is also applied:	
A	No constitutional symptoms
B	Presence of 1 or more of the following: (1) unexplained fevers (temperature >38°C), (2) drenching night sweats, and (3) unexplained weight loss of more than 10% in the preceding 6 months

TABLE 32.3 International prognostic index

Variable	Score 0	Score 1
Age	≤60 years	>60 years
Stage	I or II	III or IV
No of extranodal sites	≤1	>1
Performance status	0 or 1	≥2
LDH	Normal	>Normal

Risk groups	No of risk factors	5-year survival (%)
Low risk	0 or 1	73
Low intermediate risk	2	51
High intermediate risk	3	43
High risk	4 or 5	26

MANAGEMENT

Treatment of NHL varies greatly depending on tumour stage, grade, symptoms, performance status, patient's age, and co-morbidities. The IPI is a helpful tool for the decision-making process.

LOW GRADE (INDOLENT LYMPHOMA) NHL

Follicular lymphoma of the centroblastic-centrocytic type represents the vast majority of this group.

Stage I and II

Only 15–20% present with localised nodal disease and these patients can be treated with involved field radiotherapy alone (e.g. 30 Gy in 15 fractions over 3 weeks) with a 10-year disease-free survival rate of 60% for stage I and 25% for stage II disease.

Stage III and IV

Unfortunately, the majority of patients have advanced disease (stage III and IV) and treatment is palliative. Patients with advanced stage disease but a modest tumour burden can have cytotoxic chemotherapy deferred until disease progression because this approach does not have a negative impact on survival. For patients with significant tumour burden, symptomatic disease or vital organ involvement, chlorambucil and prednisolone produces clinical remission in 65% of cases and is a commonly used regimen. Combination chemotherapy produces higher complete response rates but does not improve overall survival. Other options include the use of fludarabine, which offers 70% remission rates as first line treatment and 50% as second line. Patients less than 60 may benefit from myeloablative therapy with autologous stem cell support and should be offered entry into appropriate clinical trials.

Relapsed disease

Patients with relapsed disease with more than one year of remission may be treated with the same initial chemotherapy. If the remission lasted less than a year then second line agents such as fludarabine or rituximab (anti-CD20 antibody) can be used or entry into a clinical trial should be considered.

HIGH GRADE (AGGRESSIVE) NHL

Diffuse large B-cell lymphoma (DLBCL) is the commonest type of high grade NHL. Patients who are high risk according to the IPI should be considered for clinical trials of myeloablative therapy with autologous stem cell support.

Traditionally, this disease has been treated with CHOP chemotherapy (3-weekly cyclophosphamide, doxorubicin, vincristine, prednisolone), but there is now good evidence that the addition of the anti-CD20 antibody rituximab improves the outlook of patients with DLBCL. (CD-20 is an antigen expressed on the surface of most B-cell lymphomas.) The National Institute for Clinical Excellence now recommends that CHOP-rituximab is the first line treatment of choice in patients with stage II–IV CD20-positive DLBCL. Patients will normally receive six to eight cycles of this combination and those with stage II disease may in addition also receive involved field radiotherapy to the sites of disease.

In patients with stage I disease, standard therapy remains three cycles of CHOP followed by involved field radiotherapy. Five-year survival is >80%.

Relapsed DLBCL
If fit enough, these patients are candidates for high dose myeloablative
chemotherapy with autologous stem cell support and clinical trials.

OTHER NHLs

Mantle cell lymphoma
This is difficult to treat and often disseminated to the gut, marrow and blood
at presentation. The median survival is 30–50 months and there is no current
consensus on management. Most were treated with CHOP, but FC
(fludarabine, cyclophosphamide)-rituximab is now commonly used first line.

Extranodal marginal zone lymphomas
These represent the commonest primary extranodal lymphoma and in most
cases the disease is localised. Prognosis at all sites is excellent. Local RT and
chlorambucil are the mainstay of treatment for most sites. Local RT alone is
used for primary cutaneous disease. There is good evidence that many
patients with stage IE gastric disease may be treated with anti-*Helicobacter*
therapy alone with careful endoscopic follow-up. Non-responders or those
with invasive disease may receive single agent chlorambucil.

Burkitt's and Burkitt-like lymphoma
These account for less than 10% of adult diffuse NHL. Burkitt's lymphoma is
usually extranodal, mainly affecting the GI tract, and also has a propensity for
the CNS involvement (20–30% lifetime risk). The Burkitt-like lymphomas are
a heterogeneous group, some of which are HIV-associated. Despite their
differences, treatment outcomes are similar for Burkitt's and Burkitt-like
lymphomas. Chemotherapy regimens are based on paediatric protocols and
include intrathecal chemotherapy for CNS prophylaxis. The prognosis is
good, with 5-year disease-free survival rates of 60% in advanced disease.

Mature T-cell lymphomas
These have broadly similar outcome to DLBCL and are usually widely
disseminated with extranodal disease at presentation. CHOP is the standard
treatment.

Cutaneous lymphomas
Eighty per cent are of T-cell origin. Mycosis fungoides (MF) is the
commonest cutaneous lymphoma and is of T-cell origin. It is characterised
by gradually progressive skin lesions that develop into plaques and tumours
over many years. Lymph node, visceral and blood involvement occurs late
on and signifies the end stages of the disease. Plaque disease can be treated
with PUVA (psoralen plus ultraviolet light A), local RT, and topical alkylating
agents or steroids. Widespread plaque disease can be treated with total
skin electron therapy (TSET). Systemic disease is treated with single

agent alkylators, purine analogues, interferon or steroids. The disease is incurable but overall 5-year survival is 87%. Sézary syndrome is a variant of cutaneous T-cell lymphoma characterised by exfoliative erythroderma, peripheral blood involvement and disabling pruritus. Five-year survival is ~10%.

FUTURE PERSPECTIVES

There are several exciting developments in the management of NHLs. Several anti-CD20 antibodies (e.g. rituximab) continue to be evaluated. Conjugation of these antibodies to radioactive isotopes (radioimmunotherapy) is an especially important development and very encouraging results have been seen with tositumomab and iodine-131. This agent has now been approved for use in the USA by the FDA for treatment of patients with CD20-positive follicular non-Hodgkin's lymphoma whose disease is refractory to rituximab and has relapsed following chemotherapy. Other anti-CD20 antibodies have been conjugated with yttrium-90. Anti-angiogenesis agents such as bevacizumab, an anti-vascular endothelial growth factor (anti-VEGF) agent, are also being evaluated. Other active areas of research include tumour vaccines and Bcl-2 antisense therapy.

   Incorporating these new treatments into a multimodality strategy, combining or sequencing with chemotherapy, and combining with other monoclonal antibodies or cytokines, or following with a vaccine or some other approach will be the main challenge over the next exciting few years in the management of NHLs.

PROBLEMS IN ADVANCED DISEASE

1. Bone marrow suppression. Severe bone marrow involvement causes pancytopenia, resulting in transfusion-dependent anaemia, thrombocytopenia and bleeding complications, and neutropenia and lymphopenia causing increased risk of bacterial and viral infections. Blood and platelets should be transfused and infections treated if these measures are appropriate. Note: anaemia may also be caused by autoimmune haemolytic anaemia, which is seen in some forms of NHL.
2. Painful bulky lymph nodes. These may ulcerate if large and are best treated with local radiotherapy.
3. Ascites and effusions (see Chs 52, 54 and 55 on malignant ascites, pericardial/pleural effusions).
4. Lymphoedema. May respond to local radiotherapy if caused by bulky nodal disease.

5. Dyspnoea. May result from pleural effusions, massive mediastinal disease, SVCO, parenchymal lesions, *Pneumocystis carinii* infection or treatment-related pneumonitis (e.g. RT).
6. Obstructive jaundice. Can occur due to bulky nodes at the porta hepatis. Local RT or placement of stent may help.
7. Constitutional symptoms. May respond to dexamethasone.
8. Tumour lysis syndrome (see Ch. 56 on metabolic problems in cancer).
9. GI obstruction, perforation and bleeding. May occur in GI lymphomas and also following chemotherapy. A surgical opinion should be sought urgently.
10. Spinal cord compression.

FURTHER READING

Hancock B W, Selby P J, Maclennan K A, Armitage J O (eds) 2000 Malignant lymphoma. Edward Arnold, London

Reiser M R, Diehl V 2002 Current treatment of follicular non-Hodgkin's lymphoma. European Journal of Cancer 38:1167–1172

Whittaker S J, Marsden J R, Spittle M, Russell Jones R 2003 Joint British Association of Dermatologists and UK Cutaneous Lymphoma Group guidelines for the management of primary cutaneous T-cell lymphomas. British Journal of Dermatology 149(6):1095–1107

CHAPTER 33

Oesophageal cancer

BACKGROUND INFORMATION

Oesophageal cancer is the fifth commonest cause of cancer death in the UK, resulting in 7250 deaths registered in 2002 (5% of all cancer deaths). It is commoner in men (incidence rate 14/100 000) than women (9/100 000) and the incidence increases with age, peaking in the seventh decade. There are approximately 7000 new cases per year, which closely matches the number of deaths per year, thus emphasising the poor outlook of this disease. The overall 5-year survival rate is 8%, with a median survival of 9 months. There are marked geographical variations in incidence, with very high rates seen in China and the Far East.

Major aetiological factors include smoking, alcohol consumption, malnutrition (β-carotene, B vitamins, vitamin C and E, selenium) and Barrett's oesophagus (5% progress to adenocarcinoma within 5 years). Other factors include asbestos exposure, metal dust (chromium and nickel) exposure, chronic inflammation, gastro-oesophageal reflux disease, achalasia, Plummer–Vinson syndrome and previous radiation injury. Hereditary factors play little role in the development of oesophageal cancer, but 95% of people with the rare condition of congenital palmar/plantar tylosis will develop the disease before the age of 65. Molecular abnormalities with the p53, Rb, APC and DCC tumour suppressor genes as well as chromosomal breaks and deletions (3, 5, 9, 13, 17, 18) are commonly found.

Pathologically, the two main histological subtypes are squamous cell carcinoma (SCC) and adenocarcinoma. Until recently, the vast majority of oesophageal cancers were squamous cell carcinomas, but over the last 20–30 years, the incidence of adenocarcinomas has continued to increase in the West to such an extent that they now represent 65–70% of histological subtypes. SCC tends to affect the upper two-thirds, and adenocarcinoma the lower third of the oesophagus. Tumours spread locally in a craniocaudal and circumferential manner. Early lymphatic spread is aided by the rich supply of lymphatics in the oesophagus and the risk of nodal spread increases with increasing depth of tumour invasion through the oesophageal wall. Haematogenous spread to the liver, bone, lung and brain usually occurs later in the disease.

PRESENTATION

Progressive dysphagia is the commonest symptom, initially of solids then later of liquids. Anorexia and weight loss are also common. Complete obstruction may lead to regurgitation, aspiration, coughing and pneumonias. Voice hoarseness may occur due to involvement of the recurrent laryngeal nerve. Clinical examination may reveal signs of weight loss and occasionally palpable cervical lymph nodes or a liver edge.

DIAGNOSIS AND STAGING

Investigations include history and examination; FBC; renal and liver function tests; calcium levels; double-contrast barium swallow. Flexible endoscopy with biopsy is the main method of obtaining a histological diagnosis (and also allows opportunity to dilate or stent strictures if necessary). FNA of enlarged neck

TABLE 33.1 2002 TNM staging of oesophageal cancer

T1	Tumour invades lamina propria or submucosa
T2	Tumour invades muscularis propria
T3	Tumour invades adventitia
T4	Tumour invades adjacent structures
N0	No nodes
N1	Regional nodes
M0	No distant metastases
Lower third oesophagus	
M1a	Coeliac nodes
M1b	Other distant metastases
Upper third oesophagus	
M1a	Cervical nodes
M1b	Other distant metastases
Middle third oesophagus	
M1b	Distant metastases including non-regional nodes
Staging	
Stage I	T1, N0, M0
Stage IIA	T2–3, N0, M0
Stage IIB	T1–2, N1, M0
Stage III	T3, N1, M0; or T4, any N, M0
Stage IV	Any T, any N, M1

nodes may also be helpful for diagnostic purposes. Trans-oesophageal endoscopic ultrasound (EUS) is the most sensitive test for assessing the depth of tumour invasion (T stage) and may also demonstrate regional lymphadenopathy. CT scanning of the neck, chest and abdomen offers complementary information for T staging and nodal staging and may demonstrate the presence of distant metastatic disease. If radical surgery is being contemplated for adenocarcinomas occurring at or near the oesophagogastric junction, laparoscopy to assess for peritoneal disease is recommended if there is any evidence of gastric extension. Tracheo-bronchoscopy should be performed if laryngeal or airway involvement is suspected.

Oesophageal cancer is staged using the 2002 TNM system (Table 33.1).

MANAGEMENT

BARRETT'S OESOPHAGUS

The annual risk of progression to invasive adenocarcinoma is only 1.3% and surveillance every 1–2 years is recommended for patients without associated dysplasia. Patients with associated high grade dysplasia have a 40–50% risk of progressing to invasive cancer within 5 years and these patients should be offered surgical resection.

EARLY AND LOCALLY ADVANCED DISEASE

Much controversy exists regarding the choice of surgical operation, the use of neoadjuvant or primary chemoradiotherapy and the use of neoadjuvant chemotherapy. For many patients these decisions are made on a case-by-case basis or by entry into a clinical trial. Treatment should be supported by high quality staging and undertaken in specialist centres.

Surgery and chemoradiation are the mainstays of treatment and may offer the chance of cure to patients with clinically localised oesophageal cancer (only 40–60% of patients present with localised disease). There is no current consensus on optimum management of oesophageal cancer. Surgery and chemoradiotherapy produce similar results, but there is some evidence that chemoradiation is more effective for locally advanced squamous cell carcinomas.

Surgery

Extensive transthoracic surgery (at least total oesophagectomy and two- or three-field lymphadenectomy) is needed because wide margins of clearance are required due to the diffuse patterns of submucosal and lymph node spread. In addition, patients with this disease are often elderly and malnourished and therefore need careful medical assessment and nutritional support prior to any radical treatment. Despite these measures, surgical mortality rates are

5–10% even in specialised centres. Surgical reconstruction of the alimentary tract can be performed by gastric pull-up, or by insertion of pedicled isoperistaltic colonic/jejunal loops. Surgery is associated with significant effects on quality of life, especially within the first year following treatment.

Chemoradiotherapy
Primary chemoradiotherapy in many centres is based on similar schedules to the Herskovic regimen (e.g. 50 Gy in 25 fractions over 5 weeks in combination with two to four cycles of cisplatin and 5FU). This produces 5-year survival rates of approximately 20–25%. Chemoradiotherapy has also been used in the neoadjuvant setting prior to surgery, but further trials are needed to confirm its benefits. Toxicity may be significant in up to 40% of patients, with symptoms of radiation oesophagitis, nausea/vomiting and problems associated with myelosuppression. There is a 10–20% risk of fibrotic stricture formation that may require treatment with dilatations.

Chemotherapy
Neoadjuvant chemotherapy with two cycles of cisplatin and 5FU has recently been shown to improve survival in the MRC OE02 study, which randomised over 800 patients with various stages of oesophageal adenocarcinoma and squamous carcinomas. The 2-year survival rates were 43% in the group that received neoadjuvant chemotherapy and 34% in the surgery alone group. Previous trials had not convincingly shown any survival benefits.

TREATMENT BY STAGE

Stage I (mucosal) disease
Endoscopic mucosal resection is the treatment of choice for these lesions and carcinoma in situ. Cure rates approach 100%.

Stage I (submucosal) and II disease
Surgery with total oesophagectomy and lymphadenectomy is the treatment of choice for most patients with good performance status and minimal medical co-morbidity. Node-positive patients may be offered two cycles of neoadjuvant cisplatin and 5FU chemotherapy. Chemoradiotherapy alone with the option of salvage surgery may be an option, especially for patients with disease of the cervical oesophagus, as surgery for this group of patients often requires pharyngectomy and laryngectomy, which may cause serious morbidity. Five-year survival for stage I disease is 50%, falling to 10–30% for stage II disease.

Stage III disease
Definitive chemoradiation or surgery with neoadjuvant chemotherapy (two cycles of cisplatin and 5FU) are the main options depending on the clinical scenario.

Patients with resectable adenocarcinomas may be offered neoadjuvant chemotherapy followed by surgical resection. Good performance status patients with non-resectable adenocarcinomas <8 cm in length can still be cured with definitive chemoradiotherapy. Patients with squamous cell carcinomas are generally offered chemoradiotherapy, especially for disease above the carina, but surgery is an option for disease below the carina.

Patients with large (>8 cm in length) unresectable tumours may receive palliative radiotherapy. This may be high dose (e.g. 50–55 Gy in 20 fractions over 4 weeks) if the patient is fit and it is technically possible, or low dose (e.g. 20 Gy in five fractions) for poor performance status patients. Oesophageal brachytherapy is another palliative option.

Patients should also be offered entry into clinical trials assessing the role of neoadjuvant chemoradiation.

Overall 5-year survival for patients with stage III oesophageal cancer is less than 20%.

Metastatic disease (stage IV disease)

Approximately 50% of patients present with stage IV disease and 5-year survival is rare. Palliative chemotherapy with ECF (epirubicin, cisplatin and 5FU) produces response rates of 50–60%, but median survival is less than a year. Chemotherapy may produce significant side effects and requires patients to be of a good performance status. Other active agents include doxorubicin, methotrexate and etoposide. See section on problems in advanced disease, below.

FUTURE PERSPECTIVES

The main focus of research is centred on new combinations of drugs and radiotherapy in the primary, neoadjuvant and palliative settings. In the concurrent chemoradiotherapy setting, the agents being investigated are irinotecan, taxanes, capecitabine, carboplatin and oxaliplatin. Some of these agents are also being studied in the palliative chemotherapy alone setting.

PROBLEMS IN ADVANCED DISEASE

(See also section on problems related to advanced head and neck cancer in Ch. 23.)

1. Dysphagia. Usually caused by luminal obstruction by the primary tumour. However, may also be caused by extrinsic compression by nodal disease, or by stricture formation secondary to surgery or chemoradiation. Reflux symptoms, thrush, xerostomia (secondary to dehydration and/or

radiotherapy) and nerve infiltration can also contribute to, or cause, the problem. Simple initial measures include rehydration and treatment of thrush or acid reflux (e.g. fluconazole 50 mg o.d., proton pump inhibitors). Several treatment options exist. Palliative external beam radiotherapy (EBRT) 20 Gy in five fractions may relieve dysphagia in up to 80% of cases, although this is usually short-lived (3–6 months). Higher dose schedules may be offered to fitter patients. EBRT is not without side effects (oesophagitis, risk of strictures/fistulas) and should not be used when there is total obstruction. Radiotherapy can also be given by intraluminal brachytherapy, which involves passing an afterloading catheter via a nasogastric tube into the oesophagus. A single 10–15 Gy dose can then be administered. Palliative dilatation is simple, cheap and effective, although its benefits are short-lived (2–4 weeks). Repeated treatments or the use of other methods are usually required. Endoscopic stenting is used for obstructing stenosing tumours and for patients in poor general condition. It is not possible for most proximal cervical oesophageal tumours. The procedure is relatively safe and 70% get functional improvement, with 10–50% being able to eat solids. More recently, self-expanding metallic stents have been introduced which are much easier to place and can be passed through almost all strictures, resulting in 90% functional success. Potential complications of stenting include perforation, bleeding and pressure necrosis. The Nd:YAG laser is ideal for fungating, non-stricturing tumours of the mid-distal oesophagus. It is effective in 70–80% of cases. Other methods used include photodynamic therapy and electrocoagulation.

2. Pain. May be due to heartburn or direct infiltration of tumour. The vertebrae and pleura may also be invaded. Radiotherapy (20 Gy in five fractions) is helpful; otherwise strong analgesia with opiates is required.

3. Malnutrition. Common problem. Early referral to dietician. Liquid or liquidised foods may be required. Nasogastric feeding is sometimes needed due to severe dysphagia.

4. Tracheo-oesophageal fistula. Usually a pre-terminal event. It causes coughing after drinking or eating. Covered self-expanding stents are useful for palliation.

5. Aspiration pneumonia. Patients with fistulas and regurgitation problems are at high risk. Antibiotics should be given where appropriate.

6. Hoarseness. Caused by compression/infiltration of the larynx or recurrent laryngeal nerve. A Teflon injection may be helpful.

7. Pericardial infiltration (see Ch. 54 on malignant pericardial effusions).

FURTHER READING

Benhidjeb T, Hohenberger P 2002 Oesophageal cancer. In: Souhami R L, Tannock I, Hohenberger P, Horiot J-C (eds) The Oxford textbook of oncology, 2nd edn. OUP, Oxford

Oesophageal cancer. START. Available at: www.startoncology.net

CHAPTER 34

Ovarian cancer

BACKGROUND INFORMATION

Ovarian cancer is the fourth commonest cause of cancer death in women and the leading cause of gynaecological cancer death. In the UK, there were 4690 deaths attributable to ovarian cancer in 2002. The incidence rate is 23/100 000, with 6730 new cases registered in 2000. The median age at diagnosis is 59 years although the highest incidence is seen in women in their mid to late seventies. Unfortunately 75% present with advanced disease and therefore only a minority of patients will have surgically curable localised disease. As ovarian cancer is a chemosensitive disease, surgery and platinum-based chemotherapy are the mainstay of treatment. However, despite high response rates (60–80%) to chemotherapy, the majority relapse (55–75%) within 2 years of treatment and overall 5-year survival is around 30%.

The exact aetiology of the disease is unknown. Approximately 5–10% of cases result from an inherited predisposition (e.g. BRCA 1 and 2, hereditary non-polyposis colon cancer (HNPCC or Lynch 2 syndrome)). Risk factors include low parity and infertility, high dietary fat intake and family history. The oral contraceptive pill (OCP) reduces risk.

Epithelial ovarian cancer accounts for 90% of cases and includes mucinous, serous, endometrioid, clear cell, Brenner, mixed epithelial and undifferentiated cancers. There is little significance prognostically to cell type, with the exception of clear cell carcinoma, which has a particularly aggressive course. Bilateral tumours are not uncommon (e.g. 40% of endometrioid and 20% of mucinous adenocarcinomas). The non-epithelial cancers include sex cord stromal, germ cell, metastatic and miscellaneous tumours. Also of interest are the tumours of borderline malignancy (or low malignant potential – LMP), which have cytological features of malignancy but lack invasive properties. They account for 4–14% of all ovarian malignancies.

The commonest sites of metastatic spread are to: (1) the peritoneum including the omentum, pelvic and abdominal viscera (by the transcoelomic route), (2) the pelvic lymph nodes and occasionally the inguinal nodes, (3) lungs and pleura.

PRESENTATION

Unfortunately early stage disease produces few or no symptoms, hence the reputation as the 'silent killer'. Some patients may experience urinary or rectal symptoms due to local pressure from tumour. Early tumours are usually discovered fortuitously on routine examinations. Late disease often presents with abdominal fullness and discomfort due to ascites, omental cake or bowel obstruction. Occasionally, patients present with symptoms and signs of distant metastatic disease, e.g. dyspnoea due to pleural effusions/lung metastases.

DIAGNOSIS AND STAGING

Investigations include full history and examination (including pelvic examination); ultrasound scan; CT scan of the abdomen and pelvis; CXR;

TABLE 34.1 FIGO staging of ovarian cancer

Stage I	Limited to ovaries
Ia	Limited to one ovary with capsule intact, no tumour on external surface of ovary, no malignant ascites
Ib	Limited to both ovaries with capsule intact, no tumour on external surface of ovary, no malignant ascites
Ic	Capsule breached or tumour on external surface of ovary or malignant ascites, or positive peritoneal washings
Stage II	Disease involves one or both ovaries with pelvic extension
IIa	Extends to uterus and/or tubes
IIb	Extends to other pelvic tissues
IIc	IIa or IIb disease with tumour on external surface of ovary or capsular rupture or malignant ascites or positive washings
Stage III	Disease involves one or both ovaries with histologically confirmed peritoneal implants outside the pelvis and/or positive retroperitoneal or inguinal nodes. Includes superficial liver metastases
IIIa	Tumour grossly limited to true pelvis, negative nodes, but with microscopic peritoneal seedlings
IIIb	Tumour of one or both ovaries, peritoneal implants of abdominal surfaces not exceeding 2 cm. Nodes negative
IIIc	Peritoneal metastases >2 cm in size beyond the pelvis and/or positive peritoneal or inguinal nodes
Stage IV	Distant metastases

routine bloods; tumour markers – CA125 (elevated in >90% with advanced disease and 50% with early disease – but non-specific). AFP and β-HCG may be performed if there is suspicion of a germ cell malignancy.

Ovarian cancer is staged surgically. The surgical procedure should include complete evaluation of all visceral and parietal surfaces within the peritoneal cavity, omentectomy, retroperitoneal lymph node biopsy, and total abdominal hysterectomy and bilateral salpingo-oophorectomy (TAH BSO). All suspected sites of involvement should be biopsied. Pleural effusions should be aspirated for cytology.

In patients with early stage disease suggested by preoperative imaging, contralateral ovarian and uterine preservation may be appropriate for some patients wishing to remain fertile.

Staging is by the FIGO system (Table 34.1).

SCREENING

At present, there is no conclusive evidence that screening (CA125, pelvic examination, transvaginal ultrasound) for ovarian cancer is beneficial even for women with two or more first-degree relatives.

MANAGEMENT

Surgery is the mainstay of treatment for ovarian cancer. It is vital for staging and diagnosis as well as treatment. However, because most patients present with advanced/disseminated disease, additional treatment with chemotherapy is required. The current standard first line chemotherapy regimen approved by the National Institute for Clinical Excellence (NICE) for ovarian carcinoma is paclitaxel (Taxol) in combination with carboplatin or cisplatin, or single agent platinum-based therapy. Carboplatin is generally preferred to cisplatin because it has a better safety profile in terms of non-haematological toxicity (less renal impairment, ototoxicity, neurotoxicity). Intraperitoneal chemotherapy is also effective, but due to technical difficulties has not become standard practice in the UK.

STAGE I DISEASE

For stage Ia and Ib patients with well-differentiated tumours, surgery alone is usually adequate with 5-year survival rates of 90–100%. For patients with grade 3 poorly differentiated tumours, stage Ic disease or clear cell histology, the 5-year survival with surgery is less good and these patients are offered adjuvant chemotherapy. The ICON1 and ACTION trials showed an improvement in absolute survival of 7% and a reduction in the risk of recurrence by 30% in patients with early stage disease.

STAGE II DISEASE

All macroscopic disease should be resected if possible (TAH BSO, omentectomy and staging biopsies). Patients should then receive chemotherapy. Five-year survival is around 50%.

STAGE III DISEASE

TAH BSO, omentectomy and maximum debulking (cytoreduction) is attempted. There is a lot of evidence that the volume of disease left at completion of primary surgery is related to survival. Patients with a residual tumour volume of less than $2\,cm^3$ have a significant survival advantage compared to patients with larger residual volumes and therefore the primary aim of surgery is to debulk disease to less than $1\,cm^3$ residual. Unfortunately only around 50% of women with stage III disease achieve optimal debulking. Six cycles of postoperative chemotherapy should be offered. The median survival with optimal debulking and chemotherapy is 39 months compared to 17 months with suboptimal debulking and chemotherapy.

Overall 5-year survival for stage III disease is 15–25%.

STAGE IV DISEASE

Patients may undergo debulking surgery, but whether this definitely improves survival is still under scrutiny. Unfortunately many are truly non-operable because of extensive disease or poor medical condition. Those fit enough should receive paclitaxel and/or platinum-based chemotherapy according to NICE guidance or be offered entry into clinical trials. Patients who are of poor performance status may tolerate single agent carboplatin or oral etoposide. Some patients may do well, but overall 5-year survival is only 5–10%.

INOPERABLE STAGE III AND IV DISEASE

In a significant number of patients, debulking is often very difficult, especially if there is disease in the supra-omental region or around the stomach and spleen. Primary surgery should generally be avoided if a large amount of disease is going to be left or if it is thought to be too risky. Primary chemotherapy can be offered instead and this may render the patient operable after two to three cycles. Chemotherapy can also be used for suboptimally resected tumours to allow further debulking surgery at a later date. This is known as interval debulking but it is somewhat controversial and further trials are required to assess its efficacy.

RECURRENT DISEASE

Secondary debulking surgery is performed in some centres, but no clear survival advantage has been proven and its role is therefore controversial. Surgery may be performed to relieve bowel obstruction. Chemotherapy as per NICE guidance should be offered to patients who are chemo-naive. Patients initially treated with chemotherapy who had a good and prolonged response may receive the same regimen again. Once failure occurs with the first line regimen, second line regimens should be considered.

Patients who relapse within 6 months of platinum based-chemotherapy are considered platinum resistant and those who do not respond at all are considered platinum refractory. These patients may be offered second line chemotherapy and there are currently six drugs licensed in the UK for this use: paclitaxel, liposomal doxorubicin, topotecan, altretamine, treosulfan and chlorambucil. Gemcitabine and etoposide are also used but are unlicensed at present. If paclitaxel was not used in the first line setting, then it is the second line drug of choice. Otherwise, current NICE guidelines recommend the use of single agent liposomal doxorubicin or topotecan in the second line treatment of ovarian cancer. They have similar efficacy, with response rates of ~20% and progression-free survival of ~4–5 months. Hormonal therapy with tamoxifen 20 mg b.d. is another option (response rate ~18%). Patients who relapse after 6 months may be retreated with the same chemotherapy regimen (response rates are 20–30%). The quality and duration of response are related to the preceding disease-free interval.

CA125 LEVELS

Although raised CA125 levels are not specific to ovarian cancer, monitoring serial changes during chemotherapy and follow-up is useful, especially in those patients who had elevated levels prior to treatment. Raised levels may precede symptoms, physical findings or even radiologically detected disease.

FUTURE PERSPECTIVES

Current trials are addressing unresolved issues such as optimal doses and schedules of chemotherapy, incorporation of new active agents into primary therapy, intraperitoneal chemotherapy, biological therapies (growth factor inhibitors, monoclonal antibodies, vaccines, cytokines), gene therapy, and the role of high dose chemotherapy with stem cell support.

PROBLEMS IN ADVANCED DISEASE

1. See Chapter 58 on problems in advanced pelvic malignancy.
2. Psychosexual problems. Radical treatment leads to problems including fatigue, nausea, change in body image due to surgical scars and loss of oestrogenic stimulus, painful intercourse, loss of libido, and relationship problems. Counselling including sexual aspects should be offered to patients and spouses. Oestrogen replacement therapy may be offered to those women with difficult menopausal symptoms.

FURTHER READING

Bristow R E 2000 Surgical standards in the management of ovarian cancer. Current Opinion in Oncology 12:474–480

Christian J, Thomas H 2001 Ovarian cancer chemotherapy. Cancer Treatment Reviews 27:99–109

Lawton F, Friedlander M, Thomas G (eds) 1998 Essentials of gynaecological cancer. Chapman and Hall Medical, London

NICE technology appraisals for ovarian cancer. www.nice.org.uk

Ozols R F et al 2000 Management of advanced ovarian cancer. Consensus Summary. Seminars in Oncology 27(3, Suppl 7):47–49

Stratton J F, Tidy J A, Paterson M E L 2001 The surgical management of ovarian cancer. Cancer Treatment Reviews 27:111–118

CHAPTER 35

Paediatric oncology

BACKGROUND INFORMATION

Childhood cancer is rare, but it is still the second commonest cause of death in the under-15 age group. In 2001, around 300 children died from cancer in the UK. There are 1400 new cases per year, with one child in 600 developing cancer before the age of 15.

The types of tumours seen in the paediatric population differ widely from adult tumours (Table 35.1). This is due to the fact that most childhood tumours arise from embryonal or mesenchymal tissue and not epithelial

TABLE 35.1 Incidence of paediatric tumours in the UK (UKCCSG Registrations 1995)

	Total number	Percentage
Leukaemias	467	30.1
CNS tumours	343	22.1
NHL	94	6
Neuroblastoma	92	5.9
Wilms'	68	4.4
Rhabdomyosarcoma	68	4.4
Hodgkin's	65	4.2
Osteosarcoma	44	2.8
Other sarcomas	41	2.6
Ewing's	28	1.8
Peripheral PNET (primitive neuro-ectodermal tumour)	13	0.8
Others	244	15
TOTAL	1554	100

tissue. The molecular genetic events leading to the development of malignancy also differ between childhood and adult tumours. The epithelial malignancies are therefore extremely rare in children.

The treatment for childhood cancers has improved dramatically over the last few decades and the overall cure rate is now approximately 65–70%. There are now 25 000 adult survivors of childhood cancer in the UK, but many suffer from long-term complications of treatment such as growth abnormalities, endocrine dysfunction and second malignancies and careful long-term follow-up of these patients is required (see section on complications of cancer treatment, below).

Due to the rarity of childhood cancer, the vast majority of children are managed in specialist centres and entered into national or international clinical trials. The main organisations that conduct clinical trials in the UK are the United Kingdom Children's Cancer Study Group (UKCCSG) and the International Society of Paediatric Oncology (SIOP).

As this is such a specialist area, this chapter only aims to give a very brief overview of the main childhood cancers and the complications of treatment.

GENERAL CONSIDERATIONS

There are some important general considerations in paediatric cancer:

1. Because of the rarity of childhood cancer, the diagnosis is often perceived to be 'delayed' by parents. This is due to the fact that parents always know when something is wrong with their child and subtle early symptoms may initially be missed by healthcare professionals. This can lead to frustration and upset.
2. All family members including siblings are affected by the diagnosis and management should therefore be 'family centred'.
3. Parents often feel that it is 'unnatural' for their child to have cancer and 'wish' they could swap places with their child and have the cancer themselves.
4. There are often significant difficulties when parents go through the agonies of having to make treatment decisions on behalf of their child.

LEUKAEMIAS

Leukaemias are the commonest type of cancer in childhood, representing 30% of all cases. Acute lymphoblastic leukaemia (ALL) is by far the commonest type (80%), followed by acute myeloid leukaemia (AML) (see Chs 26 and 27 on leukaemias).

LYMPHOMAS

The outlook for children with Hodgkin's disease is excellent, with up to 90% achieving cure. The mainstay of treatment is chemotherapy and involved field radiotherapy. Due to long-term side effects of treatment, modern trial protocols aim to reduce the doses of chemotherapy and radiotherapy without compromising cure rates.

The commonest types of NHL seen in children are high grade T-cell lymphoblastic, anaplastic large cell and Burkitt/Burkitt-like B-cell lymphomas. Overall survival rates are good (80% cure rate). The mainstay of treatment is similar to that of ALL with intensive combination chemotherapy.

BRAIN TUMOURS

(See also Ch. 15 on brain tumours.)

Brain tumours represent the second commonest type of childhood cancer, comprising 20% of all cases. There are a wide variety of tumour types and in contrast to adult brain tumours, over two-thirds of tumours arise infratentorially (posterior fossa) and only one-third supratentorially (Table 35.2). Paediatric gliomas are the commonest subtype and fortunately tend to be low grade rather than high grade.

Surgery, radiotherapy and chemotherapy are the mainstays of treatment. Radiotherapy is generally avoided in children under 3 years due to increased risk of neurological toxicity. The overall 5-year survival rate is 50%, but prognosis varies dramatically depending on the type of tumour, e.g. nearly all patients with germinomas are cured, but median survival for high grade brainstem gliomas is measured in months. Long-term neuropsychiatric complications from surgery and radiotherapy can be very significant.

TABLE 35.2 Infratentorial (posterior fossa) and supratentorial brain tumours in childhood

Infratentorial	Supratentorial
Cerebellar astrocytoma	Astrocytomas (all grades)
Medulloblastoma	Ependymomas
Brainstem gliomas	Oligodendroglioma
Ependymomas	Germ cell tumours (germinoma, teratoma)
	Pineoblastoma
	Optic gliomas
	Craniopharyngiomas and pituitary tumours
	PNET (primitive neuro-ectodermal tumour)
	Meningioma
	Choroid plexus tumour

Low grade astrocytomas represent the commonest group of brain tumours in children. Maximal surgical resection followed by observation is the mainstay of treatment. Patients with progressive disease may receive radiotherapy if aged more than 5 years or chemotherapy (if less than 5 years old) in order to delay the need for radiotherapy. Overall 5-year survival is ~85%, but late relapses are not uncommon.

High grade astrocytomas have a poor prognosis. Maximal debulking surgery followed by radiotherapy is the mainstay of treatment. Five-year survival is ~20%.

Ependymomas are treated by resection followed by radiotherapy. Five-year survival is ~50%.

Cerebellar astrocytomas are usually low grade. The outlook is favourable following complete resection with 10-year survival rates of 70–90%. The role of radiotherapy following incomplete resection is controversial.

Medulloblastomas are the commonest type of PNET (primitive neuro-ectodermal tumour), arise in the cerebellum and have a tendency to seed throughout the CNS. Treatment is by surgical resection followed by whole craniospinal axis irradiation and chemotherapy. Five-year survival is 50–60%. Beyond 5 years, the chance of relapse is less than 10%.

Brainstem gliomas represent ~10% of childhood brain tumours. Unfortunately, most are diffuse pontine high grade astrocytomas and have a very poor outlook. MRI appearances are diagnostic. (Biopsy is contraindicated.) Radiotherapy (e.g. 54 Gy in 30 fractions over 6 weeks) is the only proven treatment, but is palliative and median survival is only 9 months.

Intracranial germ cell tumours (GCTs) can be classified as germinomatous and non-germinomatous. Germinomas are the equivalent of testicular seminomas and usually occur in the suprasellar or pineal regions. They are treated by craniospinal radiotherapy following resection or biopsy, and are highly curable. Non-germinomatous GCTs usually occur in the pineal region and often produce the tumour markers alpha-fetoprotein (AFP) and human chorionic gonadotrophin (HCG). They are treated with chemotherapy and radiotherapy and may also require surgery. They have a poorer outlook than germinomas, but cure rates are still high.

NEUROBLASTOMA

These malignant tumours arise from the neural crest tissue of the sympathetic nervous system and can therefore arise from the adrenal glands and anywhere along the sympathetic chain from the neck to the pelvis.

Most children are less than 4 years old, with one-third of all cases occurring in those less than 1 year old. The overall survival rate of 45% is poor because the disease is often metastatic at presentation. However, there is a wide spectrum of tumour behaviour and some subgroups of patients can do extremely well. For example, children less than 1 year have a better outlook than older children. Poor prognostic factors include high disease stage, amplification of the *N-myc* oncogene, and presence of the chromosome 1p deletion. Most neuroblastomas take up MIBG (meta-iodobenzyl guanidine) and radiolabelled ^{131}I-MIBG can be used for diagnostic and therapeutic purposes.

Presenting features are often non-specific and generalised and may include malaise, fever, weight loss, abdominal swelling, vomiting and failure to thrive. Pain may occur virtually anywhere due to either the local effects of the primary tumour or to bone metastases. Tumour secretion of catecholamines may cause sweating attacks and palpitations.

Due to the diverse nature of neuroblastomas, treatment is stratified according to risk groups based on stage and other prognostic factors such as the *N-myc* amplification. Treatment may vary from surgery alone for good prognosis early localised disease (90% survival rate) to multimodality therapy for poor prognosis advanced metastatic disease (10–15% survival rate) including surgery, chemotherapy (high dose chemotherapy with stem cell rescue), radiotherapy and ^{131}I-MIBG. Observation alone is usually sufficient for children with stage 4S 'special' disease without *N-myc* amplification, because these tumours usually spontaneously regress (85% of cases). (Stage 4S disease is defined as children aged 1 year or less with a localised primary tumour and metastases limited to the liver, skin and bone marrow.)

WILMS' TUMOUR (NEPHROBLASTOMA)

Wilms' tumour is the most common childhood malignant primary tumour of the kidney. The majority occur in children less than 5 years of age with a mean of 3–4 years and in approximately 5% of cases the disease is bilateral. Wilms' tumour is associated with various rare congenital abnormalities such as the Beckwith–Wiedemann syndrome, hemi-hypertrophy, aniridia and renal tract abnormalities.

Pathologically, the classic Wilms' tumour is a triphasic tumour with blastemal, stromal and epithelial components, but there are a wide variety of histological appearances. The triphasic tumour represents a prognostically favourable appearance and anaplastic tumours represent an unfavourable histology. Rhabdoid tumours and clear cell sarcomas are also unfavourable histologies, but are not strictly classified as Wilms' tumours.

Most children present with abdominal swelling and discomfort. Gross haematuria, fever and hypertension are other frequent features.

In terms of management, patients are stratified into risk groups based on tumour stage and histology. Patients with early stage favourable histology are treated with surgery and chemotherapy with 5-year survival of 80–95%. More advanced disease requires postoperative flank radiotherapy to the tumour bed in addition to more intensive chemotherapy. Whole lung radiotherapy is offered to patients with persistent unresectable lung metastases following chemotherapy.

BONE SARCOMAS

Sarcomas of bone, including Ewing's sarcoma, are discussed in Chapter 40.

RHABDOMYOSARCOMA

Rhabdomyosarcoma (RMS) is the commonest malignant mesenchymal tumour in children and accounts for ~4–5% of all childhood malignancies. The median age at diagnosis is 5 years, and boys are more commonly affected than girls. There is an association with the Li–Fraumeni familial cancer syndrome. Overall survival at 5 years is now ~70%.

RMS arises from striated muscle and may occur at any site in the body. The commonest sites are the head and neck region (including the orbits, nasopharynx and parameningeal tissues), genitourinary tract, and the trunk and limbs. Pathologically, RMS is classified according to the International classification system for childhood RMS (Table 35.3).

Most children present with a rapidly growing asymptomatic mass. Symptoms and signs if present are usually related to the primary site of disease, e.g. haematuria, epistaxis, visual disturbance. Generalised symptoms of widespread metastatic disease are not common at presentation.

The management plan requires stratification of patients into risk groups based on the histological type, stage and site of the tumour. Low risk patients are treated by 9 weeks of chemotherapy and surgical resection of the tumour. Prognosis for these patients is excellent, with cure rates of 85%. Higher risk

TABLE 35.3 International classification system for childhood rhabdomyosarcoma

Prognostic group	Histology
I: Superior prognosis	Botryoid
	Spindle cell
II: Intermediate prognosis	Embryonal
III: Poor prognosis	Alveolar
	Undifferentiated
IV: Uncertain prognosis	Rhabdoid features

patients require more intensive chemotherapy and may also require further surgery or radiotherapy to sites of residual disease. The outlook for those with metastatic disease is poor, with 5-year survival of ~25%.

PRIMARY HEPATIC TUMOURS

Primary malignant tumours of the liver are rare accounting for only 1.2–5% of all paediatric neoplasms. There are two main types – hepatoblastoma and hepatocellular carcinoma (HCC).

Hepatoblastoma is an embryonic tumour of very young children with a median age at presentation of 12–16 months. It usually presents as an asymptomatic abdominal mass and over 90% of patients will have an elevated AFP. Anaemia and thrombocytosis are common.

HCC is a disease of older children, with a peak incidence of 10–14 years. Patients present with an abdominal mass or distension. Systemic symptoms of anorexia, nausea, fever and weight loss may be present. AFP is raised in 60–90% of cases.

The only chance of cure for both types of tumour is complete surgical resection. Unfortunately, over 50% of patients with hepatoblastoma and 70–80% with HCC are unresectable at diagnosis. However, hepatoblastoma is a chemosensitive disease and cisplatin/anthracycline-based combination chemotherapy has dramatically increased complete resection rates and improved overall survival rates to 79% at 3 years. HCC is less chemosensitive and overall 3-year survival is approximately 40%.

RETINOBLASTOMA

Retinoblastoma is the commonest malignant intraocular tumour of childhood and can occur sporadically or be inherited. About 40–50% of patients have the genetic form of the disease, which is inherited as autosomal dominant, but is autosomal recessive at the molecular level (requires inactivation of both alleles). The inherited form presents earlier and is more likely to be bilateral/multifocal than the sporadic form. In addition, patients with the inherited form have a significant risk of developing a second malignancy later in life.

Unilateral retinoblastoma presents on average at 24 months of age while bilateral disease presents at 12 months. The prognosis for this disease is now excellent, with current overall survival of approximately 95% at 5 years.

Patients present with strabismus, reduced visual acuity and red eye, but by far the most important sign is leucokoria (white pupillary reflex). The main diagnostic tools are ophthalmoscopy, ultrasonography, CT and MRI. Biopsy is avoided in order to prevent spread outside of the eye.

Treatment requires a multidisciplinary approach with involvement of the paediatric oncologist, ophthalmologist, geneticist, radiologist, radiotherapist and orthoptist. Wherever possible the eye is preserved.

Small tumours may be treated with focal laser therapy, cryotherapy, plaque radiotherapy (with local applicators) and thermotherapy. Larger tumours can be treated with chemotherapy followed by focal therapies if the tumour shrinks significantly. Tumours that do not shrink with chemotherapy can be treated with plaque radiotherapy (with local applicators) or external beam radiotherapy.

Surgical enucleation is the treatment of choice if there is glaucoma, extensive involvement of the optic nerve, tumour filling the globe and when focal therapy has failed. Adjuvant chemotherapy and radiotherapy is offered if there is evidence of disease in the cut end of the optic nerve.

MALIGNANT GERM CELL TUMOURS (MGCTs)

Malignant germ cell tumours of childhood are rare, representing only 3% of all childhood malignancies. There is a bimodal age distribution with a peak in under 3-year-olds and a second peak over the age of 12. There is an increased incidence of these tumours in children with dysgenic gonads and congenital abnormalities such as defects in the urogenital system, sacral agenesis and cryptorchidism.

Except for the gonads, MGCTs usually arise in midline structures such as the midbrain, mediastinum, retroperitoneum and sacrococcygeal region. This is because these structures lie along the normal migration pathway of germ cells during embryogenesis.

There are significant differences between childhood and adult MGCTs both in composition and in distribution. In prepubertal children extragonadal tumours are much commoner and most MGCTs contain yolk sac elements. See Table 35.4 for the relative incidence according to age, sites and pathological subtypes of the MGCTs of childhood.

INDIVIDUAL TUMOUR SITES

Sacrococcygeal tumours

Almost half of these lesions occur in neonates, mainly girls, and most are benign. However, up to one-third of tumours with extensive intra-abdominal or intraspinal extension contain malignant tissue (invariably yolk sac tumour). Treatment is usually by surgical excision. Primary chemotherapy (bleomycin, etoposide, cisplatin-BEP) is used for unresectable malignant tumours. Recurrence can be detected by measurement of serum AFP levels.

TABLE 35.4 Relative incidence of paediatric germ cell tumours according to age and pathology

Site	Relative incidence (%)	Age	Pathology
Sacrococcyx	35	Neonate	Teratoma: Mature 65% Immature 5% Malignant 10–30%
Ovary	25	Early teens	Teratoma: Mature 65% Immature 5% Malignant 30% (yolk sac 30%, mixed 30%)
Testis	20	Infant and adolescent	Teratoma: Mature 20% Malignant 80% (yolk sac 90%, germinoma 10%, embryonal carcinoma 1–5%)
Cranium	5	Child	Germinoma 20–50% Embryonal carcinoma 20–50% Mature teratomas 20–30%
Mediastinum	5	Adolescent	Teratoma: Mature 60% Mixed 20% Embryonal carcinoma 20%
Retroperitoneum	5	Infant	Teratoma: mature or immature, rarely malignant
Head and neck	3	Infant and neonate	Usually mature teratoma, immature rarely malignant
Vagina	2	Infant	Usually yolk sac

Reproduced with permission of Elsevier from Pinkerton C R 1997 Malignant germ cell tumours of childhood. European Journal of Cancer 33(6):895–902.

Mediastinal tumours

These occur in the anterior mediastinum and usually present with tracheal or bronchial obstruction. They are more common in adolescent males. AFP and β-HCG levels may be raised. If the tumour is malignant then primary chemotherapy is the treatment of choice followed by surgical resection of any residual tumour.

Ovarian tumours

Most are benign, but approximately one-third contain malignant elements and these tumours may spread transcoelomically to cause ascites and peritoneal implants. The lymph nodes, liver and lung are the usual sites of distant metastases. AFP and β-HCG levels may be raised. Surgical excision is curative for localised disease. Primary chemotherapy is required for unresectable and metastatic disease. This may be followed by excision of the primary tumour.

Testicular tumours

Approximately 80% of childhood testicular tumours are malignant. The lymph nodes and lungs are the commonest site of distant metastases. AFP and β-HCG levels may be raised. Treatment is by radical orchidectomy via the high inguinal route. Chemotherapy is used to treat metastatic disease. Overall event-free survival is over 90%.

Intracranial disease

See section on brain tumours, above.

COMPLICATIONS OF CANCER TREATMENT IN CHILDREN

The success of treatment of childhood cancers comes at the price of acute toxicity and more importantly long-term side effects.

CHEMOTHERAPY

The main acute side effects include nausea, vomiting, risk of neutropenic sepsis, hair loss and failure to thrive.

Long-term effects include cardiotoxicity (anthracyclines), renal impairment (cisplatin), infertility (alkylating agents) and increased risk of second malignancies with alkylating agents (especially leukaemia).

RADIOTHERAPY

Side effects may be enhanced if combination chemotherapy has also been used.

Acute general side effects include fatigue and skin soreness. Other effects are related to the site irradiated (see section on side effects of radiotherapy in Ch. 5).

Long-term effects depend on the site irradiated.

1. Brain. Neuropsychiatric sequelae including reduction in IQ.
2. Musculoskeletal system. Growth abnormalities, tissue hypoplasia, and risk of radiation-induced sarcoma.
3. Endocrine system. Hormone replacement therapy is often required. Infertility results from gonadal irradiation.

4. Kidney. Renal impairment – related to total dose and volume of kidney irradiated.
5. Heart. Increased risk of cardiovascular disease. Exacerbated if anthracyclines have also been administered.
6. Lung. Radiation pneumonitis and fibrosis. Chemotherapy (e.g. actinomycin D, cyclophosphamide) reduces the threshold for damage.
7. Gut. Risk of radiation enteritis.
8. Dental. Poor development of teeth. Problems are exacerbated by xerostomia and hypoplasia of the jaw and maxilla.
9. Second malignancies. This is a multifactorial process and not fully understood. Some children have a genetic predisposition and have a higher risk of second cancer. Sarcomas are the commonest type of second malignancy.

FURTHER READING

Pinkerton C R, Plowman P N (eds) 1997 Paediatric oncology. Clinical practice and controversies, 2nd edn. Chapman and Hall Medical, London
Pinkerton C R, Michalski A J, Veys PA (eds) 1999 Clinical challenges in paediatric oncology. Martin Dunitz, London

Pancreatic cancer

BACKGROUND INFORMATION

Pancreatic cancer is the sixth commonest cause of cancer death in the UK. In 2002, there were 6880 deaths, representing 4% of all cancer deaths. There is equal incidence in men and women (11/100 000) accounting for approximately 7000 new cases per year. This is similar to the death rate, confirming the very poor prognosis of this disease. The peak incidence is the seventh decade of life. Over 80% of patients present with metastatic disease and of the small number who have resectable disease, only 20% will survive 2 years. It is not surprising therefore, that the overall 5-year survival is 3%, with median survival of 9–12 months. Most patients with metastatic disease die within 90 days.

The aetiology of pancreatic cancer is unknown, but there are several risk factors. Smoking increases risk 2-fold. Black males have a 30–40% increased risk. Other possible but unproven factors are ingestion of N-nitroso compounds (found in processed meats), caffeine, alcohol, obesity, chronic pancreatitis and diabetes mellitus. Molecular genetic factors are very important in this disease, with over 80% of cancers expressing mutations in the K-ras oncogene. However, familial pancreatic cancer is rare and accounts for less than 5% of cases.

Pathologically, adenocarcinoma (arising from exocrine ducts) and its variants represent 90% of all of the numerous histological subtypes, which also include acinar cell carcinoma, sarcomas and neuroendocrine tumours (see Ch. 17 on carcinoid and other neuroendocrine tumours). Approximately 65% of adenocarcinomas arise in the head of the pancreas, with 25–30% in the body and 5–10% in the tail. These tumours usually produce an intense fibrotic reaction and spread by the perineural, lymphatic and vascular routes, with most patients having lymph node involvement at presentation. Metastatic spread to the peritoneum, liver and lung is common.

PRESENTATION

Initial symptoms are often non-specific and include abdominal pain radiating to the mid and lower back, anorexia and weight loss, nausea, vomiting, abdominal distension and change in bowel habit. The pain is due to invasion of the splanchnic plexus and retroperitoneum and it is characteristically severe, gnawing, dull and persistent. Obstructive jaundice occurs in 70% (90% if head of pancreas involved) of patients but usually occurs later in the disease. Clinically there are often few signs, but patients may have cachexia, hepatomegaly, jaundice, a palpable gallbladder (Courvoisier's sign), migratory superficial phlebitis (Trousseau's sign), an epigastric mass, or a peri-umbilical mass (Sister Joseph's nodule). The occasional patient may present with glucose intolerance or diabetes. Unfortunately, most present with inoperable disease.

DIAGNOSIS AND STAGING

Investigations used in the diagnosis of pancreatic cancer include history and examination; CXR; routine bloods (FBC, renal and liver function tests, calcium, glucose); CA19.9; CEA tumour markers. CA19.9 can be significantly raised in obstructive jaundice.

Abdominal ultrasound ± guided biopsy may be used. Biopsy may also be obtained under CT-guidance. Endoscopic ultrasound (EUS) is useful in selected cases for assessment of small tumours and nodal and/or portal vein involvement. In the presence of jaundice with dilated bile ducts, endoscopic retrograde cholangiopancreatography (ERCP) outlines the ducts and allows biopsy and insertion of stents to relieve bile outflow obstruction. Percutaneous transhepatic cholangiography (PTC) is another option allowing biopsy, delineation of where the obstruction is, and stenting.

Spiral CT scanning of the abdomen provides useful information regarding resectability of the primary tumour and can evaluate hepatic or other distant metastases, enlargement of regional lymph nodes, invasion of retroperitoneal structures and intraperitoneal dissemination. Laparoscopy is useful for staging patients with potentially operable disease as 25% in this group will be found to have intra-abdominal disease that precludes curative resection. The role of positron emission tomography (PET) scanning remains under evaluation.

Staging is by the 2002 TNM system (Table 36.1).

MANAGEMENT

As outcomes are so poor in pancreatic cancer, patients who are fit enough should be offered entry into clinical trials for all stages of the disease.

TABLE 36.1 TNM 2002 staging for pancreatic cancer (summary)

T1	Tumour ≤2 cm, limited to pancreas
T2	Tumour >2 cm, limited to pancreas
T3	Tumour beyond pancreas, but without coeliac axis or superior mesenteric artery
T4	Tumour involves coeliac axis or superior mesenteric artery
Stage IA	T1, N0, M0
Stage IB	T2, N0, M0
Stage IIA	T3, N0, M0
Stage IIB	T1–3, N1, M0
Stage III	T4, any N, M0
Stage IV	Any T, any N, M1

The only potentially curative treatment is surgery, but over 90% of patients are unresectable at diagnosis due to the presence of locally advanced or metastatic disease. The importance of good palliative and supportive care in patients with pancreatic cancer cannot be overemphasised.

SURGERY

Patients who have a positive resection margin at the time of surgery have similar outcomes to patients receiving palliative treatment with chemo-radiation. The goal of surgery is therefore complete resection, so accurate preoperative staging is vital. Patients are considered resectable if on CT scanning, there is: (1) no evidence of extrapancreatic disease and (2) no involvement of the superior mesenteric vessels or the portal vein. Unfortunately only 10–15% are operable at diagnosis.

Traditionally, the Whipple's procedure (pancreatoduodenectomy) has been the operation of choice, but more recently the pylorus-preserving Whipple (PPW) pancreatoduodenectomy has been increasingly employed as this reduces nutritional problems following surgery. Surgery should be undertaken in centres with a specialist interest in pancreatic surgery with a high volume of cases (>20 cases per surgeon per year), as this has been shown to improve outcomes. Operative mortality is now less than 5% in such centres. The 5-year survival for patients who have operable disease is only 15–20%, with median survival of 15–19 months. There is evidence that adjuvant chemotherapy offers a small but significant survival advantage (ESPAC-1 trial), but entry into neoadjuvant/adjuvant clinical trials should still be encouraged.

Surgery also has roles in the palliative setting. Biliary-enteric bypasses may be performed in patients found to be unresectable at laparotomy. ERCP/PTC and stenting is used for common bile duct obstruction. Gastrojejunostomy or endoscopic stenting can relieve gastric outflow obstruction.

CHEMORADIOTHERAPY

Postoperative adjuvant chemoradiotherapy (CRT) is standard treatment in the USA. The GITSG trial, which compared surgery alone to surgery + CRT, showed an improvement in median survival from 11 months to 21 months and 2-year survival from 18% to 43% favouring the surgery + CRT group. Stomatitis, neutropenia and diarrhoea are common side effects of this treatment. In Europe, however, a large multicentre trial (ESPAC-1) has shown no benefit for adjuvant chemoradiotherapy and it is has not become standard practice in Europe.

Neoadjuvant chemoradiotherapy has been proposed to improve resectability rates and decrease local recurrences, and studies are ongoing in this field.

In patients with inoperable locally advanced disease, chemoradiotherapy has been shown to improve local control compared to radiotherapy alone. One-year survival of 40–47% and median survival of 10–11 months has been demonstrated. This approach should only be considered in good performance status patients and balanced against potential toxicity.

CHEMOTHERAPY

The role of chemotherapy in the adjuvant setting has been discussed above.

The role of chemotherapy in advanced disease needs to be carefully considered with patients on an individual basis. Combination regimens such as FAM (5FU, doxorubicin, mitomycin C) offer no significant survival advantage over 5FU alone. However, a recent trial has shown significant clinical benefit of gemcitabine over 5FU (24% versus 5%). There was also a significant survival advantage but this was small (5.65 months versus 4.41 months and 1 year survival of 18% versus 2%). The National Institute for Clinical Excellence (NICE) has recommended that gemcitabine may be used in the first line setting for patients with advanced or metastatic disease.

FUTURE PERSPECTIVES

Much research is focused on improving chemoradiation regimens by optimising radiation delivery and using newer agents such as gemcitabine, which is also being assessed in combination chemotherapy trials. The role of adjuvant chemotherapy continues to be evaluated (e.g. ESPAC-3 trial is assessing adjuvant 5FU versus gemcitabine). Recent results from trials of matrix metalloproteinase inhibitors and farnesyl transferase inhibitors have been disappointing. However, there is much current interest in the use of pancreatic cancer vaccine therapy with some early encouraging results.

PROBLEMS IN ADVANCED DISEASE

Advanced pancreatic cancer may cause severely debilitating symptoms and early referral to the palliative care and pain teams is very important.

1. Pain. This is a common problem (occurs in 85%). Classically epigastric, radiating to the back. Due to coeliac plexus involvement. Patients with opioid-resistant pain may be offered a coeliac plexus block with 100% alcohol. This may be administered either intraoperatively or percutaneously and produces effective pain relief for over 3 months in 60–75% of patients. Palliative chemoradiotherapy or radiotherapy alone may have a limited role. Postprandial abdominal pain caused by malignant stricture of the main pancreatic duct may occur in up to 15% of patients. Placing a pancreatic stent across the stricture can relieve this problem.

2. Obstructive jaundice. Prolonged biliary obstruction may lead to malabsorption, malnutrition, pruritus, malaise, anorexia, recurrent cholangitis and hepatic dysfunction. Patients with bile duct obstruction who are inoperable can have stenting performed by ERCP or PTC. Relief of obstruction is obtained in >90% of patients. Metallic stents stay patent for longer than polyethylene stents, but as they are more expensive, they tend to be used in patients with life expectancy greater than 3 months. If the disease was unresectable at laparotomy then a surgical biliary-enteric bypass can be performed (e.g. choledochojejunostomy). Simple external biliary drainage is useful only for short-term decompression.

3. Obstructive vomiting. This usually occurs secondary to duodenal or gastric outlet invasion and occurs in 10–20% of patients. A palliative gastrojejunostomy remains the standard treatment, but this has a mortality rate of 10%. Another possibility is the use of self-expandable metallic stents for selected cases.

4. Ascites. A common problem due to peritoneal disease and/or hypoalbuminaemia (see Ch. 52 on malignant ascites).

5. Steatorrhoea and malabsorption. Caused by blockage of the pancreatic duct leading to loss of pancreatic enzymes to below 10% of normal. Steatorrhoea is not controlled well by standard anti-diarrhoeal agents, but does respond to pancreatic enzyme replacement, e.g. Creon 10 000, 1–2 capsules per meal.

6. Cachexia and anorexia. Cachexia is involuntary weight loss of >10% and is associated with muscle loss and hypoproteinaemia. Anorexia is loss of appetite. Both can have a very detrimental effect on quality of life and response and tolerance to treatment. The following four-step approach may be helpful. (1) Treat potentially reversible cause of anorexia, e.g. anxiety, depression, constipation, nausea, vomiting, and pain; (2) if early satiety or evidence of gastroparesis, try metoclopramide 10–20 mg pre-meals; (3) add megestrol acetate 160 mg o.d. (increasing to 800 mg) or dexamethasone 2 mg o.d.; (4) try thalidomide 100 mg at night, or melatonin 20–40 mg a day.

7. Neuropsychiatric disturbance. Anxiety, depression and emotional disturbance are particularly common in this disease. Counselling and referral to psychiatry team for treatment may be appropriate.
8. Liver metastases. Tender hepatomegaly often responds to steroids, e.g. dexamethasone 8–16 mg o.d. Prognosis is particularly poor.
9. Superficial migratory thrombophlebitis (Trousseau' s syndrome) and disseminated intravascular coagulation (DIC). Coagulopathies are a common problem in pancreatic cancer, leading to recurrent episodes of thrombophlebitis, venous and arterial thrombosis, and bleeding episodes. Treatment of thrombophlebitis requires anti-inflammatories and TED (anti-thromboembolic) stockings. DIC is very difficult to manage, but sometimes responds to treatment of the primary tumour.

FURTHER READING

Evans D, Abbruzzuse J L, Pisters P W (eds) 2001 Pancreatic cancer. Springer-Verlag, Berlin
Kuvshinoff B W, Bryer M P 2000 Treatment of resectable and locally advanced pancreatic cancer. Cancer Control 7(5):428–436
Reber H A (ed) 1998 Pancreatic cancer: pathogenesis, diagnosis and treatment. Humana Press, Totowa, NJ

CHAPTER 37

Penile cancer

BACKGROUND INFORMATION

Cancer of the penis is uncommon, with an incidence of 1 in 100 000 men in Western countries. There were under 300 new cases diagnosed in the UK in 1999. It is typically a disease of older men, the highest incidence being in the seventh decade. Risk factors include poor hygiene, phimosis, infection with the human papilloma virus (HPV – mainly types 16 and 18) and smoking. Circumcision at birth confers almost 100% protection.

Pathologically, 95% of penile cancers are squamous cell carcinomas. Other histological types include melanoma, basal cell carcinoma, sarcomas and lymphoma. The majority occur on the glans, coronal sulcus or on the prepuce. Premalignant conditions such as Bowen's disease, erythroplasia of Queyrat (carcinoma in situ), leucoplakia and Paget's disease all predispose to penile cancer. Lymphatic spread occurs to femoral, superficial and deep inguinal nodes and then to pelvic nodes. The grade and depth of invasion of the primary tumour and the presence of metastatic spread to the inguinal nodes are the most important prognostic factors.

The overall 5-year survival is approximately 50%, with 5-year disease-specific survival reported at 66% with node-negative and 27% with node-positive cases. Patients usually die of locoregional complications, as distant metastases are relatively unusual.

PRESENTATION

Most men present with an ulcerated or exophytic lesion that does not heal. The majority of lesions are seen on the glans (50–70%), followed by the prepuce (20–30%), coronal sulcus (6%) and shaft (2%). Phimotic patients may have swelling and discharge. Enlarged groin nodes are a common presenting feature.

TABLE 37.1 2002 TNM staging of penile cancer (summary)

Tis	In situ
Ta	Non-invasive verrucous carcinoma
T1	Subepithelial connective tissue
T2	Corpus spongiosum, cavernosum
T3	Urethra, prostate
T4	Other adjacent structures
N1	One superficial inguinal node
N2	Multiple or bilateral superficial inguinal
N3	Deep inguinal or pelvic

TABLE 37.2 Jackson staging system for penile cancer

Stage 1	Confined to foreskin/glans
Stage 2	Invasion of shaft
Stage 3	Operable inguinal nodes
Stage 4	Invasion of scrotum/perineum, inoperable nodes or distant metastases

DIAGNOSIS AND STAGING

Clinical examination should include careful attention to the inguinal nodes. Routine bloods including FBC, renal and liver function, and calcium are required. Biopsy for histological diagnosis is essential. Ultrasound can help define depth of invasion, particularly with regard to corpus cavernosum infiltration. Other investigations include CXR; CT scan of abdomen and pelvis to assess for metastatic disease; FNA or core biopsy of clinically palpable nodes.

Staging is by the 2002 TNM classification, although the Jackson system is also used (Tables 37.1 and 37.2).

MANAGEMENT

Premalignant conditions can be treated with local excision, Moh's surgery, laser excision, cryosurgery, or superficial RT. The options for treating invasive penile cancer include surgery, laser therapy, radiotherapy and chemotherapy. Decisions are based on the stage of the cancer and patient choice.

EARLY DISEASE (Ta–T2)

Early disease can be treated with surgery, laser therapy or radiotherapy. Lesions confined to the foreskin may require only circumcision. Laser therapy for low grade Ta–T1 tumours offers good cosmetic results. Partial penectomy with a clear margin of 2 cm (aiming to leave a functional penis, i.e. adequate micturition and penetration) is commonly performed for T1–2 tumours. Alternatively, radiotherapy may be used, particularly if sexual function is important to the patient. External beam radiotherapy (50–60 Gy in 4–6 weeks) has excellent local control rates but can cause severe skin and urethral reactions and up to 30% may develop a urethral stricture. Brachytherapy with iridium-192 wire implants is also effective. The patient should be circumcised prior to radiotherapy. Those who fail radiotherapy may be salvaged surgically. Radiotherapy is not recommended for lesions >4 cm.

The 5-year survival rates for patients with node-negative localised disease are 80%+. Concurrent chemoradiotherapy is still under evaluation and looks promising.

LOCALLY ADVANCED DISEASE (T3–4)

Total penectomy with perineal urethrostomy is usually offered to patients with proximal tumours and T3 disease. Radiotherapy may be an option for selected T3 disease. Total emasculation is performed if there is T4 disease. Neo adjuvant chemotherapy may improve outcome. Inoperable bulky disease may respond well to palliative radiotherapy and chemotherapy (cisplatin, methotrexate, bleomycin (PMB)).

MANAGEMENT OF LYMPH NODES

Decisions regarding the management of lymph nodes are highly controversial and based on the clinical involvement of inguinal nodes and the stage and grade of the primary. Around 50% of patients have palpable nodes at presentation, but only half turn out to be malignant. This is due to the high incidence of coexisting inflammatory and infective conditions that cause lymphadenopathy. Radical lymph node dissection has a mortality rate of ~3% and morbidity is high (e.g. wound infections, skin necrosis and lymphoedema).

Clinically N0 disease

Between 10% and 20% of patients with clinically negative nodes have occult micrometastatic disease. In general, patients with early stage, low grade tumours should be kept under close observation and salvaged with bilateral node dissection if necessary. Those with advanced primaries and high grade histology should undergo bilateral inguinal lymphadenectomy as these patients have the highest risk of occult disease. Prophylactic groin irradiation has not been definitely shown to prevent subsequent groin metastases.

Clinically positive nodes

These patients should undergo bilateral radical node dissection, although some surgeons prefer to treat with a course of antibiotics first to exclude infection. The role of additional pelvic node dissection remains controversial because only a few patients with positive pelvic nodes will survive long term. Patients with two or more positive nodes or nodal extracapsular spread may be offered adjuvant chemotherapy or radiotherapy in the context of clinical trials.

Fixed and inoperable nodes may be treated with neoadjuvant chemotherapy or radiotherapy followed by radical ilio-inguinal lymphadenectomy in those who respond well. Gross inoperable groin nodes sometimes respond well to palliative radiotherapy or chemotherapy.

METASTATIC DISEASE

Despite high response rates (55–70%) to PMB (cisplatin, methotrexate, bleomycin) or cisplatin and 5-FU chemotherapy, median survival is only 10 months.

FUTURE PERSPECTIVES

Current research is focused on the use of concurrent chemoradiation, new chemotherapy and immunotherapy combinations, and the role of sentinel node biopsy.

PROBLEMS IN ADVANCED PENILE CANCER

1. See Chapter 58 on problems in advanced pelvic malignancy.
2. Fungating and bleeding groin nodes. These can be very painful and distressing, but can respond well to palliative radiotherapy (e.g. 30 Gy in 10 fractions). Chemotherapy may also be of benefit. Regular dressings and antibiotics orally or topically (e.g. metronidazole gel) also help.
3. Lymphoedema. Genital and limb swelling may be gross and referral to the lymphoedema team should be made.
4. Urinary outflow obstruction. May require long-term catheterisation. Sometimes suprapubic catheterisation is required.
5. Psychological distress. Patients may need psychosexual counselling. Loss of sexual function is very common following surgery. Anxiety and depression are also common.

FURTHER READING

Hakenberg O W, Wirth M P 1999 Issues in the treatment of penile carcinoma. A short review. Urology International 62:229–233
Mobilio G M, Ficarra V 2001 Genital treatment of penile carcinoma. Current Opinion in Urology 11:299–304

CHAPTER 38

Prostate cancer

BACKGROUND INFORMATION

In the UK, prostate cancer is responsible for approximately 10 000 male deaths per year, representing the fourth largest cause of death from cancer after lung, breast and bowel cancer. In 2000, there were 27 150 new cases diagnosed in the UK. It is predominantly a disease of older age, with 85% of cases occurring over the age of 65 years. There is strong evidence suggesting an increasing incidence in the UK over the last 50 years, which cannot be explained by the ageing population alone.

The exact aetiology is unknown, but involves complex environmental and genetic factors. Black African-Americans have some of the highest prostate cancer rates in the world and are also more likely to be diagnosed with metastatic disease and have a worse stage-for-stage prognosis than Caucasians. Chinese and Japanese races have the lowest incidence. Inheritance of prostate cancer-susceptible genes (e.g. HPC-1 – hereditary prostate cancer-1 locus) is thought to account for approximately 10% of all prostate cancer cases. Occupational exposure to various chemicals may also increase prostate cancer risk, but there are few convincing examples. The role of diet is controversial, but it seems likely that the Western diet, which is high in animal fats and low in vegetables, increases the risk of prostate cancer. Vitamin E has recently been shown to have a protective effect, but the role of vitamin A remains uncertain. There is no convincing evidence that smoking or alcohol increases risk. Low testosterone levels may convey a protective effect, but the exact role of hormones in the pathogenesis of prostate cancer is unclear.

Prostatic intraepithelial neoplasia (PIN) is considered a premalignant lesion and the main precursor of carcinoma of the prostate. High grade PIN has clearly been associated with the concomitant or subsequent presence of invasive carcinoma.

Approximately 95% of prostate cancers are adenocarcinomas and most develop in the periphery of the prostate gland. Histological grading is based on the Gleason sum score. This is based on classifying the histology into five histological patterns (graded 1–5) that may vary in multiple biopsies of individual tumours. The two most prominent patterns are added together to give the Gleason score, which gives significant prognostic information. Values vary from 2 to 10, where 2 corresponds to a very well-differentiated tumour and 10 corresponds to a very poorly differentiated tumour. Patients with high scores have a much worse prognosis than those with low scores. For example, those with lower grade lesions (Gleason scores 2–4) have 2.1% yearly rate of developing metastases and 15-year survival of 94%, whereas those with higher grade lesions (Gleason scores 7–10) have a 13.5% yearly rate of developing metastases and 15-year survival of 13–58%.

Prostate cancer may spread locally to the seminal vesicles, bladder base, urethra and through the prostatic capsule into periprostatic tissue. Rectal involvement is rare due to presence of a separating fascia (Denonvilliers' fascia). Lymph node spread usually occurs initially to the obturator nodes, and then to other pelvic nodes and eventually into the para-aortic chain. Haematogenous spread most commonly involves the bones, followed by liver and lung metastases. The vast majority of bone metastases are osteoblastic (80%), with the axial skeleton most at risk.

Other primary tumour types are rare and include mucinous adenocarcinoma, transitional cell carcinoma, squamous cell carcinoma, adenosquamous carcinoma, small cell carcinomas, carcinosarcomas, lymphomas, germ cell tumours and sarcomas. Melanoma and lung cancer are the commonest cancers that metastasise to the prostate.

The natural history of prostate cancer is highly variable, often unpredictable and poorly understood. Post-mortem studies of men over 50 years dying from other diseases have revealed that 30% have microfoci of prostate cancer. However, only 10% of men will be diagnosed with prostate cancer in their lifetime and only 3% will die from the disease. It is therefore clear that many men have a latent form of prostate cancer and will not develop clinically significant disease in their lifetime and this raises important questions regarding screening and early detection of prostate cancer, and the potential for overtreatment with its associated morbidity and mortality. Parameters such as the Gleason score, initial tumour stage and PSA can help to predict those cancers that are most likely to be clinically significant and therefore require some form of treatment. Other factors such as age, potential life expectancy, co-morbidity and patient choice also need to be taken into account.

PRESENTATION AND CLINICAL FEATURES

Asymptomatic patients are increasingly being diagnosed because of increased awareness of prostate cancer and demands for PSA testing. A small number of patients (10%) are also diagnosed incidentally following transurethral resection of the prostate (TURP) for presumed benign prostatic hypertrophy (BPH). In symptomatic men the commonest presentation is with urinary outflow obstruction, i.e. increased frequency, incomplete emptying, intermittency, urgency, weak stream, straining and nocturia. Frank haematuria, incontinence, haemospermia, rectal symptoms, impotence, lymphoedema and loin pain (due to ureteric obstruction and hydronephrosis) are usually symptoms of more locally advanced disease. Bone pain, anorexia and weight loss are features of metastatic disease. Occasionally, spinal cord compression is the mode of presentation.

General examination may reveal the presence of bladder distension, lymphoedema and groin nodes. Local disease may be palpable on digital rectal examination (DRE), which can detect approximately 55% of prostate cancers. Findings may vary from palpation of a small firm peripheral nodule (T2a disease) to a grossly enlarged hard craggy fixed mass (T4 disease).

DIAGNOSIS AND STAGING

Investigations should include full clinical examination including DRE, PSA (prostate specific antigen – normal range less than 4 ng/ml), transrectal ultrasound and biopsy (covered with appropriate antibiotics), CT/MRI imaging of the abdomen and pelvis, and isotope bone scanning if PSA is greater than 20 ng/ml or Gleason grade is ⩾8. If the disease is obviously metastatic at presentation with a high PSA (e.g. >200 ng/ml), then biopsy of the prostate may be omitted.

Measurement of PSA levels is useful in diagnosis and staging, as well as monitoring for recurrent/progressive disease and response to treatment. Assays do vary as there is currently no gold standard test, but the normal range is usually 0–4 ng/ml, although slightly higher levels are normal with increasing age. PSA is not specific to prostate cancer and may be elevated in benign conditions such as prostatic hyperplasia and prostatitis. Following successful radical prostatectomy, PSA levels should be undetectable within 3–4 weeks. If PSA levels remain detectable following surgery then treatment failure is highly likely. Following radical radiotherapy, the PSA may take several months to reach its nadir. Patients that achieve a PSA nadir of less than 1–1.5 ng/ml are more likely to become long-term disease-free survivors. Following hormonal manipulation of metastatic disease, those patients who achieve a nadir PSA of less than 4 ng/ml have a significantly longer duration of remission than those who do not reach this level.

Great controversy still exists regarding screening for prostate cancer with PSA testing and transrectal ultrasound. It remains subject to large European clinical trials.

Staging is by the 2002 TNM system (Table 38.1).

TABLE 38.1 2002 TNM staging of prostate cancer

T1	Clinically inapparent, not palpable or visible on imaging
T1a	Incidental finding, involving ≤5% of resected tissue
T1b	Incidental finding, involving >5% of resected tissue
T1c	Needle biopsy positive
T2	Tumour confined to prostate
T2a	One half of one lobe involved
T2b	More than one half of one lobe involved
T2c	Both lobes involved
T3	Tumour invades through prostatic capsule
T3a	Extracapsular spread
T3b	Invasion of seminal vesicle(s)
T4	Tumour fixed or invades adjacent structures other than seminal vesicles (bladder neck, external sphincter, rectum, levator muscles or pelvic wall)
N1	Regional node(s), i.e. below bifurcation of common iliac arteries
M1a	Non-regional node(s)
M1b	Bone(s)
M1c	Other site(s)

MANAGEMENT

EARLY LOCALISED DISEASE (T1–2 (SOME T3), N0, M0)

The management of early prostate cancer is one of the most controversial topics in oncology and accurate diagnosis and staging are required to help select the most appropriate treatment modality. Over the past decade, there has been a significant downward shift in the stage of presentation of prostate cancer, mainly due to increased awareness and increased use of the serum marker PSA. Many patients are now presenting at an earlier stage with clinically localised disease.

On the current available evidence from the literature, the optimum treatment policy for early localised prostate cancer is unknown. The four main options include:

1. Surgery – radical prostatectomy
2. Radiotherapy – radical external beam radiotherapy or brachytherapy
3. Surveillance – (a) 'watchful waiting', or (b) active surveillance
4. Hormone therapy.

Important considerations in deciding the type of treatment include the clinical stage and grade of the tumour, PSA level, and patient factors such as performance status, age, medical co-morbidity, prostate size, erectile function and personal choice. Treatment failure is more likely in patients with higher pretreatment Gleason scores, PSA scores and clinical stages (Table 38.2).

The patient needs to be fully informed about the possible options and made aware of the potential side effects of all the management modalities.

TABLE 38.2 Risk of recurrent disease following local therapy based on pretreatment Gleason score, PSA and stage

Risk group	Recurrence rate following local therapy (%)
Low. PSA <10, Gleason ≤6, T1, 2a	6–20
Intermediate. PSA 10–20, Gleason 7, T2b, T3a	34–60
High. PSA >20, Gleason 8–10, T3b	50–100

Surveillance

Most men diagnosed with early prostate cancer will die from other causes. For example, the predicted 15-year prostate cancer mortality for men with Gleason score 6 tumours is approximately 10%, whereas the mortality rate from other causes is 40–76%. Immediate radical treatment is therefore only likely to have a small impact on survival, but may cause significant long-term side effects. For this reason, surveillance rather than immediate radical treatment should be a management option. There are two main approaches to surveillance: (a) 'watchful waiting' and (b) active surveillance.

(a) 'Watchful waiting' Patients with factors such as older age (>70 years), low Gleason scores (≤7), medical co-morbidity and life expectancy of less than 10–15 years are likely to be offered a conservative watch and wait policy rather than radical treatment. The aim of this approach is to avoid any treatment if possible. Palliative treatment (e.g. hormonal therapy and palliative radiotherapy) is offered for those who develop symptomatic progressive disease.

(b) Active surveillance This is a relatively new concept with the aim of trying to individualise treatment. It is a suitable option for patients aged 50–80, otherwise fit for radical treatment, who have early stage disease (T1–2), Gleason scores ≤7, and initial PSA <15. Patients are carefully monitored with frequent PSA testing, DRE and repeat prostate biopsies. Those with short PSA doubling times or upgraded histology (i.e. higher Gleason scores) are offered early radical treatment. It is estimated that this approach may spare up to two-thirds of early prostate cancer patients from radical treatment without affecting overall survival. However, as the optimum active surveillance policy is unknown, further research is ongoing in this field.

Surgery – radical prostatectomy

Surgery is an option for men with T1–2, N0 tumours with low–moderate Gleason scores and a life expectancy of 10 years or more. Occasionally, highly selected patients with T3 disease or minimal local lymph node metastases are also offered surgery. Radical retropubic prostatectomy is the most widely used technique and involves complete excision of the prostate, seminal vesicles and adjacent tissue. A bilateral pelvic lymphadenectomy is also generally performed. Newer nerve-sparing techniques, as pioneered by

Walsh, are safer and reduce blood loss, impotence and incontinence rates. Surgery carries a mortality rate of 0.3%, incontinence rate of 10–20%, and impotence rate of 10–90% – with average of 30% (depending on age, stage and surgical centre). Before the Walsh technique was developed, impotence rates approached 100%. Other complications include urethral stricture (2–5%), rectal injury (<1%) and bleeding.

The 10-year crude survival following radical prostatectomy is 70–84% with a cause-specific survival of 90–94%. Disease-free survival at 10 years is 72–78%. PSA progression-free survival at 5 years is 59–83% and at 10 years is 47–74%. The role of adjuvant hormonal therapy and adjuvant radiotherapy is uncertain at present.

External beam radiotherapy (EBRT)

In the UK, EBRT is the most frequently used modality for treatment of localised prostate cancer. The development of CT-planned conformal radiotherapy has allowed more accurate targeting of the prostate and has reduced the volume of excess normal tissues treated by 50% compared to older techniques, and this has translated clinically into reduced side effects. Current schedules in the UK use 55–70 Gy in 20–35 fractions over 4–7 weeks, but there are ongoing multicentre studies assessing higher doses (70–78 Gy) in view of the improved side effect profile of conformal radiotherapy and encouraging dose–response effects seen in earlier studies. A recent dose escalation study using intensity-modulated radiotherapy (IMRT) confirmed a low rate of complications using doses up to 81 Gy.

Another recent development has been in the use of neoadjuvant and adjuvant hormonal therapy with radiotherapy. Improvements in survival have been seen for patients with poorly differentiated tumours (Gleason 8–10), T3 tumours and node-positive disease. It has therefore become common practice to offer hormonal therapy neoadjuvantly for 3–6 months and adjuvantly for up to 3 years, to these higher risk patient groups. The optimum duration of adjuvant hormone therapy is unknown.

The 10-year disease-specific survival for localised prostate cancer following RT is ~60–85%.

Acute side effects of EBRT include fatigue, proctitis causing increased frequency of bowel movements, and urinary frequency and urgency. EBRT also carries an incontinence risk of <1% and impotence risk of 30–50% (depends on age and other risk factors including diabetes and hypertension). Sildenafil (Viagra) is often helpful for impotence following EBRT. Late chronic radiation proctitis occurs in less than 5% of patients with only 1–2% developing severe symptoms. Other uncommon late complications include chronic cystitis, haematuria and urethral strictures.

Prostate brachytherapy

Prostate brachytherapy involves placing radioactive implants into the prostate gland. This may be achieved using permanent radioactive seeds (the most commonly used method) or temporary implants via a microselectron machine. This type of therapy offers the obvious advantage of delivering a very high dose to the prostate gland whilst sparing adjacent tissues.

Permanent radioactive seeds are inserted by the transperineal route under transrectal ultrasound guidance. The usual radioactive source is iodine-125 in the UK, but palladium-103 can also be used. The minimum dose delivered to the prostate capsule plus a margin of 2–3 mm is 145 Gy. Approximately 50% of the prostate may receive more than 150% of this dose.

The procedure is most suitable for prostate cancer patients with the following characteristics: (1) Gleason scores ≤6, (2) PSA <10 ng/ml, (3) stage T1–2, (4) good urinary function and (5) prostate volumes less than 40 ml. Outcomes for this group of patients are excellent, with freedom from PSA relapse of 80% at 5 years and 70% at 10 years.

Side effects of brachytherapy include transient urethritis in all patients, impotence (30%), incontinence (1%) and proctitis (usually transient). Approximately 15% will develop acute retention of urine following the procedure, requiring temporary catheterisation. About 2–3% of patients still have significant urinary symptoms at 1 year.

Hormone therapy alone

Early hormonal therapy can delay local interventions for prostate cancer (e.g. the need for radiotherapy), but is not curative when used alone. Hormone therapy alone is most likely to be offered to patients with higher presenting PSA levels and Gleason scores of 8–10.

LOCALLY ADVANCED DISEASE (T3–4, N0–1, M0)

The main options include: external beam radiotherapy with neoadjuvant and adjuvant hormone therapy (see above), hormone therapy only, surveillance, or entry into clinical trials. Surgery may also be an option for selected patients with T3 disease.

The 10-year survival rates for patients with T3 disease treated with radiotherapy and hormonal therapy are approximately 35%. The survival for T4 disease is less impressive with 15% 10-year survival.

METASTATIC DISEASE (T ANY, N1 OR M1)

Approximately 75–80% of patients with metastatic prostate cancer will respond to hormone therapy. Asymptomatic patients with a PSA greater than 50 should also be considered for therapy. The median response time is 18–24 months for first line therapy and 6–10 months for second line therapy, although more recent data have suggested longer response times. Overall, patients with metastatic disease have a median survival of 3–4 years and 30% are still alive at 5 years.

First line treatment is with androgen deprivation. Medical castration by luteinising hormone releasing hormone (LHRH) agonists is currently the most common way of achieving androgen deprivation, but bilateral orchidectomy is another equally effective option. LHRH agonists initially cause stimulation of hypothalamic LHRH secretion before downregulating hypothalamic receptors. This leads to the initial tumour flare response (noticed clinically in 1.2% of patients), which may be avoided by starting an anti-androgen a week before and continuing for 2 weeks after commencing the LHRH agonist.

Non-steroidal anti-androgens include flutamide (250 mg t.d.s.) and bicalutamide (50 mg o.d.) and both are licensed for use in conjunction with LHRH agonists in the treatment of metastatic disease. Flutamide is also licensed for use as monotherapy. These drugs block androgen receptors so LH production continues, causing testosterone levels to actually increase. Many patients can therefore retain libido and potency if not already on LHRH agonists. However, due to high oestradiol levels, gynaecomastia may be a problem. Withdrawal of anti-androgens should be considered in patients with progressive disease because this action produces a PSA reduction in 20% of patients with a median response time of 3.5–5 months.

The steroidal anti-androgen cyproterone acetate (200–300 mg daily) is a progesterone derivative that blocks and decreases the number of androgen receptors. It is now less frequently used due to its potential hepatotoxicity. Side effects include decreased libido, impotence and fluid retention.

Oestrogen derivatives are also used in metastatic disease and include diethylstilbestrol (1–3 mg o.d.) and fosfestrol. They cause negative feedback on the hypothalamus, leading to diminished LH production. Unfortunately, although extremely effective in high dosage, they can cause an excess of cardiovascular fatal and non-fatal events as well as gynaecomastia (40% of patients) and they are generally reserved as second and third line therapy. They are often combined with aspirin to reduce thrombotic risk.

Maximum androgen blockade (MAB) refers to the combination of LHRH agonists with anti-androgens with the aim of decreasing testosterone production at both the testicular and adrenal levels. However, the survival benefits of this approach are marginal and mainly seen in younger patients with a lower tumour burden. It has not become standard practice.

Intermittent androgen blockade. This involves withdrawal of androgen blockade following a clinical response with reintroduction of therapy on clinical progression. The aim is to delay the onset of androgen refractoriness and reduce side effects of treatment. It is not standard practice at present as it is still undergoing clinical trials.

(See also section on problems in advanced prostate cancer, below.)

HORMONE REFRACTORY PROSTATE CANCER (HRPC)

HRPC refers to progressive disease despite castrate levels of serum testosterone. HRPC sometimes responds to dexamethasone (1.5–2 mg), prednisolone (5 mg o.d.) or hydrocortisone (30 mg daily). Chemotherapy is of limited value. Mitoxantrone and prednisolone are sometimes used in symptomatic patients with good performance status and produce palliation of symptoms in ~30% of cases with a median response time of 10 months. Taxanes have also been used with limited success. Median survival for patients with HRPC is only 1 year (see section on problems in advanced prostate cancer, below).

FUTURE PERSPECTIVES

The role of chemoprevention is still in its infancy, but clinical trials with 5α-reductase inhibitors (e.g. finasteride), selenium, vitamin E and aromatase inhibitors are ongoing. Radiotherapy dose escalation studies with conformal and IMRT techniques continue. Some centres are now combining external beam radiotherapy with brachytherapy to obtain further dose intensification. In high risk localised prostate cancer, the role of pelvic nodal irradiation and the role of hormone therapy in relation to radiotherapy continues to be evaluated (e.g. MRC PR07 trial). In the metastatic setting, intermittent hormone therapy trials are currently maturing and early results are encouraging. Newer chemotherapy agents such as the taxanes and molecular targeted therapies are also being evaluated.

PROBLEMS IN ADVANCED PROSTATE CANCER

1. Bone pain (see also Ch. 48 on bone metastases). Can be treated with external beam radiotherapy to very good effect with a response rate of 80%. Widespread pain can be treated with strontium-89 injections (which may be repeated) or wide field irradiation (requiring anti-emetic cover). IV bisphosphonates or IV fosfestrol for 5 days may also be helpful.
2. Urinary prostatism. Starting hormonal treatment may help; otherwise consider using alpha blockers (e.g. tamsulosin hydrochloride 400 μg o.d.) if there are urinary obstructive symptoms or antimuscarinics if there are problems with incontinence and urinary frequency (e.g. oxybutynin 5 mg b.d.–t.d.s.). TURP may be required if symptoms are very severe. If patient has had brachytherapy, TURP should be avoided if possible or delayed for at least 1 year due to the risk of urinary incontinence.
3. Impotence. Very common after treatment for prostate cancer. Consider using non-steroidal anti-androgens instead of LHRH analogues. Try sildenafil (Viagra) 25–100 mg 1 hour prior to intercourse. Other options include apomorphine (2 mg sublingually) and intracavernosal or intraurethral injection of prostaglandin E1 (alprostadil).

4. Anaemia and thrombocytopenia. Due to marrow infiltration or gross haematuria. May need repeated transfusions.
5. Haematuria and perineal pain. Can be treated with palliative radiotherapy, e.g. single 10 Gy, 20 Gy in 5 fractions, or 30 Gy in 10 fractions.
6. Lymphoedema. Due to extensive nodal disease, may be treated with compression therapy (bandaging, elastic stockings, exercises, skin massage). Nodal disease may be treated with radiotherapy.
7. Spinal cord compression (see Ch. 60 on spinal cord compression).
8. Pathological fractures (see also Ch. 48 on bone metastases). Plain X-rays should be taken of long bones which have shown increased uptake on isotope bone scans. Prophylactic nailing may prevent fractures of unstable or lytic lesions. IV bisphosphonates have also been shown to reduce the risk of pathological fracture.
9. Hypercalcaemia (see also Ch. 56 on metabolic problems). Very uncommon in prostate cancer despite high prevalence of bone metastases.
10. Obstructive uropathy. Treat with urethral Foley catheter if possible, otherwise consider suprapubic catheter. Stenting or nephrostomy may be required if there is obstruction of the ureters, but this may not be appropriate in extremely advanced and distressing disease.
11. Hot flushes. Due to androgen withdrawal, may be treated with megestrol acetate 20 mg b.d. with up to 80% of men reporting at least a 50% reduction in hot flushes. Transdermal estradiol patches (50 μg/24 hours) or cyproterone acetate 50–100 mg b.d. may also be helpful. Clonidine and venlafaxine have also been used.
12. Gynaecomastia. Caused by disturbances between the ratio of oestrogens and androgens within the body and is most commonly encountered with the use of the non-steroidal anti-androgens and diethylstilbestrol. It is often associated with mastodynia (painful breast). Low dose radiotherapy (single 8 Gy fraction of electrons to the breast bud) is commonly used for treatment and prophylaxis. Prophylactic RT reduced the frequency of gynaecomastia from 67% to 28% in a recent large flutamide trial. Radiotherapy treatment of established gynaecomastia reduces pain and discomfort in most patients, but has little effect on breast size. Surgery (mammoplasty) is reserved for patients with advanced gynaecomastia, with fibrosis and chronic or irreversible changes of breast tissue.
13. Inflammatory syndrome. This is an end-stage syndrome of fever and weight loss. Corticosteroids and diethylstilbestrol may be of some palliative benefit.

FURTHER READING

COIN/BAUS. Guidelines on the management of prostate cancer. Available at: www.rcr.ac.uk
Jani A B, Hellman S 2003 Early prostate cancer: clinical decision making. Lancet 361(22 March):1045–1053

Kantoff P, Wishnow K I, Loughlin K R (eds) 1997 Prostate cancer. A multidisciplinary guide. Blackwell Science, Oxford

Kirkby R S, Christmas T J, Brawer M K 2001 Prostate cancer, 2nd edn. Mosby, Edinburgh

Parker C 2003 The natural history of early prostate cancer and the rationale for active surveillance. Cancer Topics 11(12):10–12

Wallace D M, Oliver R T D, Ash D, Miles A 2002 UK key advances in clinical practice series. The effective management of prostate cancer. Aesculapius Medical Press, London

Renal cancer

BACKGROUND INFORMATION

Renal cancer accounts for 2–3% of all cancers in the UK with 6200 new cases registered in 2000. In 2002, there were 3360 deaths attributable to this disease. It is more common in men than women (2 : 1 ratio) and is predominantly seen after the age of 50 with a mean age at diagnosis of 70 years. There has been a constant increase in incidence over the last 50 years mainly due to enhanced detection of tumours by greater use of imaging modalities such as ultrasound and CT.

Early stage renal cancer is localised and resectable, with a 10-year disease-free survival rate of ~40%. Unfortunately, 40–50% present with advanced regional or metastatic disease with a 5-year survival of no more than 35% depending on the stage of disease. Renal cancer is one of the few tumours that may undergo spontaneous remission, but this is very rare and usually occurs post-nephrectomy. Bilateral tumours account for 2–3% of cases.

The aetiology of renal cancer is not clear, but it is associated with smoking (×5 risk), obesity, hypertension and Von Hippel–Lindau (VHL) disease. Advances in molecular medicine have shown the importance of the VHL tumour suppressor gene, which is located on chromosome 3. In more than 90% of renal tumours, there are deletions or translocations involving chromosome 3 in the region of the VHL gene.

Pathologically, renal cell (clear cell) carcinoma (RCC) accounts for ~80% of renal cancer. Other cell types are granular, sarcomatoid, papillary and chromophobe. Urothelial transitional cell carcinoma of the renal pelvis accounts for 5–10% of primary renal cancers. RCC characteristically grows into the renal veins and may extend as tumour thrombus into the vena cava and even up into the right atrium. Invasion of renal veins is associated with remote metastases in 75% of cases. The commonest sites for metastatic spread are bone, lung, brain, liver and skin.

PRESENTATION

Most patients present with painless haematuria, but up to 40% of patients are now diagnosed incidentally following ultrasound examination or CT scanning. Microcytic anaemia due to haematuria or haemolysis is common. The classic triad of haematuria, loin pain and a renal mass is uncommon (<10%).

About 10% of patients present with paraneoplastic syndromes that include hypertension, polycythaemia, hypercalcaemia, anaemia, pyrexias and hormone secretion (e.g. Cushing's, excess gonadotrophins causing masculinisation or feminisation). Approximately 25% present with metastatic disease and so may have symptoms and signs related to distant metastases.

DIAGNOSIS AND STAGING

Investigations should include: history/examination, renal and liver function tests, calcium, FBC, ESR, CXR to assess pulmonary spread. Intravenous urogram (IVU) is commonly used in the initial investigation of haematuria. Renal ultrasound (US) is helpful in differentiating between cysts and solid masses. Abdominal CT scanning with and without contrast is the imaging modality of choice for renal cancer diagnosis and staging. MRI or inferior vena cava venography may be helpful when there is uncertainty regarding the degree of vena cava involvement, which may be crucial for surgical

TABLE 39.1 2002 TNM staging of renal cancer

T1	≤7 cm, limited to kidney
T1a	≤4 cm
T1b	>4 cm ≤7 cm
T2	>7 cm, limited to kidney
T3	Into major veins, adrenal or perinephric invasion, but not beyond Gerota's fascia
T3a	Invades adrenal or perinephric tissues
T3b	Extends into renal vein or vena cava below diaphragm
T3c	Extends into vena cava above diaphragm
T4	Invades beyond Gerota's fascia
N1	Single regional node
N2	More than one regional node
M1	Distant metastases
Stage I	T1, N0
Stage II	T2, N0
Stage III	T1/2/3, N1; or T3, N0
Stage IV	T4; or any T, N2; or any T, any N, M1

planning. Biopsy of the primary tumour is generally avoided because of the risk of severe haemorrhage and tumour seeding.

Other investigations such as bone scans and chest CT are only required if there is clinical suspicion of metastatic disease.

Staging is based on the 2002 TNM classification (Table 39.1).

MANAGEMENT

LOCALISED DISEASE (STAGES I–III)

Surgery offers the only chance of cure in localised disease. Radical nephrectomy with or without lymphadenectomy is the treatment of choice and offers 5-year survival of approximately 65%. This involves removal of the kidney, adrenal gland, perinephric fat and Gerota's fascia. In more locally advanced tumours, renal vein and vena cava resection is also employed. The effectiveness of lymphadenectomy has not been proven and this practice varies between centres. In selected cases partial nephrectomy can be performed (e.g. small tumours <4 cm, bilateral tumours, poor renal function, patients with one kidney). Those medically or technically unfit for surgery may receive arterial embolisation.

There is no proven effective adjuvant therapy, but trials with immuno-modulating drugs such as interferon (IFN) and interleukin-2 (IL-2) are ongoing. The role of adjuvant radiotherapy for high-risk patients requires further evaluation.

ADVANCED DISEASE (STAGE IV)

Nearly all of these patients are incurable. Median survival in this group is 12–24 months, although the range of survival is wide. Nephrectomy, radiotherapy and embolisation can aid in palliation of local symptoms and related paraneoplastic syndromes such as ectopic hormone secretion. There is some evidence that nephrectomy may induce regression of distant metastases, but this is a rare event. Another potential benefit of nephrectomy in the metastatic setting is to reduce tumour burden prior to immunotherapy.

Selected patients with solitary metastases may undergo nephrectomy and metastasectomy to achieve prolonged survival. The chances of benefit improve if there is a long disease-free interval between nephrectomy and the development of the metastasis. Five-year survival of over 20% has been reported.

Unfortunately, renal cancer is a chemoresistant disease (in part due to high expression of the MDR (multidrug resistance) gene product) and response rates to various schedules do not exceed 10%. For this reason and because of the occasional spontaneous regressions, immunotherapy has been the main focus in renal cancer trials. Single agent interferon alpha (5–20 MU s.c. three times per week) is commonly used and has response rates of 15–20%. The main side effects are fatigue and a flu-like syndrome that may be extremely debilitating for some patients. Single agent interleukin-2 (IL-2) also has response rates of 10–20%. Combinations of IFN and IL-2 have shown response rates of up to 32%. IL-2 has also been combined with lymphokine activated killer (LAK) cells to produce response rates of 33%. However, IL-2 (especially when given intravenously) has toxic side effects, which include a capillary leak syndrome that may lead to shock and multi-organ failure. Another regimen, described by Atzpodien, involves an 8-week course of treatment with IFN, IL-2 and 5FU and showed a response rate of 39%. This regimen is being evaluated further in the MRC RE04 trial. Highest responses are generally seen in patients with low tumour burden and no CNS or bone metastases.

Hormone manipulation is also used in renal cancer. Megestrol acetate has response rates of less than 10%, but is often used in patients thought too unwell to tolerate immunotherapy. It can increase the feeling of well-being and improve appetite.

Radiotherapy is used in the palliative setting only.

FUTURE PERSPECTIVES

The current MRC RE04 trial is a randomised phase III trial of IFN-α, IL-2 and 5FU versus IFN-α alone in metastatic renal cancer. There are ongoing trials with angiogenesis inhibitors including thalidomide. Other studies in the metastatic setting are evaluating antibody and tumour vaccine therapies. Adjuvant studies with chemo-immunotherapy are ongoing (e.g. EORTC 30955). Possibly one of the most interesting approaches is the use of non-myeloablative allogenic peripheral-blood stem-cell transplantation in metastatic disease, which essentially induces a graft-versus-tumour effect. Response rates of 53% were seen in one small trial in patients who had not responded to conventional treatment and further evaluation is required.

PROBLEMS IN ADVANCED DISEASE

1. Localised symptoms from primary tumour. May be controlled by either surgical resection, tumour embolisation or occasionally local radiotherapy.
2. Haematuria. Can respond to palliative radiotherapy to kidney, e.g. single 8 Gy fraction. Tranexamic acid may also be helpful.

3. Bone pain (see Ch. 48 on bone metastases). Responds well to palliative radiotherapy.
4. Post-infarction syndrome. Following embolisation, patients may experience severe pain, fever, leucocytosis and paralytic ileus. This usually settles after a few days with supportive measures (analgesics, anti-pyretics).
5. Brain metastases (see Ch. 49 on brain metastases).
6. Hypercalcaemia (see Ch. 56 on metabolic problems in cancer). Treat with IV fluids and bisphosphonates.

FURTHER READING

Childs R, Chernoff A, Contentin N et al 2000 Regression of metastatic renal cell carcinoma after non-myeloablative allogenic peripheral blood stem-cell transplantation. New England Journal of Medicine 343:750–758
Wolchok J D, Motzer R J 2000 Management of renal cell cancer. Oncology 14(1):29–34

Sarcomas of bone

BACKGROUND INFORMATION

Bone sarcomas are very rare tumours, which are seen more commonly in children than in adults. There are approximately 350 new cases per year in the UK. Osteosarcoma is the commonest bone sarcoma, accounting for 20% of this group of tumours, with an incidence of 3 per million population. Its highest incidence is in adolescence and old age. Causal risk factors include Paget's disease or previously irradiated tissue. Chondrosarcomas and fibrosarcoma/ malignant fibrous histiocytoma (MFH) are the other main types seen in adults.

Low grade tumours generally have a good prognosis (~90% 5-year survival), whilst those with high grade disease have a 5-year survival of 50–75% with multi-modality therapy. Patients who develop a sarcoma associated with Paget's disease have a particularly poor prognosis. Resectability is the most important prognostic factor and therefore tumours of the axial skeleton have the worst prognosis. The lung is the initial site for metastatic disease in 90% of cases.

Ewing's sarcoma (a primitive neuroectodermal tumour – PNET) is mainly seen in adolescents and is treated with multi-modality therapy.

PRESENTATION

Most patients present with local pain and swelling, which may be associated with a joint effusion. Any unexplained pain or swelling in the limb of a teenager must arouse suspicion. Mobility may be affected. Pathological fracture is occasionally the presenting complaint.

DIAGNOSIS AND STAGING

Investigations should include history and examination; CXR; plain X-rays of affected bone; CT of the primary lesion and chest. MRI is useful for

TABLE 40.1 Musculoskeletal Tumour Society (Enneking) staging system for bone sarcomas (does not include Ewing's)

Stage	Grade	Site
IA	Low grade	Intracompartmental
IB	Low grade	Extracompartmental
IIA	High grade	Intracompartmental
IIB	High grade	Extracompartmental
III	Local or distant metastases	Any

delineating soft tissue extension and presence of skip metastases, as is bone scan to assess for distant metastases. Percutaneous Trucut or open biopsy may be used to obtain histological diagnosis.

There is no universally accepted staging system, but the Musculoskeletal Tumour Society (Enneking) system is one example in clinical use (Table 40.1).

MANAGEMENT

A multi-modality approach is required for high grade lesions. Neoadjuvant chemotherapy (cisplatin/doxorubicin) followed by surgical resection and then further chemotherapy is the mainstay of treatment. Wide excision of the tumour, preferably with limb salvage (often requiring metallic endoprostheses or bone allografts), will offer good local control. Limb salvage can be offered in 70–80% of cases. Patients with a limited number of lung metastases may undergo primary treatment and metastasectomy with 5-year survival of 15–20%. Patients with advanced disease at presentation should be offered chemotherapy and then surgery if a good response is seen. Radiotherapy has a limited role, as these tumours are very radioresistant. It may be used for disease that is incompletely resected or in the palliative setting for painful bony metastases.

Chondrosarcomas are both chemo- and radioresistant and surgery alone is the mainstay of treatment.

EWING'S SARCOMA

Ewing's sarcoma is a rare bone tumour with a peak incidence in the early teenage years. Pathologically it is closely related to the primitive neuroectodermal tumour (PNET) family of tumours. Ewing's sarcoma arising in soft tissue is known as a peripheral primitive neuroectodermal tumour (PPNET) and is treated in the same way.

The majority occur in the long bones (60%), with the remaining 40% occurring in the flat bones, ribs and vertebrae. The commonest presenting symptom is pain and swelling of the affected area. Generalised symptoms of weight loss, fever and fatigue may also occur. Around a quarter of patients have detectable metastases (usually lung) at presentation.

Treatment requires a multidisciplinary approach with chemotherapy, surgery and radiotherapy. Combination chemotherapy is used both neoadjuvantly and following surgery and radiotherapy. Enhanced endoprosthetic surgical techniques have improved functional outcome. Patients with inoperable tumours or positive resection margins require radiotherapy. Whole lung radiotherapy is also used for patients with lung metastases.

Overall 5-year survival is around 55–65%. Those with localised disease have a 75–90% survival rate compared to 10–20% for those with metastatic disease.

FUTURE PERSPECTIVES

Current research is focused on high dose chemotherapy regimens with bone marrow or stem cell transplantation, the use of trastuzumab (Herceptin) in HER-2 expressing tumours, and improving surgical techniques in limb sparing surgery.

PROBLEMS IN ADVANCED DISEASE

1. Loss of limb function. Mainly due to the painful effects of local disease and as a result of previous surgery. Palliative radiotherapy is useful for pain control.
2. Lung metastases (see Ch. 59 on pulmonary metastases).

FURTHER READING

Dorfman H D, Czerniak B 1997 Bone cancers. Cancer 75:203–210

CHAPTER 41

Sarcomas of soft tissue – adult

BACKGROUND INFORMATION

Adult soft tissue sarcomas represent a rare and heterogeneous group of tumours, which has made the study and understanding of this disease difficult. There are around 1000 new cases in the UK per year with an incidence of 2 per 100 000. Around 50% of these patients will die of the disease.

Sarcomas mostly arise from mesenchymal tissue and therefore can occur in any site throughout the body. Around 50% arise in the extremities (two-thirds lower limbs, one-third upper limbs), 30% intra-abdominally (visceral and retroperitoneal), 10% trunk and 10% in other sites. The aetiology is not clear and most cases are sporadic. However, alterations in tumour suppressor genes (p53 and RB-1) are common in sarcomas, suggesting abnormalities in cell cycle regulation are important. Chromosomal aberrations are seen in virtually all sarcomas. They are also more common in genetic diseases such as neurofibromatosis and Li–Fraumeni syndrome. Ionising radiation and chemicals such as dioxins and vinyl chloride are known risk factors.

Pathologically, there are many histological types of sarcoma, but the commonest include malignant fibrous histiocytoma (MFH) (30%), liposarcoma (12%), leiomyosarcoma (10%), synovial sarcoma (6%), fibrosarcoma (5%) and rhabdomyosarcoma (more common in children) (5%). There is no universally accepted grading system, but in Europe, the Trojani grading system is commonly employed. This uses three grades (1–3), which correspond to low, intermediate and high grade depending on the degree of necrosis, mitotic index and degree of morphological differentiation. Sarcomas tend to be locally invasive and spread along fascial planes. Distant spread is by the haematogenous route and lung metastases are the commonest metastatic site. Lymph node metastases are uncommon.

Poor prognostic factors include age >60 years, tumour size >5 cm, high histological grade and advanced stage. Retroperitoneal sarcomas often have a worse prognosis due to their location and later presentation (and therefore often larger size), leading to greater difficulty in complete surgical resection.

PRESENTATION

Soft tissue sarcomas most commonly present as painless, enlarging masses. Unfortunately misdiagnosis and late presentation is common probably because of the fact that the ratio of benign to malignant masses is 100:1. Deepness, firmness, fixity, rapid growth and size >5 cm are worrying signs. If symptoms do occur they are usually related to mass effects such as nerve and vascular compression producing pain, venous engorgement and lymphoedema, or visceral compression causing ureteric or bowel obstruction etc.

DIAGNOSIS AND STAGING

Investigations should include: history and examination; CXR; ultrasound of primary lesion; MRI/CT of primary lesion. MRI gives better definition

TABLE 41.1 2002 TNM staging of soft tissue sarcomas	
TX	Primary tumour cannot be assessed
T0	No evidence of primary tumour
T1	Tumour 5.0 cm or less in greatest dimension
T1a	Superficial tumour
T1b	Deep tumour[a]
T2	Tumour more than 5.0 cm in greatest dimension
T2a	Superficial tumour
T2b	Deep tumour[a]
NX	Regional lymph nodes cannot be assessed
N0	No regional lymph node metastases
N1	Regional lymph node metastases
MX	Presence of distant metastases cannot be assessed
M0	No distant metastases
M1	Distant metastases
Stage IA	T1a/b, N0, M0, low grade
Stage IB	T2a/b, N0, M0 low grade
Stage IIA	T1a/b, N0, M0 high grade
Stage IIB	T2a, N0, M0 high grade
Stage III	T2b, N0, M0, high grade
Stage IV	Any T, N1, any grade; or any T, any N, M1, any grade

[a] Deep tumours are either beneath superficial fascia or invade through fascia. Retroperitoneal, mediastinal and pelvic sarcomas are classified as deep tumours.

between muscles, fat and vessels. CT of the chest should be done to exclude pulmonary metastases. Incisional open biopsy or Trucut core biopsy are preferred to FNA for obtaining a histological diagnosis.

Staging is based on the 2002 TNM system (Table 41.1) and incorporates the histological tumour grade.

MANAGEMENT

Patients should be referred to a specialist multidisciplinary centre.

SURGERY

Surgery is the mainstay of treatment. For low grade localised tumours (stage I), adequate complete wide en bloc surgical excision alone gives >90% 5-year survival. The need for amputation is now rare, with limb-sparing operations with reconstruction (e.g. free flaps) being possible in 95% of operable cases. In higher grade tumours (stages II/III), the local recurrence rates are much higher for limb-preserving surgery alone and therefore these patients should have postoperative radiotherapy.

The 5-year survival rates for stage II disease are 70%, but only 20–50% for stage III. In patients with local nodal disease (stage IIIA), surgical resection of the primary and lymphadenectomy followed by radiotherapy is the treatment of choice if technically feasible. Five-year survival in this group of patients is poor (<20%). Patients with stage IVB pulmonary disease at presentation with operable lung metastases have a chance (~30%) of cure and should be offered surgery. The role of surgery for liver metastases is less clear in terms of survival benefits.

RADIOTHERAPY

Postoperative radiotherapy plays a major role as an adjunct to surgery in improving local tumour control compared to surgery alone. For completely resected tumours, the local recurrence rate is reduced from approximately 30–40% to 10%, with some evidence that this is also translated into a small overall survival benefit. This approach is regarded as an alternative to amputation. The general indications for postoperative radiotherapy include all grade 2 and 3 sarcomas and incompletely resected disease. A dose of 60–64 Gy in 30–32 fractions over 6–7 weeks is usually given. Careful CT planning and a 'shrinking field' technique minimise the risk of late side effects, such as lymphoedema and fibrosis.

Occasionally primary radical radiotherapy may be offered to medically inoperable patients with curative intent. Technically inoperable tumours may benefit from palliative radiotherapy. Radiotherapy is also employed for treatment of locally recurrent grade 1 disease.

CHEMOTHERAPY

The most active agents are doxorubicin, ifosfamide and DTIC, with single agent response rates of 20–30%. The role of adjuvant chemotherapy is controversial and is not standard practice at present. A large multicentre study is currently re-addressing this issue. The main role of chemotherapy is in the palliative setting. Both single agent and combination chemotherapy (e.g. doxorubicin + ifosfamide) regimens can be used. Current practice is to use single agent doxorubicin as there is no survival advantage gained with combination therapy. However, better partial response rates are seen with combination therapy and this may be useful in situations where bulk disease is directly contributing to the patient's symptoms. Patients should be offered entry into clinical trials assessing new agents and combinations.

RECURRENT DISEASE

This does not preclude cure. In locally recurrent disease, further resection followed by radiotherapy if possible is the treatment of choice. Patients who develop resectable lung metastases (up to five lesions) have a 5-year survival of 20–35%. Prognostic factors include completeness of resection, number of nodules, histology and disease-free interval. Repeated metastasectomy also offers the chance of cure in selected patients.

HEAD AND NECK DISEASE

Although patients often present with smaller tumours in the head and neck, they are not amenable to wide excisions due to anatomical constraints. For this reason adjuvant radiotherapy is required to improve local control. Five-year survival is ~50%, and despite radiotherapy, most patients die from local disease.

RETROPERITONEAL SARCOMA

These tumours are often large and slow growing. Complete surgical resection is the treatment of choice but is possible in less than 50% of cases. High grade lesions have a high risk of local (and distant) recurrence. Adjuvant radiotherapy is difficult to administer due to the high risk of bowel toxicity and the often large volumes that need to be treated. Insertion of tissue expanders at surgery can reduce the amount of bowel in the radiation field. Overall prognosis in this group of patients is poor.

FUTURE PERSPECTIVES

Current research is centred on the role of adjuvant and neoadjuvant chemotherapy. Biological therapies with cytokines, angiogenesis inhibitors and inhibitors of cell signal pathways are undergoing clinical trials. Improved radiotherapy techniques and advances in surgical reconstruction emphasise the multi-modality approach to treatment.

PROBLEMS IN ADVANCED DISEASE

Since sarcomas can arise anywhere in the body, they can cause many problems common to other cancers. Particular problems include:

1. Loss of limb function. This may be due to effects of local disease causing pain, nerve compression, vascular compression and lymphoedema. Surgery may lead to loss of important muscle groups and radiation can lead to skin and muscle atrophy which both compromise limb function. Adequate analgesia, physiotherapy and treatment of the lymphoedema may help.
2. Lymphoedema. A common problem. Requires good skin care, to avoid infection. Mainstay of treatment is compression therapy with bandaging, compression pumps, elastic support and exercises.
3. Lung metastases (see Ch. 59 on pulmonary metastases). Many patients may still be cured following resection of lung metastases. If complete resection is achieved, 5-year survival is ~30%. Most recurrences occur in the lung and reoperation can still offer cure. Poor prognostic factors include disease-free interval <2.5 years, high histological grade, incomplete resection and age >40 years.

FURTHER READING

Brennan M F, Lewis J J 2001 Diagnosis and management of soft tissue sarcoma. Isis Medical Media, Oxford

Dirix L Y, Somville J, Van Oosterom A T 1996 Diagnosis and treatment of soft tissue sarcomas in adults. Current Opinion in Oncology 8(4):289–298

Enzinger F M, Weiss S W 1995 Soft tissue tumors, 3rd edn. Mosby, St Louis

START oncology guidelines. Soft tissue sarcomas. Available at: www.startoncology.net

CHAPTER 42

Skin cancer – non-melanoma

BACKGROUND INFORMATION

Non-melanoma skin cancer (NMSC) is by far the most common form of cancer and the incidence continues to increase. In 1997, there were 40 151 cases of NMSC diagnosed in the UK. Fortunately, the mortality rate is very low (400 deaths in the UK reported in 1998) as most of these cancers are diagnosed early and are easily treated.

The vast majority of NMSCs are basal cell carcinomas (BCC) and squamous cell carcinomas (SCC). Other types are uncommon and are listed in the Table 42.1.

The most important risk factor for the development of most NMSCs is chronic exposure to sunlight. UVB (290–320 nm) is the main carcinogenic wavelength, but UVA (320–400 nm) adds to the risk. Other risk factors include exposure to ionising radiation, precursor lesions (e.g. actinic keratoses), chemical carcinogens, immunosuppression (e.g. transplant patients and HIV AIDS), chronic ulcers, and genetic conditions (e.g. xeroderma pigmentosum).

BASAL CELL CARCINOMAS

BCCs are by far the commonest type of NMSC. The commonest sites involved are the nose, eyelids, inner canthi and post-auricular areas. There are various

TABLE 42.1 Uncommon types of NMSC

Carcinomas	Merkel cell carcinoma, eccrine porocarcinoma, microcystic adnexal carcinoma
Sarcomas	Angiosarcoma, dermatofibrosarcoma protuberans, Kaposi's sarcoma, leiomyosarcoma
Lymphomas	T-cell lymphomas (mycosis fungoides), B-cell lymphomas
Skin metastases	Especially lung and renal cancer

histological types of BCCs. The commonest type is the nodular BCC, which characteristically has a raised pearly edge with associated telangiectasia and central ulceration (rodent ulcer). Other BCC variants include cystic, superficial, morphoeic, keratotic and pigmented types.

BCCs very rarely metastasise and the prognosis is usually excellent. However, if left untreated, some may cause severe local tissue destruction including infiltration through bone into other structures such as the brain.

SQUAMOUS CELL CARCINOMAS

SCCs most commonly affect the head and neck region followed by the trunk. They tend to form erythematous papular lesions or plaques and may ulcerate. They commonly arise from precursor lesions such as actinic keratoses and can evolve from in situ carcinomas (e.g. Bowen's disease and Paget's disease).

Invasive SCCs have the potential to recur locally and metastasise, but this occurs uncommonly. Five-year rates of local recurrence and metastasis are 8% and 5% respectively. Risk factors for local recurrence and metastasis include: size >2 cm, tumour depth >4 mm, lip and ear lesions, poor differentiation and perineural invasion.

The prognosis for most patients with primary invasive SCC is excellent, but the outlook for those with regional lymph node metastases or distant metastases is poor, with 10-year survival of <20% and <10% respectively. Distant metastatic sites most commonly involved are the lungs, liver, brain, skin and bone.

Variants of SCCs include: (1) verrucous carcinoma – a locally aggressive, indolent, cauliflower-shaped tumour with a low propensity for metastatic spread and (2) keratoacanthoma – fast growing, very well differentiated SCC that may spontaneously involute.

DIAGNOSIS AND STAGING

Skin examination should be performed under good light. Regional nodes should be examined. Punch biopsy under local anaesthetic is the usual method employed to gain a histological diagnosis.

Skin cancer is staged according to the 2002 TNM classification (Table 42.2).

MANAGEMENT OF NMSC

Surgical excision is the mainstay of treatment for SCCs and BCCs and also provides histological characterisation of the tumour. Other treatment options include radiotherapy, cryotherapy, electrodesiccation and curettage, laser therapy, photodynamic therapy, and Moh's micrographic surgery.

TABLE 42.2 TNM staging of NMSC (only applies to carcinomas and does not include eyelid, vulva or penis)

Tis	Carcinoma in situ
T1	Tumour $\leq$2 cm
T2	Tumour >2 cm $\leq$5 cm
T3	Tumour >5 cm
T4	Tumour invades deep extradermal structures, i.e. cartilage, muscle or bone
N0	No nodes
N1	Regional nodes
M0	No distant metastases
M1	Distant metastases

TABLE 42.3 Examples of radiotherapy regimens for NMSCs

Small lesions <5 cm²
20 Gy single fraction (one visit, convenient for elderly patients with lesions less than 2.5 cm diameter – worse cosmesis though)
35 Gy in 5 fractions over 1 week
42.5–45 Gy in 10 fractions over 2–3 weeks
50–52.5 Gy in 15 fractions

Larger lesions[a]
50–55 Gy in 15–20 fractions over 3–4 weeks
60 Gy in 20–30 fractions over 4–6 weeks

[a] Local control rates for radiotherapy fall dramatically for lesions more than 5 cm in diameter.

The choice of therapy depends on the situation. Small (<1 cm) low-risk tumours can be treated with any of the above methods. Larger lesions (>1 cm) are generally best treated with surgical excision as this method produces the highest local control rates (especially Moh's micrographic surgery – 5-year local control of 97% for SCCs). However, radiotherapy may be preferred for patients with (1) lesions arising in the lips, ear and nose for better cosmetic effect, (2) deeply infiltrating lesions, (3) lesions where surgery is likely to lead to functional loss, (4) elderly patients unfit for surgery, (5) unresectable lesions.

Radiotherapy may be delivered using electrons and superficial X-rays for superficial lesions, brachytherapy for lesions affecting curved planes (e.g. lip) or megavoltage X-rays for deep lesions. Fractionation schedules vary widely and some examples are given in Table 42.3.

Local lymph node disease from SCC should be surgically resected if possible. Postoperative radiotherapy is usually offered when there is a high risk of recurrence (e.g. presence of extracapsular spread, >1 node or node >3 cm, close or involved margins, skin infiltration). Radical radiotherapy

TABLE 42.4 Results for treatment of BCC

T stage	5-year local control rates (%)
T1	95
T2	88
T3	50
T4	50

TABLE 42.5 Results for treatment of SCC

T stage/nodal status	5-year survival (%)
T stage	Disease-free
T1	95–99
T2	60–85
T3	60–75
T4	<40
Nodal status	Overall
1 node	50
2 nodes	30
3+ nodes	<15

alone may be offered for medically inoperable patients. Palliative radiotherapy may be helpful for painful ulcerating lesions.

Distant metastatic disease may be treated with cisplatin-based combination chemotherapy, but the outlook is generally very poor. Radiotherapy may be useful to palliate bone and brain metastases.

Typical results for treatment of BCCs and SCCs are shown in Tables 42.4 and 42.5.

PROBLEMS IN ADVANCED DISEASE

1. Fungating lesions. If radical therapy is not possible or inappropriate, palliative radiotherapy (e.g. single 8 Gy or 20 Gy in five fractions) may useful, especially if there is bleeding.
2. Infection. Systemic and topical antibiotics should be used. Topical metronidazole gel is effective for offensive anaerobic infections.

FURTHER READING

Alam M, Ratner D 2001 Cutaneous squamous cell carcinoma. Review article. New England Journal of Medicine 344(13):975–983

Motley R, Kersey P, Lawrence C 2002 Multiprofessional guidelines for the management of the patient with primary cutaneous squamous cell carcinoma. British Journal of Dermatology 146:18–25

Sober A J, Haluska F G (eds) 2001 American Cancer Society. Atlas of clinical oncology. Skin cancer. BC Decker, Hamilton, Ontario

Telfer N R, Colver G B, Bowers P W 1999 Guidelines for the management of basal cell carcinoma. British Journal of Dermatology 141:415–423

Small bowel cancer

BACKGROUND INFORMATION

Small bowel cancers are rare, accounting for less than 2% of all gastro-intestinal (GI) tract cancers. In 1997, there were only 502 small bowel cancers registered in the UK. The incidence is 1/100 000 population with a slight male predominance and the average age at diagnosis is 60 years.

The explanation for the low incidence of malignancy in the small bowel (which represents 75% of the total length of the GI tract and 90% of the mucosal surface) is unclear, but may in part be due to the following factors:

1. Large volumes of alkaline juices increase transit through the bowel, decreasing exposure time to carcinogens. Alkaline juice and enzymes may also detoxify some carcinogens.
2. High levels of immunoglobulin A (IgA) may be protective.
3. Low levels of bacteria resulting in decreased conversion of bile acids into potential carcinogens.

There are four main types of primary small bowel cancer: adenocarcinomas (45%), carcinoids (30%), sarcomas (10%) and lymphomas (15%). Metastatic lesions of the small intestine are more common than primary tumours and may occur from direct invasion or by intraperitoneal seeding (colon, ovary, uterus and stomach cancer), or by haematogenous spread (melanoma, breast and lung cancer).

The vast majority of adenocarcinomas arise in the proximal duodenum and jejunum. The ampulla of Vater is the most common site. The most important risk factor is the presence of pre-existing single or multiple adenomas. Patients with familial adenomatous polyposis have a 5% risk of developing small bowel adenocarcinoma. Other predisposing factors include alcohol, Crohn's disease, coeliac disease, neurofibromatosis and urinary diversions (e.g. ileal conduits). Overall 5-year disease-specific survival for adenocarcinoma of the small bowel is 30% (median survival 20 months).

The majority of small bowel sarcomas are gastrointestinal stromal tumours (GISTs). These tumours express the tyrosine kinase receptor, kit (CD117), and can respond well to treatment with the kit tyrosine kinase receptor inhibitor, imatinib mesylate (Glivec).

Carcinoid tumours and lymphomas are discussed in other chapters.

PRESENTATION

Non-specific symptoms such as abdominal pain, anaemia, nausea, bleeding and weight loss are common. Obstructive jaundice may occur with peri-ampullary tumours. Occasionally, patients may present as a surgical emergency with an acute abdomen (e.g. complete obstruction, perforation). Unfortunately, many patients have metastatic disease at diagnosis.

DIAGNOSIS AND STAGING

Investigations should include: full history and examination; baseline bloods for FBC, renal and liver function; CXR. Plain X-rays of small bowel may reveal obstruction. Small bowel follow-through may be useful, but enteroclysis (double contrast X-ray study with insufflation of barium and methylcellulose) offers greater sensitivity (90% versus 30%) for detecting small bowel tumours. CT may identify the primary tumour mass, but is more useful for preoperative staging purposes and detecting metastatic disease. Endoscopic ultrasound (EUS) is particularly useful in evaluating ampullary tumours, and submucosal tumours such as GISTs and carcinoids. Small bowel endoscopy may be used to obtain a biopsy and ablate tumours and bleeding lesions, but is limited by inability to visualise the distal jejunum and ileum. Angiography is occasionally useful.

Staging is by the TNM 2002 system (Table 43.1).

MANAGEMENT

ADENOCARCINOMA

Surgery is the mainstay of treatment and offers the only realistic chance of cure. Up to two-thirds of patients have potentially operable disease at presentation. Tumours of the first and second parts of the duodenum often require pancreaticoduodenectomy. In other sites, resection of the small bowel with wide margins and the corresponding mesentery is adequate. Unfortunately, despite aggressive surgical resection, many patients relapse

TABLE 43.1 2002 TNM staging of small bowel carcinoma	
T0	No evidence of primary tumour
Tis	Carcinoma in situ
T1	Tumour invades lamina propria or submucosa
T2	Tumour invades muscularis propria
T3	Tumour invades into subserosa or into non-peritonealised peri-muscular tissue with <2 cm extension
T4	Tumour perforates visceral peritoneum or directly invades other organs or structures (including mesentery/retroperitoneum >2 cm extension)
N0	No nodes
N1	Regional nodes
M0	No metastases
M1	Distant metastases

with metastatic disease. There is no proven adjuvant therapy at present. In the palliative setting, 5FU-based chemotherapy is used, but data on its efficacy is somewhat lacking. Palliative surgical resections and bypass procedures may be a very useful intervention for selected patients. Overall disease-specific 5-year survival is 30%.

CARCINOIDS

See Chapter 17.

GISTs

GISTs may arise anywhere in the GI tract with ~20% occurring in the small bowel. Traditionally these tumours have had a very poor outlook, with 5-year survival of around 30%. Surgery is the mainstay of treatment, but 35–50% are unresectable at diagnosis. There is no role for adjuvant chemotherapy or radiotherapy at present. Recently, the kit tyrosine kinase receptor inhibitor, imatinib mesylate, has achieved response rates of over 65% in patients with metastatic GISTs. This is now the standard treatment in the metastatic setting and may eventually have a role in the adjuvant/neoadjuvant setting.

FUTURE PERSPECTIVES

New agents such as irinotecan and oxaliplatin are being assessed in metastatic small bowel adenocarcinoma. The role of imatinib in GISTs continues to evolve.

PROBLEMS IN ADVANCED DISEASE

1. Gastric outflow obstruction. Can cause severe nausea and vomiting. Usually due to proximal duodenal tumours. A gastroduodenal stent may offer very effective palliation with up to 90% of patients achieving clinical benefit.
2. Obstructive jaundice. Most common with ampullary tumours. Treatment options include stenting, endoscopic laser photocoagulation and palliative bypass procedures. NB: stenting of both the duodenum and the bile duct is possible.
3. Ascites (see Ch. 52 on malignant ascites).
4. Liver metastases (see Ch. 51 on liver metastases).
5. GI bleeding. May be severe and life-threatening, in which case options (depending on the clinical scenario) include: (1) palliation only, with sedation, (2) endoscopic ablation of bleeding tumour, (3) laparotomy and surgical intervention. Mild bleeding causing symptomatic anaemia may be treated with iron sulphate and tranexamic acid.

FURTHER READING

Gill S S, Heuman D M, Mihas A A 2001 Small intestinal neoplasms. Journal of Clinical Gastroenterology 33(4):267–282

CHAPTER 44

Testicular cancer

BACKGROUND INFORMATION

Testicular tumours are relatively rare but are the most common cancers in men aged 20–30. Approximately 85% of cases are diagnosed between the ages of 20 and 49 years. Incidence rates are rising, with a 40% increase between 1970 and 1987. In 2000, there were 2010 new cases registered in the UK. Fortunately the results of modern treatment are excellent and the vast majority of patients can expect to be cured.

Germ cell tumours (GCTs) account for 95% of malignant testicular neoplasms, with lymphomas, Leydig cell tumours, Sertoli cell tumours and sarcomas making up the remainder. GCTs are generally subdivided into seminomas and non-seminiferous germ cell tumours (NSGCTs – including teratomas), although mixed tumours are not uncommon. NSGCTs have a lower peak incidence age (mid 20s) than seminomas (mid 30s). There are two main pathological classifications in use: the British and WHO classifications (Table 44.1).

TABLE 44.1 Classification of testicular tumours

British classification	WHO classification
Intratubular germ cell neoplasia	Intratubular uncommitted malignant germ cell
Seminoma	Seminoma
Spermatocytic seminoma	Spermatocytic seminoma
Teratoma:	Non-seminomatous germ cell tumour:
teratoma differentiated	mature teratoma
malignant teratoma intermediate (MTI)	embryonal carcinoma with teratoma (teratocarcinoma)
malignant teratoma undifferentiated (MTU)	embryonal carcinoma
Yolk sac tumour	Yolk sac tumour
Malignant teratoma trophoblastic	Choriocarcinoma

All GCTs with the exception of spermatocytic seminoma arise from carcinoma in situ, also known as intratubular germ cell neoplasia (ITGCN). Approximately 5% of men with testicular cancer have ITGCN in the contralateral testis and this will progress to invasive cancer in 50% at 5 years and virtually 100% at 10 years.

The best-known risk factor for testicular cancer is a history of testicular maldescent (cryptorchidism), which produces a 10-fold increased risk. Other risk factors include a positive family history of testicular cancer in first-degree relatives, genital abnormalities and testicular atrophy. There is no proven association with testicular injuries, wearing tight trousers, taking hot baths, vasectomy, smoking or alcohol. Exercise and late onset of puberty are associated with reduced risk.

PRESENTATION

Most patients present with a painless enlarged testicle or a lump in the testicle (85%). A decrease in testicular size may also occur. Pain (~10%) and inflammation (15%) may also be present and should not delay referral. Other features include a dragging sensation (30%) in the abdomen or groin, a recent history of trauma (10%) and backache (5%). Cancer in the undescended testis may present as an inguinal or abdominal mass. Rare presentations include hydrocele and gynaecomastia (due to very high levels of β-HCG).

DIAGNOSIS AND STAGING

Ultrasound scan of both testis and abdomen, CXR and tumour markers (AFP, β-HCG and LDH) should all be done preoperatively. Tumour markers are more useful in teratoma, in which 70% will produce elevated β-HCG and 70% AFP. Seminoma does not produce AFP, but β-HCG is mildly elevated in 20–35% of cases.

Biopsy of the contralateral testis should be considered for patients at high risk of ITGCN, i.e. <30 years with small volume testis (<16 ml).

All patients require formal staging with CT of the chest, abdomen and pelvis. CT of the brain is also required if there are multiple pulmonary metastases or β-HCG greater than 10 000 IU/l. Isotope bone scan should be carried out if there is suspicion of bone metastases.

The RMH (Royal Marsden Hospital) staging system (Table 44.2) has been commonly used in the past and is still useful, but has been superseded by the International Germ Cell Consensus Classification (IGCCC) prognostic grouping (Table 44.3).

TABLE 44.2 RMH staging system for testicular cancer

Stage I	No evidence of disease outside testis
Stage IM	As above, but persistently raised tumour markers
Stage II	Infra-diaphragmatic nodal involvement
IIA	<2 cm
IIB	2–5 cm
IIC	≥5–10 cm
IID	>10 cm
Stage III	Supra- and infra-diaphragmatic nodes (A, B, C as above)
	M+ mediastinal nodes, N+ neck nodes
Stage IV	Extranodal metastases
	L1 <3 lung metastases, L2 multiple lung metastases <2 cm, L3 multiple lung metastases >3 cm
	H+ Liver metastases. Other sites specified

TABLE 44.3 IGCCC Prognostic grouping for testicular cancer

Teratoma	Seminoma
Good prognosis	
Testis/retroperitoneal primary; no non-pulmonary visceral metastases	Any primary site; no non-pulmonary visceral metastases
AFP <1000 ng/dl	Normal AFP
β-HCG <5000 IU/l	Any β-HCG
LDH <1.5 upper limit of normal	Any LDH
56% of teratomas	90% of seminomas
5-year survival 92%	5-year survival 86%
Intermediate prognosis	
Testis/retroperitoneal primary; no non-pulmonary visceral metastases	Any primary site; non-pulmonary visceral metastases
AFP >1000 <10 000	Normal AFP
β-HCG >5000 <50 000	Any β-HCG
LDH >1.5 × N <10 × N	Any LDH
28% of teratomas	10% of seminomas
5-year survival 80%	5-year survival 73%
Poor prognosis	
Any of:	No patients in this group
mediastinal primary or non-pulmonary visceral metastases	
AFP >10 000	
β-HCG >50 000	
LDH >10 × normal	
16% of teratomas	
5-year survival 48%	

MANAGEMENT

Teratoma and seminoma have different clinical outcomes and require different clinical management.

INTRATUBULAR GERM CELL NEOPLASIA (ITGCN)

Men less than 30 years old with testis size <16 ml have a 35% risk of contralateral ITGCN and should therefore have a biopsy. If present, ITGCN should be treated with orchidectomy or external beam radiotherapy to the remaining testis (20 Gy in 10 fractions) because this reduces the subsequent risk of developing a contralateral cancer.

SEMINOMA STAGE I

Between 80 and 85% present with stage I disease and approximately 80% will be cured by orchidectomy alone, but adjuvant radiotherapy to the para-aortic strip (20 Gy in 10 fractions) will reduce the rate of relapse to ~3%. Other options include a single cycle of adjuvant carboplatin chemotherapy or a surveillance strategy with treatment on relapse.

TERATOMA STAGE I

Patients with histology that shows lymphovascular invasion have a 40% chance of relapse (usually in the first year) and should be treated with two cycles of postoperative chemotherapy (BEP regimen – bleomycin, etoposide and cisplatin). This reduces the relapse rate to 1–2%. Stage I patients with no high risk features may be managed by surveillance, which involves 'active' management with regular follow-up clinical examinations, CXRs, CT scans and tumour markers.

Patients with rising markers following surgery are staged as IM and should be treated as for metastatic disease.

SEMINOMA STAGES II, III AND IV

Patients with stage IIA disease can be treated with radiotherapy ('dog-leg' technique, 35 Gy in 15–17 fractions over 2 weeks). Stage IIB disease is usually treated with chemotherapy, but radiotherapy is an alternative. Higher stages of disease should be treated with cisplatin and etoposide combination chemotherapy.

Residual masses following chemotherapy can generally be managed by a policy of observation. Most masses less than 3 cm contain fibrous tissue only, and will shrink over time. Masses greater than 3 cm may well contain cancer and salvage chemotherapy may be required. Surgical resection is not routinely indicated because there is a significant risk of morbidity due to the highly infiltrative nature of seminoma causing lack of clear tissue planes.

TERATOMA STAGES II, III AND IV

Patients with good prognosis disease should receive three cycles of BEP chemotherapy.

Patients with intermediate/poor prognosis disease should receive four cycles of BEP chemotherapy. Bleomycin is usually omitted from the last cycle due to increased risk of pulmonary toxicity. Entry into clinical trials is encouraged for poor prognosis patients. Patients who present very unwell with high markers or significant metastatic disease should be referred for immediate chemotherapy with delayed orchidectomy.

If a complete response is achieved with chemotherapy then relapse is unlikely in good prognosis patients, occurring in <10% of patients. The relapse rate is higher in the poor prognostic group. Patients with rising markers usually need further chemotherapy unless the disease is localised and has occurred late, in which case surgery is an option. The standard salvage chemotherapy regimen is VeIP (vinblastine, ifosfamide, cisplatin), but combinations including taxanes are also used. Entry into clinical trials is encouraged (e.g. high dose chemotherapy with peripheral stem cell rescue is currently under evaluation). Overall cure rates for relapsed disease are of the order of 30%+. Surgery is the mainstay of treatment for late relapse (more than 2 years from initial treatment) and the outlook for this group of patients is better.

Residual masses can remain after chemotherapy and marker normalisation. They may contain viable tumour, differentiated teratoma or fibrosis/necrosis only. Masses >1 cm should be treated with complete surgical excision if possible. If para-aortic/retroperitoneal lymphadenopathy is performed, there is an increased risk of retrograde ejaculation. If there is incomplete excision then further chemotherapy may be offered. Radiotherapy is very rarely indicated.

FUTURE PERSPECTIVES

In stage I non-seminomatous germ cell tumours, trials are assessing the role of PET imaging in prediction of relapse, and whether less intensive surveillance with CT scanning is possible without compromising outcome.

For patients with intermediate risk metastatic germ cell tumours, a large phase III trial is about to assess BEP plus paclitaxel versus BEP alone.

In advanced poor prognosis disease, the role of high dose chemotherapy with stem cell rescue continues to be evaluated.

PROBLEMS IN ADVANCED DISEASE

1. Brain metastases (see also Ch. 49 on brain metastases). Brain metastases occurring at initial presentation (30–40% 5-year survival) have a much better prognosis than brain metastases on relapse (2–5% 5-year survival) or as part of progressive chemoresistant disease. Haemorrhage into metastases may occur following chemotherapy and so surgical resection if technically feasible should be considered as the initial treatment. The role of radiotherapy is unclear but it may be given as a part of the treatment of relapsed disease.
2. Gynaecomastia. May occur in 25% with advanced disease (usually regresses if patient responds to chemotherapy). If painful or distressing then danazol 100 mg q.d.s. or radiotherapy to the breast buds may help (e.g. 8 Gy single fraction).
3. Bulky lymph node disease. May cause abdominal pain and swelling, back pain, ureteric obstruction and lymphoedema. Radiotherapy may be helpful in the palliative setting.
4. Respiratory distress. Patients with chemoresistant disease in the lungs may suffer increasing respiratory compromise, cough and stridor. Steroids, morphine and midazolam may be indicated. Respiratory distress may also occur in patients with multiple lung metastases following chemotherapy treatment.
5. Psychosocial and sexual problems. As most patients are young, psychological morbidity is a particular problem so psychological support should be offered. Most patients will have been in employment and will suffer financial losses with obvious consequences for the family, so additional support services should be addressed as necessary. Fertility worries are also an issue and sperm banking should be discussed. A testicular prosthesis can be offered if required and is best performed at the time of primary orchidectomy.

FURTHER READING

Bosl G J, Motzer R J 1997 Testicular germ-cell cancer. New England Journal of Medicine 337:242–253

COIN/Scottish Intercollegiate Guidelines Network (SIGN). Management of Adult Testicular Germ Cell Tumours. A National Clinical Guideline. Available at: http://show.cee.hw.ac.uk/sign/home.htm or www.rcr.ac.uk

Einhorn L H, Donohue J P 1998 Advanced testicular cancer: Update for urologists. Journal of Urology 160:1964–1969

Javved M, Makhoul I. Germ cell tumours. Available at: http://www.emedicine.com/med/topic863.htm

Thyroid cancer

BACKGROUND INFORMATION

Thyroid cancer is the commonest endocrine malignancy, but represents less than 1% of all malignant disease in the UK, with approximately 1000 new cases per year. There were 336 deaths in the UK attributed to thyroid cancer in 1998. The disease is commoner in women than men, with a 3:1 ratio and the majority of cases occur between the ages of 25 and 65 years.

There are four main types of thyroid cancer: papillary, follicular, medullary and anaplastic. Papillary (70%) and follicular (15%) carcinomas are referred to as differentiated thyroid cancer (DTC) and are highly treatable and curable with overall 10-year survival of 85–93%. Good prognostic indicators are age 15–45 years, female sex, tumour <4 cm diameter, no extrathyroid extension and no distant metastases. Medullary carcinoma (4%) has an intermediate prognosis with 10-year survival rates of 65–90%. Anaplastic (1–2%) thyroid cancer is highly aggressive and 75% of patients develop distant metastases (usually lung metastases). The prognosis is very poor, with median survival of 3–4 months. Thyroid lymphomas account for <5% of primary thyroid cancers. Other rare tumours are teratomas, squamous cell carcinomas and sarcomas.

The aetiology of DTC is unknown, but previous exposure to radiation in childhood is a definite risk factor. The mean latency period between exposure and the development of thyroid malignancy is 25–30 years. The majority (80%) of medullary cancers are sporadic, but there are three hereditary forms: MEN 2A, MEN 2B (MEN = multiple endocrine neoplasia) and familial medullary thyroid cancer. These all involve mutation of the *RET* proto-oncogene which encodes a receptor tyrosine kinase. A thorough family history should be taken.

Pathologically, papillary cancers arise from follicular cells and are often multifocal. They tend to spread by the lymphatic route and therefore lymph nodes are commonly involved (35–40%). Follicular cancers commonly exhibit vascular invasion and tend to spread by the haematogenous route to bone and lung. Nodal disease is less common. Hürthle cell carcinoma is a rare variant and tends to behave more aggressively. Both papillary and follicular cancers produce thyroglobulin, which acts as a very useful tumour marker.

Medullary cancers arise from the parafollicular C-cells and secrete calcitonin. Extrathyroid invasion and nodal metastases are common, with ~15% presenting with distant metastatic disease.

PRESENTATION

Most patients present with a lump in the neck due either to a palpable thyroid nodule or to cervical lymphadenopathy (40% of patients with papillary carcinoma present with palpable neck nodes). The voice may change due to local pressure effects or recurrent laryngeal nerve involvement. Rarely, a patient with follicular carcinoma will present with symptoms of bone metastases.

Anaplastic tumours are typically seen in old age and present as a rapidly enlarging goitre with associated neck node masses, causing dysphagia, dysphonia and stridor.

Most patients are euthyroid. Clinically, it may be difficult to distinguish a cancerous mass from benign thyroid nodules, which happen to be very common in the general population (4–6% incidence). Only 5% of thyroid nodules turn out to be cancerous. However, a nodule that is large (>4 cm), hard, firm or fixed should raise suspicion.

DIAGNOSIS AND STAGING

Investigations should include: history and examination, including preoperative vocal cord examination; thyroid function tests and autoantibody status; FNA of nodule/neck mass with or without neck ultrasound; CXR; routine bloods (FBC, renal and liver function, calcium), thyroglobulin levels, calcitonin levels (if medullary carcinoma suspected); CT/MRI in selected cases (e.g. for clinically fixed tumours, if limits of goitre cannot be determined or for patients with haemoptysis). CT contrast should be avoided in the assessment of DTC as it contains iodine and reduces subsequent iodine-131 uptake by thyroid tissue. Isotope studies are reserved for post-treatment imaging.

Thyroid cancer is staged by the 2002 TNM system (Table 45.1). TNM staging helps to stratify patients into prognostic groups (Table 45.2).

TABLE 45.1 2002 TNM staging for thyroid cancer (simplified)

T1	Tumour ⩽2 cm limited to thyroid
T2	Tumour >2 cm ⩽4 cm limited to thyroid
T3	Tumour >4 cm limited to thyroid, or any tumour with minimal extrathyroid extension (e.g. strap muscles)
T4a	Tumour extends beyond thyroid capsule (any size) and invades any of larynx, trachea, oesophagus, recurrent laryngeal nerve or subcutaneous tissues
T4b	Tumour invades prevertebral fascia, mediastinal vessels or encasement of carotid artery
N0	No nodes
N1a	Level 6 nodes
N1b	Unilateral, bilateral or contralateral cervical nodes, or mediastinal nodes
M0	No distant metastases
M1	Distant metastases

NB: All anaplastic tumours are considered T4.

TABLE 45.2 TNM staging and prognosis for DTC

Stage		10-year cancer specific mortality (%)
I	<45 years, tumour <1 cm, no distant metastases (any T, any N, M0) ⩾45 years, tumour <1 cm, no distant metastases (T1, N0, M0)	1.7
II	<45 years, any tumour size, including metastases (any T, any N, M1) ⩾45 years, tumour 1–4 cm, no distant metastases (T2–3, N0, M0)	15.8
III	⩾45 years with tumour extending beyond the thyroid capsule ± lymph node metastases (T4, N0, M0 or any T, N1, M0)	30
IV	⩾45 years with distant metastases (any T, any N, M1)	60.9

MANAGEMENT

Most thyroid nodules are benign, so it is important to avoid unnecessary surgery. In general, if the FNA indicates malignancy or is suspicious then surgical intervention is required.

DIFFERENTIATED THYROID CANCER (PAPILLARY AND FOLLICULAR)

Patients with low risk tumours (age <45, tumour <1 cm) can safely undergo ipsilateral thyroid lobectomy alone followed by thyroid-stimulating hormone (TSH) suppression with thyroxine. Higher risk patients should undergo total thyroidectomy with a level 6 node dissection (pre-and paratracheal nodes are removed). The recurrent laryngeal nerves should invariably be preserved (injury rates are 1–6%). Selective neck dissection is required if there is clinically palpable or suspicious lymphadenopathy. Following surgery, calcium levels are checked because 30% of patients will be hypocalcaemic and require calcium supplementation due to damage to the parathyroid glands. Fortunately, hypocalcaemia is usually transient and only 2% require calcium supplementation at 3 months following surgery.

Radioiodine (iodine-131) ablation is offered to nearly all patients with tumours >1 cm following total thyroidectomy. Postoperative radioiodine ablation therapy has five main potential benefits:

1. Destruction of residual thyroid cancer cells. Radioiodine ablation reduces local and distant recurrence rates and improves survival in the vast majority of DTC patients, especially in patients with tumours >1 cm in size.
2. Ablation of residual thyroid tissue renders patients completely devoid of thyroid tissue, so that thyroglobulin levels should be undetectable if treatment is successful. This is very helpful for follow-up purposes, as any subsequent elevation of thyroglobulin indicates disease recurrence.
3. Ablation of the residual normal thyroid tissue means that if more radioiodine is given it will be taken up by persistent or metastatic thyroid cancer and this will aid in treatment and diagnosis.
4. Ablation of all thyroid tissue will prevent occurrence of a new primary thyroid cancer in the future.
5. Whole body post-ablation gamma camera scanning may show the presence of metastatic disease.

If radioiodine ablation is planned for 3–4 weeks after surgery, then hormone replacement therapy should be deferred until after the ablation because this will allow TSH levels to rise to >30 mu/l, encouraging radioiodine uptake into thyroid tissue. If therapy is planned later than this, then tri-iodothyronine (T3) 20 μg t.d.s. p.o. should be started postoperatively and then stopped 14 days prior to ablation to allow the TSH level to rise.

The optimum radioiodine ablation dose is unknown, but doses of 3.0–3.7 GBq are commonly used in UK centres. At this dose level patients require admission to hospital for up to 5 days due to radiation protection legislation. A post-ablation whole body gamma scan is performed prior to discharge to assess the amount of residual thyroid tissue and the presence of metastatic disease. The patient can then be restarted on thyroxine.

Side effects of radioiodine therapy are generally very mild, but may include:

1. Throat discomfort and occasional neck swelling
2. Transient loss of taste and dry mouth due to salivary gland uptake. This can be minimised by sucking sweets or chewing gum

3. Nausea and vomiting from radiation gastritis due to oral administration of iodine
4. Pulmonary pneumonitis and fibrosis in patients with diffuse lung metastases – more likely with higher and repeated doses
5. Mild pancytopenias with repeated doses
6. Second malignancies. However, the risk of second malignancies (especially leukaemia) only becomes significant with high cumulative doses of radioiodine.

A further diagnostic radioiodine uptake scan is performed at 4–6 months. If the scan is negative, and thyroglobulin levels are undetectable, then the patient should continue thyroxine to suppress TSH to less than 0.1 mu/l. No further imaging is necessary if thyroglobulin levels remain undetectable. If the scan is positive, a further ablative dose of radioiodine is given and the scan repeated again. Radioiodine therapy is further repeated if there continues to be uptake on the scans and thyroglobulin levels are elevated. NB: Pregnancy must always be excluded before offering radioiodine therapy.

Recurrent disease is often curable if operable or amenable to radioiodine therapy. Recurrent neck disease is usually managed surgically. Lung metastases are treated with radioiodine therapy. Bone metastases are generally managed with a combination of surgery, radioiodine and external beam radiotherapy. Patients with a rising thyroglobulin, but a negative diagnostic iodine uptake scan, should have an ultrasound or MRI scan of the neck and a CT scan (without contrast) of the chest. If neck disease is present and operable it should be resected. If lung metastases are present then high dose radioiodine therapy (e.g. 5 GBq) should be tried. If CT and MRI are negative, a bone scan may demonstrate bone metastases. FDG-PET (fluorodeoxyglucose positron emission tomography) scanning may help to exclude potentially operable disease. If all tests remain negative, then an empirical therapeutic dose of radioiodine may be tried. If treatment is successful then thyroglobulin levels should become undetectable.

External beam radiotherapy (EBRT) is not often required, but can be given to patients with inoperable disease that does not take up radioiodine. Doses of 55–66 Gy over 4–7 weeks are employed. Palliative radiotherapy may be used to treat painful bone metastases, mediastinal disease and brain metastases.

Chemotherapy with doxorubicin and cisplatin has been reported to produce partial response rates of 10–20% when other therapies have failed.

MEDULLARY THYROID CANCER

Patients are treated with total thyroidectomy and selective neck dissection. These tumours do not take up ^{131}I. Postoperative EBRT is indicated for positive resection margins, gross residual disease and if multiple lymph nodes were involved (especially if postoperative calcitonin is raised).

Follow-up is aided with calcitonin and CEA tumour marker levels. Overall 10-year survival rates range from 65 to 90%. Patients with MEN II have a worse outlook because the disease tends to be more aggressive in this group of patients. Radiotherapy may be useful for controlling symptoms in inoperable and metastatic disease. Chemotherapy is generally ineffective, but may be considered in patients with inoperable progressive symptomatic disease. Octreotide may be very useful for controlling severe diarrhoea and other systemic symptoms of advanced disease.

NB: All patients with medullary thyroid cancer should have appropriate preoperative investigations to exclude coincident phaeochromocytoma and hyperparathyroidism.

ANAPLASTIC THYROID CANCER

Radical surgery is not possible in the vast majority of patients due to the aggressive invasive nature of the disease, but tracheostomy is often performed palliatively for obstructive symptoms. If the patient is fit enough and the tumour volume is small enough, radical EBRT (55–65 Gy over 4–7 weeks) may provide local control for a short period. Less intense treatment over 1–2 weeks may be more appropriate for poorer prognosis patients. The disease does not respond to ^{131}I.

Single agent doxorubicin chemotherapy has produced response rates of 30%, but survival is only marginally improved. Patients suitable for chemotherapy should be offered entry into clinical trials.

THYROID LYMPHOMA

This usually occurs in women over 55 years and most arise on the background of Hashimoto thyroiditis. The most common cell type is diffuse large cell lymphoma, which may arise in association with MALT lymphoma. Surgical resection of the thyroid mass is not routinely part of the management strategy. Combination chemotherapy (e.g. CHOP) and radiotherapy produces the best treatment results. Radiotherapy alone is probably adequate treatment for primary thyroid MALT lymphoma. Oral chlorambucil is also used.

FUTURE PERSPECTIVES

A new development is the use of recombinant TSH, which can be used instead of withdrawing thyroxine from patients, prior to radioiodine therapy. This may significantly reduce the morbidity of hypothyroid symptoms. Current chemotherapy trials are focused on the role of paclitaxel, liposomal doxorubicin and thalidomide. Radiolabelled therapeutic iodine-131-MIBG and indium 111-octreotide continue to be assessed in the treatment of medullary thyroid cancer. Finally, new surgical techniques such as video-assisted thyroidectomy and radiofrequency ablation of locally recurrent disease are being evaluated.

PROBLEMS IN ADVANCED DISEASE

See Chapter 23 on head and neck cancer.

FURTHER READING

British Thyroid Association and the Royal College of Physicians 2002 Guidelines for the management of thyroid cancer in adults. Available at www.british-thyroid-association.org

Kinder B K 2003 Well differentiated thyroid cancer. Current Opinion in Oncology 15:71–77

Mazzaferri E L, Kloos R T 2001 Current approaches to primary therapy for papillary and follicular thyroid cancer. Journal of Clinical Endocrinology and Metabolism 86(4):1447–1463

Pasieka J L 2003 Anaplastic thyroid cancer. Current Opinion in Oncology 15:78–83

Vini L, Harmer C 2002 Management of thyroid cancer. Lancet Oncology 13:407–414

Vaginal cancer

BACKGROUND INFORMATION

Primary vaginal cancer is rare. It accounts for only 1–2% of all gynaecological malignancies with less than 200 new cases per year in the UK. Vaginal neoplasms are usually secondary deposits from cervical, endometrial, rectal and vulval cancers. The diagnosis of primary vaginal cancer therefore often requires exclusion of these more common cancers. Fifty per cent occur in women who have previously had a hysterectomy. The commonest site for primary lesions is the posterior wall of the upper two-thirds of the vagina.

Pathologically, the vast majority of primary vaginal cancers are squamous cell carcinomas (90%), but other types include adenocarcinomas (5–10%), malignant melanoma and sarcomas. The aetiology of vaginal cancer is unknown, but the presence of HPV (human papilloma virus), vaginal intraepithelial neoplasia (VAIN) and chronic irritation are all thought to play a role. Maternal exposure to diethylstilbestrol is a risk factor for clear cell adenocarcinoma, classically seen in young women. Lymph node involvement is common and is a poor prognostic factor. Tumours in the upper two-thirds of the vagina spread to the pelvic and para-aortic nodes and lower third tumours spread to the inguinal nodes. The commonest sites of metastatic disease are the lungs, liver and skeleton.

Patients with stage I and II disease (no extension to pelvic wall) have 5-year survival between 45 and 70%, but this falls with stage III and IV disease (pelvic wall and adjacent organs involved) to 5–30%. The overall 5-year survival rate is disappointing because most women are elderly and present with later stage disease.

PRESENTATION

The commonest symptom is painless postmenopausal bleeding. Vaginal discharge, pelvic pain and urinary symptoms may also occur and are suggestive of more advanced disease.

TABLE 46.1	FIGO staging of vaginal cancer
Stage 0	In situ disease
Stage I	Limited to vaginal wall
Stage II	Involvement of subvaginal tissue, but not to pelvic side wall
Stage III	Extends to pelvic wall, and/or pelvic or inguinal nodes
Stage IVA	Invades mucosa of bladder and/or rectum, and/or beyond true pelvis
Stage IVB	Distant metastases

DIAGNOSIS AND STAGING

Investigations should include full history and examination; baseline bloods (FBC, renal and liver function, calcium); EUA and biopsy. CT/MRI scanning is used for more advanced lesions to assess nodal involvement.

Staging is by the FIGO system (Table 46.1).

MANAGEMENT

VAGINAL INTRAEPITHELIAL NEOPLASIA (VAIN)

The options for treatment include surgical excision, laser vaporisation, topical 5FU and intravaginal brachytherapy (e.g. 30 Gy to 5 mm from the surface applicator in 10 fractions given over 2 weeks).

INVASIVE DISEASE

Radiotherapy is the mainstay of treatment, but as the disease is so rare, the optimum schedule is unknown. Intravaginal brachytherapy alone may be offered to superficial stage I lesions less than 0.5 cm thick. More advanced disease requires external beam radiotherapy to the pelvis (e.g. 45 Gy in 25 fractions over 5 weeks) and a boost to the primary tumour. The inguinal nodes are included in the field if the lower third of the vagina is involved. The boost to the primary tumour may be achieved by either (i) a combination of further external beam radiotherapy to the primary and intravaginal brachytherapy or (ii) an interstitial brachytherapy implant into the vaginal mass. A total dose of at least 70–75 Gy is required. Patients with incurable disease may be treated with palliative radiotherapy (e.g. 40 Gy in 15 fractions over 3 weeks or shorter schedules for poor performance status patients).

Radical surgery is usually reserved for patients with early lesions (stage I) of the upper vagina or radiation failures. It involves radical vaginectomy, hysterectomy and lymphadenectomy. Very occasionally a pelvic exenteration (which includes removal of bladder and/or rectum) may be performed for highly selected stage IV disease or recurrent disease.

Chemotherapy has a very limited role and is usually reserved for palliation in younger patients. Platinum-based combinations are used.

PROBLEMS IN ADVANCED DISEASE

See Chapter 58 on problems in advanced pelvic malignancy.

FURTHER READING

Blake P, Lambert H, Crawford R (eds) 1998 Gynaecological oncology. A guide to clinical management. Oxford Medical Publications, Oxford

Lawton F, Friedlander M, Thomas G (eds) 1998 Essentials of gynaecological cancer. Chapman and Hall Medical, London

Vulval cancer

BACKGROUND INFORMATION

Vulval cancer is uncommon, accounting for only 4% of all gynaecological malignancies with an incidence of 3/100 000. It is mainly a disease of old age, with the majority of patients over 65 years.

The aetiology is complex, but infection with the human papilloma virus (HPV), a history of abnormal vulval skin (e.g. lichen sclerosis, squamous hyperplasia), and the presence of high grade vulval intraepithelial neoplasia (VIN) are important factors. Smoking, hypertension and obesity are associated risk factors.

Pathologically, 90% of vulval cancers are squamous cell carcinomas, the remainder being melanomas (5%), Bartholin's gland carcinomas, other adenocarcinomas, basal cell carcinomas and sarcomas. The labia majora is the commonest site of the primary lesion. Lymph node spread is common and the usual pattern of spread is initially to the inguinal nodes, followed by the femoral nodes and then to the pelvic nodes, which are considered as distant metastases. If groin nodes are involved, the risk of positive pelvic nodes is 17–34%.

Early diagnosis and prompt treatment may avoid a potentially very distressing death from uncontrolled locoregional disease. The 5-year survival is 85–97% for stage I and II disease and ~30–70% for stage III and IV disease. Overall disease specific 5-year survival is ~75%.

PRESENTATION

Most patients present with pruritus vulvae or a lump/ulcer on the vulva. Other symptoms include bleeding, discharge and pain. An enlarged groin node is occasionally the presenting feature. Vulval cancer may be asymptomatic. Warts are uncommon in the elderly woman and should, therefore, be treated with suspicion. Warts are more common in

TABLE 47.1 FIGO staging of vulval cancer

Stage 0	In situ carcinoma
Stage Ia	Confined to vulva/perineum ≤2 cm. Stromal invasion ≤1 mm
Stage Ib	Confined to vulva/perineum ≤2 cm. Stromal invasion >1 mm
Stage II	Confined to vulva/perineum >2 cm
Stage III	Tumour any size with (i) adjacent spread to lower urethra and/or vagina, or anus and/or (ii) unilateral lymph node metastases
Stage IVa	Tumour invades any of upper urethra, bladder, rectum, pelvis, bilateral regional nodes
Stage IVb	Any distant metastases including pelvic nodes

premenopausal women and should be initially managed as condylomata acuminata.

DIAGNOSIS AND STAGING

Investigations used in the diagnosis of vulval cancer include: full clinical examination including careful groin palpation and cervical smear; EUA and a full thickness biopsy; FBC, liver and renal function tests; CXR; MRI/CT of the abdomen and pelvis to assess primary tumour and nodal disease; fine needle aspiration cytology (FNAC) of palpable groin nodes.

Staging is by the FIGO system (Table 47.1). The presence of positive lymph nodes is the most important prognostic indicator.

MANAGEMENT

SURGERY

Surgery is the mainstay of treatment for vulval cancer and over the last 20 years there has been a trend towards less radical procedures. Early disease where the tumour is <2 cm and stromal invasion is less than 1 mm (stage Ia) can be treated with wide local excision alone with 1 cm margins. A greater resection is required for more advanced lesions. The extent of the resection will depend on the size and site of the tumour, depth of invasion and lymph node status.

Dissection of bilateral groin nodes should be performed when the depth of invasion is greater than 1 mm (stage Ib or worse) or greater than 2 cm in diameter (stage II or worse). However, unilateral inguinal lymphadenectomy is possible for well-lateralised primary tumours (i.e. medial edge of cancer is >2 cm from midline of vulva). If the ipsilateral nodes are shown to be positive, then lymphadenectomy or radiotherapy of the contralateral inguinal nodes is required.

Lymphoedema of the lower limbs is the main complication of surgery and may occur in 14–21% of patients. Wound infection and breakdown is now seen less commonly. Other complications include venous thromboembolism, incontinence (urinary and faecal), introital stenosis, rectoceles, lymphocysts and psychosexual problems.

RADIOTHERAPY

Radiotherapy also plays an important role. It may be used as a primary treatment (e.g. 55–65 Gy over 6–7 weeks) if a patient has advanced inoperable disease, locally recurrent disease or is medically unfit for surgery.

Preoperative RT alone (e.g. 55–60 Gy over 6–7 weeks) or concurrent chemoradiotherapy (e.g. 50.4 Gy in 28 fractions over 40 days with 5FU and mitomycin C or 5FU and cisplatin) can be used to render inoperable tumours operable.

Postoperative RT (e.g. 45–50 Gy in 25 fractions over 5 weeks) should be considered if resection margins are less than 8 mm, because the risk of local recurrence in this situation is 50%. If two or more groin nodes are positive or if there is extracapsular spread, then postoperative RT should be given to the inguinal and pelvic nodes (e.g. 45–50 Gy in 25 fractions over 5 weeks).

The side effects of external beam radiotherapy may be severe and include: (1) acute reactions such as skin desquamation and ulceration, diarrhoea, urinary frequency and incontinence and (2) late reactions such as skin fibrosis, vaginal stenosis, radiation proctitis and enteritis. These reactions are now minimised by using lower dose per fraction regimens, i.e. 1.6–1.8 Gy per fraction.

Brachytherapy with ^{192}Ir needles can be used for earlier stage lesions, especially if the lower vagina is involved.

CHEMOTHERAPY

Chemotherapy is generally used in the metastatic or recurrent disease setting. The most active agents are 5FU, cisplatin, mitomycin C, bleomycin and methotrexate. Combination chemotherapy produces response rates of 40–50% but the benefits are often short-lived and overall prognosis is poor. Toxicity is often a problem due to the older age of this group of patients.

FUTURE PERSPECTIVES

The main focus of current clinical research is on the role of concurrent chemoradiotherapy in the neoadjuvant and primary settings. In the metastatic setting, paclitaxel is being studied in phase II clinical trials.

PROBLEMS IN ADVANCED VULVAL CANCER

See Chapter 58 on problems in advanced pelvic malignancy.

FURTHER READING

Blake P, Lambert H, Crawford R (eds) 1998 Gynaecological oncology. A guide to clinical management. Oxford Medical Publications, Oxford

Lawton F, Friedlander M, Thomas G (eds) 1998 Essentials of gynaecological cancer. Chapman and Hall Medical, London

COMPLICATIONS OF CANCER AND EMERGENCIES

Bone metastases

INTRODUCTION

The skeleton is the one of the most frequent sites to be affected by metastatic disease. Moreover, recent improvements in the management of metastatic disease have led to greater survival, resulting in an increase in the number of patients developing bone metastases. It is now estimated that there are over 20 000 patients diagnosed with bone metastases per year in the UK.

The commonest tumours that metastasise to bone are prostate, breast, lung (which account for 80% of cases) followed by kidney, myeloma, thyroid, gynaecological and gastrointestinal (GI) tract cancers. The sites most commonly involved are, in order of frequency, the spine, pelvis, ribs, skull (axial skeleton) and proximal long bones. Distal or acral metastases are extremely rare and if present are usually due to lung cancer. There is significant mortality, morbidity and reduced quality of life related to a range of complications that include pain, hypercalcaemia, impending fracture, pathological fracture, spinal instability, neurological complications and bone marrow suppression. Loss of ambulatory ability is a poor prognostic sign, increasing the risk of thromboembolic disease, DIC (disseminated intra-vascular coagulation), atelectasis and pressure sores as well as exacerbating hypercalcaemia.

Cancer usually spreads to bone by haematogenous dissemination, but several factors affect the distribution of disease. These include the biological properties of the cancer cells, chemotactic factors produced by bone (e.g. growth factors, cytokines, prostaglandins), cancer cell–host cell interactions, distribution of red bone marrow, and Batson's plexus (low pressure, high volume system of valveless vertebral veins communicating with venous plexuses from pelvis to skull which allows arrest and reversal of blood flow). Cancers may cause osteolytic, osteoblastic or mixed metastatic bone lesions. Osteolytic bone metastases are the most common type. The mechanism is complex, and involves tumour cells secreting numerous paracrine factors (cytokines, growth factors, parathyroid hormone related protein (PTHrP)) that stimulate osteoclastic resorption of bone and osteoblastic new bone formation. The bone cells in turn secrete growth factors and cytokines that stimulate tumour growth. Thus, there is positive feedback interdependence between tumour cells and bone. Depending on which is the most predominant process, osteolytic, osteoblastic or mixed lesions will occur. Osteoblastic sclerotic lesions are much less common than osteolytic lesions and are mainly seen in prostate cancer. Other cancers that can cause osteoblastic sclerotic metastases include breast, kidney, thyroid and Hodgkin's disease.

Treatment is palliative in almost all cases. Therapeutic interventions include analgesics, surgery, radiotherapy, hormones, chemotherapy, bisphosphonates and vertebroplasty and therefore a multidisciplinary approach to management is required.

The overall prognosis is extremely variable depending on the site of the primary, extent of disease and the general condition of the patient. For example, patients with melanoma and lung cancer have a median survival of only a few months compared to 2–3 years for breast and prostate cancer. Bone metastases from germ cell tumours, lymphoma and thyroid cancer are potentially curable. Solitary lesions are rare but long-term survival may be possible following surgical resection in selected cases, e.g. a rib metastasis from renal cancer.

PRESENTATION

Bone metastases may be the presenting feature of malignancy, but more commonly occur later on in the course of the disease. Pain is the most frequent symptom, but it should be remembered that 30–50% patients with known bone metastases are pain free. When pain is present, it is usually related to some but not all of the metastases, it is often worse at night, and although initially relieved by activity eventually becomes worse on movement as the disease progresses. The pain has biological and mechanical components: biological pain is related to chemical mediators released by the tumour causing nerve irritation, and tumour pressure effects within bone; mechanical pain is due to loss of bone strength and stiffness and causes movement-related pain. Metastases involving joints may mimic arthritis. Other symptoms may be related to nerve involvement, spinal cord compression, fractures, hypercalcaemia and bone marrow suppression.

DIAGNOSIS

Baseline bloods should be taken including FBC, liver and renal function tests, alkaline phosphatase, calcium. Plain X-rays of painful lesions and weight-bearing bones (if hot spot seen on bone scan) should be taken. If surgery is proposed, plain X-rays should include the whole length of the bone so that all lesions can be assessed to aid planning of the operation. Bone scintigraphy is more sensitive than radiography for detecting skeletal metastases and is very useful for assessing occult bone lesions and responses to treatment. However, tumours that do not evoke an osteoblastic response (e.g. many myelomas, some lymphomas and rapidly growing destructive lung cancers and melanomas) and very small lesions may not be detected by scintigraphy. In diffuse disseminated disease, bone scintigraphy may appear to be normal when in fact there is markedly increased uptake, reducing urinary excretion of the isotope leading to a faint or absent renal appearance – this is called a 'superscan'.

Optional investigations include MRI, which is very useful for assessing spinal disease (lymphoma and myeloma especially), soft tissue extension, spinal cord compression and distinguishing osteoporotic fractures from pathological fractures. CT is useful for confirming solitary lesions when bone scan findings and plain films are equivocal, assessing bone mineral content/cortical stability and also demonstrating soft tissue extension. PET (positron emission tomography) scanning is still investigational. Bone biopsy, mammography, thyroid examination/ultrasound, tumour markers (e.g. thyroglobulin, PSA) may be helpful if the primary is unknown.

MANAGEMENT

The aims of managing patients with metastatic bone disease include relieving pain, preserving and restoring function, and preventing and treating complications. The patient's overall prognosis and life expectancy should be taken into account when deciding on treatment interventions. General measures include the pharmacological management of pain (with paracetamol, NSAIDs, opiates, antidepressants and anticonvulsants) as well as bed rest for patients with impending fractures, steroids for spinal cord compression and fluids/bisphosphonates for hypercalcaemia. Physiotherapy and rehabilitation also play very important roles. The major therapeutic modalities are surgery, radiotherapy and systemic therapy.

ORTHOPAEDIC SURGERY

The role of the surgeon falls into three main categories.

1. Prophylactic fixation of metastatic deposits where there is a risk of fracture
Recognised indications for prophylactic surgery include:

- destruction of more than 50% of cortex in a long bone (risk of fracture should be regarded as inevitable without fixation)

TABLE 48.1 Mirel's scoring system for assessing risk of pathological fracture

Variable	Score 1	Score 2	Score 3
Site	Upper limb	Lower limb	Peritrochanter
Pain	Mild	Moderate	Functional
Lesion	Blastic	Mixed	Lytic
Size (bone diameter)	<⅓ cortex destroyed	⅓–⅔ cortical destruction	>⅔ cortical destruction

Scores of 7 or less have <5% fracture risk and conservative management is appropriate.
Scores of 9 or above have a high fracture risk and prophylactic fixation is required.
Scores of 8 are intermediate risk with a 15% fracture risk and careful decision-making is required.

- large lytic metastasis in long bone (e.g. lytic lesion of femur ≥2.5 cm is at high risk of fracture)
- avulsion of the lesser tuberosity of the femur (indicates imminent hip fracture)
- pain exacerbated by movement or persistent pain despite RT.

Mirel has devised a practical scoring system for pathological fracture risk assessment (Table 48.1).

Surgical techniques for impending fractures are similar to pathological fractures (see below). Avoidance of fracture during the operation is very important as this will reduce inpatient stay and improve the overall result.

2. Stabilisation or reconstruction following pathological fracture

The main principles underlying the orthopaedic management of pathological fractures are:

- the procedure should provide immediate stability
- the surgeon must assume the fracture will not reunite
- the fixation should aim to last the patient's lifetime
- all lesions in the affected bone should, where possible, be stabilised.

Load-bearing devices are preferred and intramedullary nailing is advised in the diaphysis of long bones. Bone defects should be filled with bone cement. Load-sharing plates and screws should be avoided in the lower limb but can be utilised in the upper limb where stresses are less.

Hip fractures are the commonest type of pathological fracture and management differs from purely traumatic fractures. X-rays of the entire femur should be obtained preoperatively to exclude more distal disease. The dynamic hip screw (DHS) should be avoided. Cemented total joint replacement or hemi-arthroplasty is recommended when destruction is limited to the femoral neck or head. Acetabular lesions are filled with bone cement with threaded pins driven into remaining good bone (Harrington procedure). Endoprosthetic reconstruction is indicated for more extensive destruction of the proximal femur (or humerus). Postoperative radiotherapy should be offered to the entire surgical field and extend the length of any prosthesis or internal fixation device. A dose of 20 Gy in five fractions is usually given after the surgical wound has healed.

Metastatic lesions or fractures of the scapula and clavicle are usually best managed by radiotherapy alone, but if there is significant destruction of the humeral head, hemi-arthroplasty is the treatment of choice. In forearm fractures, plate fixation with cement augmentation is highly effective.

When life expectancy is assumed to be less than 6 weeks, careful decision-making by the multidisciplinary team is required before offering major orthopaedic surgery.

3. Decompression of spinal cord and nerve roots, followed by stabilisation of the affected vertebra

See Chapter 60 on spinal cord compression.

RADIOTHERAPY

Radiotherapy is an extremely useful modality for the management of pain from bone metastases. However, it should be noted that RT is less helpful for mechanical type pain.

Radiotherapy can be utilised in the following ways:

1. Local radiotherapy

There is a considerable body of evidence to support the use of a single 8 Gy fraction for localised bone pain. Approximately 70% of patients will experience pain relief, with 50% improving within 2 weeks and another 20% within 4 weeks. The median duration of response is 6 months. Higher dose fractionated courses (e.g. 20 Gy in five fractions or 30 Gy in 10 fractions) are usually offered when there is associated spinal cord or nerve root compression, involvement of weight-bearing bones or in the postoperative setting. Radical radiotherapy may be appropriate for highly selected patients with a solitary bone metastasis, e.g. thyroid cancer, renal cancer.

2. Wide-field radiotherapy

Larger radiation fields may be required to cover painful areas such as the lumbar spine and pelvis, which is a common site of metastases in prostate cancer. A single fraction of 8 Gy or 20 Gy in five fractions can be given to a large 'spade-shaped' field. Premedication with antiemetics (5-HT$_3$ inhibitors) is advisable.

3. Hemibody radiotherapy

For patients with multiple painful bony metastases, hemibody radiotherapy is very effective, with pain response rates of 70%. The upper body receives a single fraction of 6 Gy and the lower body a single 8 Gy fraction. If both halves of the body need irradiating, then a gap of 6–8 weeks between the upper and lower body treatments is required to allow bone marrow recovery. Antiemetics should be given prior to the radiotherapy and frail patients are admitted overnight in case of severe vomiting and dehydration, which can be treated with fluids, steroids and further antiemetics. Fewer than 50% will require further local radiotherapy for recurrent pain. Myelosuppression is a common complication and for this reason hemibody radiotherapy is generally avoided if systemic chemotherapy is likely to be offered. A full blood count should be checked prior to treatment.

4. Systemic radionuclides

This method of treatment is also very useful for treating multiple painful bone metastases and is better tolerated than hemibody radiotherapy. Strontium-89 is the most commonly used systemic radioisotope and is a pure β-emitter with a half-life of 50 days. It is metabolised in a similar manner to calcium and so preferentially concentrates at sites of new bone formation. Over 80% of prostate cancer patients achieve symptomatic benefit with strontium-89 and it has also been shown to be clinically useful in breast cancer. It can also be used in conjunction with external beam radiotherapy and repeated injections can be used (at least 4 months after initial injection) as long as blood counts are satisfactory. The main side effects are myelo-suppression (20–30% falls in white cell and platelet counts are common) and an initial acute exacerbation of pain (flare) in 10–15% that actually predicts for a good response. Other radionuclides that are available include samarium-153 and rhenium-186. Iodine-131 is useful in the treatment of bone metastases from thyroid cancer.

SYSTEMIC THERAPY

The selection of appropriate systemic therapies mainly depends on the type of tumour, the likely prognosis and the performance status of the patient. Options include chemotherapy, hormone therapy, immunotherapy and bisphosphonates.

I. Chemotherapy

Combination chemotherapy may be curative for patients with bone involvement from lymphoma or germ cell tumours, but is palliative for other tumour types. Bone metastases from breast cancer may respond extremely well to chemotherapy, but it is generally reserved for hormone-insensitive tumours and/or aggressive life-threatening disease.

2. Hormone therapy

Hormone-sensitive breast cancer has a predilection for spread to bone and hormone therapy is effective in 60% of patients. Tamoxifen 20 mg o.d.

is used in premenopausal women and anastrozole 1 mg o.d. in postmenopausal women. Androgen ablation in prostate cancer produces pain relief as well as an improvement in 30–50% of bone scans and normalisation of PSA in 70%.

3. Immunotherapy

Interferon and/or interleukin-2 offer little benefit to renal cancer and melanoma patients with bone metastases and are more effective for soft tissue disease.

4. Bisphosphonates

These drugs inhibit osteoclastic bone resorption. In patients with bone metastases, they are useful for pain relief, hypercalcaemia (see section on hypercalcaemia in Ch. 56 – Metabolic problems in cancer), and prevention of skeletal related events. Most studies using these drugs have been in breast cancer. Radiotherapy is still the treatment of choice for painful bone metastases, but bisphosphonates are a useful additional option. Regular bisphosphonates decrease skeletal related events (fractures, bone pain, requirement for radiotherapy, hypercalcaemia) in breast cancer (by 25–50%), myeloma, prostate cancer and other tumours. The most commonly used agents are monthly intravenous pamidronate (90 mg IV) and oral clodronate (800 mg b.d. p.o. 30 minutes before food). Zoledronic acid is a promising new highly potent third generation bisphosphonate and has recently been shown to produce a more rapid and complete control of hypercalcaemia than pamidronate. It is also the first bisphosphonate to be proven to be effective in delaying and reducing the complications of the predominantly osteoblastic lesions seen in prostate cancer.

Bisphosphonates may also prevent or at least delay the development of skeletal metastases although further studies are ongoing. Data suggesting a survival benefit in the metastatic setting with the use of bisphosphonates is controversial. In the adjuvant setting, a recent phase III breast cancer study did show a significant survival benefit for patients who received bisphosphonate therapy, but further data are needed to confirm this.

VERTEBROPLASTY

This new technique involves the injection of low viscosity polymethyl-methacrylate cement into metastatic lytic vertebral bodies that have been extensively destroyed by tumour and are causing mechanical symptoms. A pain relief success rate of 97% has been reported with a complication rate of 2–3% mainly due to leakage of the cement. An associated fracture is a contraindication to the technique due to the risk of cement leakage, which can lead to catastrophic neurological injury.

FURTHER READING

BASO Guidelines 1999 The management of metastatic bone disease in the United Kingdom. European Journal of Surgical Oncology 25:3–23

Coleman R E 2000 Management of bone metastases. Oncologist 5:463–470. Available at: www.theoncologist.com

Coleman R E 2001 Metastatic bone disease: Clinical features, pathophysiology and treatment strategies. Cancer Treatment Reviews 27:165–176

Schachar N S 2001 An update on the nonoperative treatment of patients with metastatic bone disease. Clinical Orthopaedics and Related Research 382:75–81

Brain metastases

INTRODUCTION

Brain metastases are the most common intracranial tumours in adults and are estimated to occur in 20–30% of cancer patients. They represent an increasingly common problem because of more effective treatment and control of cancer as well as increased detection with CT and MRI scanning.

The commonest primary tumours that metastasise to the brain are lung cancer (48%), breast cancer (15%), melanoma (9%) and colon cancer (5%), with other known primary (13%) and unknown primary (11%) tumours making up the rest. In young adults, sarcomas and germ cell tumours are the commonest types. Approximately 80% of brain metastases are located in the cerebral hemispheres, 15% in the cerebellum, and 5% in the brainstem. At diagnosis 65–75% have multiple brain metastases. Colon, breast and renal metastases often lead to single brain metastases, whereas lung and melanoma usually produce multiple lesions. Cerebellar lesions have a worse prognosis.

The overall prognosis of patients with brain metastases is poor, with a median survival of 3–4 months. Median survival of untreated patients is 4 weeks. Only half of patients will die from systemic disease and therefore the goal of treatment is to achieve local control. Prognostic factors can help identify patients with a better prognosis who may benefit from more intensive treatments. Factors that are prognostically favourable include: good performance status (Karnofsky (KPS) >70), good neurological function, solitary brain metastasis, absence of extracranial disease, younger age and a controlled primary tumour. The Radiotherapy and Oncology Group (RTOG) have developed a useful prognostic guide based on recursive partitioning analysis (RPA) of a large database containing hundreds of patients with brain metastases (Table 49.1).

A few patients may enjoy long-term survival. In one large study of over 700 patients with brain metastases, 8.1% of patients were alive at 2 years and 2.4% alive at 5 years. Not surprisingly, younger age, a single metastasis, and treatment with surgical resection, whole brain radiotherapy (WBRT) and chemotherapy were factors associated with the best chance of long-term survival.

TABLE 49.1 RPA prognostic guide for patients with brain metastases

RPA class	Criteria	Median survival
I	All of the following: KPS >70, age <65 years, controlled primary, no extracranial disease	7.1 months
II	KPS >70 and at least one of the following: >65 years, uncontrolled synchronous primary, extracranial disease	4.2 months
III	KPS <70	2.3 months

KPS, Karnofsky performance status; RPA, recursive partitioning analysis.

CLINICAL PRESENTATION

Over 80% of brain metastases are discovered after diagnosis of systemic cancer has been made and most are symptomatic.

The commonest symptoms are headache (42%), mental change (32%), gradual onset focal weakness (27%), seizures (20–25%), speech disturbance (10%), ataxia (17%) and sensory disturbance (6%). Headaches tend to be diffuse and mild or bi-frontal but may occasionally be localised over the site of the lesion. A worsening throbbing morning headache associated with increasing drowsiness and confusion suggests raised intracranial pressure due to CSF obstruction or extensive tumour mass. An acute onset of symptoms may be due to bleeding into a metastasis, tumour embolisation, vascular invasion/occlusion by tumour, or seizures.

The commonest signs are hemiparesis (44%), altered mental state (35%), ataxia (13%), papilloedema (9%), and hemisensory loss (9%).

DIAGNOSIS

Gadolinium-enhanced MRI is more sensitive than CT for demonstration of intracranial metastases. At the time of diagnosis, 50% will have a solitary metastasis shown on CT, whereas less than 30% will have only one lesion on MRI.

Imaging features that suggest metastases rather than primary brain tumours include the presence of multiple lesions, grey–white matter junction location, lesser degree of margin irregularity, and a small tumour with a large area of surrounding vasogenic oedema.

If the primary is unknown, a CXR will reveal a mass in 60%. If the CXR is negative, then CT of the chest and abdomen may be useful. Mammography and blood tests for PSA, β-HCG and AFP may be appropriate as breast cancer, prostate cancer and testicular tumours may be very responsive to therapy. However, further investigations are not usually helpful if nothing is suggestive on clinical history and examination.

MANAGEMENT

Initial management may require urgent treatment of raised intracranial pressure (ICP) if this is compromising consciousness and respiratory function. This may be achieved with steroids, mannitol and, if necessary and indicated, sedation, intubation and hyperventilation (low pCO_2 decreases raised ICP). Virtually all patients should receive steroids, and dexamethasone IV or p.o. is the steroid of choice due to its minimal mineralocorticoid activity and low tendency to induce psychosis.

Over 70% of patients will improve symptomatically on steroids and responses are usually seen within 6–24 hours, reaching a maximum effect at 3–7 days. Focal symptoms respond less well than generalised neurological symptoms. The optimum dose is unknown, but a dose of 8–16 mg of dexamethasone is commonly used. Median survival is improved from 1 to 2 months with steroids alone.

Seizures should be treated with appropriate anticonvulsants. There is no evidence for using anticonvulsants in the prophylactic setting.

Possible further management includes surgery, radiosurgery, radiotherapy, chemotherapy, biological therapy, or best supportive care only. This will depend on several factors including histological diagnosis, performance status, age, single or multiple metastases and presence of active extracranial disease.

There is a subgroup of patients with a very short life expectancy for whom active treatment with WBRT is inappropriate. They include patients with poor performance status and active extracranial disease. Patients over 60 or with non-small cell lung cancer also have a poor outlook and the decision to offer WBRT needs careful consideration.

SOLITARY METASTASIS

Patients with a solitary metastasis, good performance status and inactive extracranial disease may have a much better outlook. Surgical resection results in immediate decompression of the brain as well as removing the source of the brain oedema leading to the resolution of headache, nausea and vomiting, and reduction in steroid requirements. Not infrequently, there is improvement in peri-tumoral brain function with amelioration of focal neurological deficits, psychomotor slowing and seizures. Postoperative WBRT has little impact on overall survival due to high incidence of deaths due to progressive systemic disease. However, it significantly reduces the number of neurological deaths and is therefore offered in many centres. Median survival is approximately 12 months.

For surgically inaccessible lesions (e.g. brainstem), stereotactic radiosurgery using a multi-source cobalt unit (gamma knife) or multiple arc linear accelerators can be used to deliver a high single dose to a small treatment volume with minimal damage to surrounding normal brain tissue. Single doses of 15–25 Gy produce 12 month local progression-free survival of approximately 60–80% and median survival of 6–7 months. However, radiosurgery is not widely available in the UK and is limited to lesions less than 4 cm in size. The addition of WBRT following radiosurgery is controversial.

MULTIPLE BRAIN METASTASES

WBRT is the treatment of choice for most patients under 60 with good performance status (KPS >70), and without active extracranial disease. The optimal schedule for WBRT is unknown, but commonly used regimens are 30 Gy in 10 fractions (2 weeks), 20 Gy in 5 fractions (1 week) or 12 Gy in 2 fractions (2 days). In general, the shorter schedules are used for the poorer prognostic patients. Median survival after WBRT is 3–7 months. The palliative efficacy of WBRT remains uncertain, but approximately 50% of patients will experience relief and improvement of symptoms.

The role of systemic chemotherapy is not clearly defined but may be initially more appropriate for patients with germ cell tumours, breast cancer, small cell lung cancer, ovarian cancer, choriocarcinoma and lymphomas.

Approximately 50–60% of breast cancer patients will have an objective response to chemotherapy. Median survival in responders is 12 months, but less than 3 months in non-responders. Anecdotally, brain metastases from breast cancer may respond to hormonal therapy such as tamoxifen. The role of biotherapy is investigational.

RECURRENT BRAIN METASTASES

There is some evidence that local treatment (surgery or radiosurgery) of recurrent solitary metastases may be of benefit, but careful patient selection is required. Reirradiation with WBRT is controversial, but some clinicians would consider it for good performance status patients without active extracranial disease who have deteriorated neurologically 4 months or more after a good response to initial radiotherapy. The optimum schedule is unknown, but 20 Gy over 2 weeks is well tolerated. Median survival following reirradiation varies between 3.5 and 5 months. Brain tolerance may be exceeded, but this is very unlikely to pose a clinical problem due to poor overall prognosis.

FURTHER READING

Consensus Statement (2nd Workshop on palliative radiotherapy and symptom control, London 2000) 2001 Radiotherapy for brain metastases. Clinical Oncology 13:91–94

Editorial 1998 Treatment of a single brain metastasis. The role of radiation following surgical resection. JAMA 280(17):1527–1529

van de Bent M J 2001 The diagnosis and management of brain metastases. Current Opinion in Neurology 14:717–723

CHAPTER 50

Leptomeningeal carcinomatosis

INTRODUCTION

Leptomeningeal carcinomatosis (LC), also known as carcinomatous meningitis, occurs in approximately 5% of all cancer patients, but is being diagnosed more frequently due to longer overall survival of cancer patients and advances in neuroimaging.

It is a disease of the entire neuro-axis and several mechanisms have been proposed to explain how malignant cells gain access to the leptomeninges. These mechanisms include: (1) infiltration via arachnoid vessels or the choroid plexus following haematogenous dissemination; (2) direct extension from pre-existing CNS tumours (primary brain tumours such as ependymomas, medulloblastomas and pineoblastomas frequently seed into the CSF); (3) direct extension from bone metastases; (4) migration from systemic tumour spreading along perineural or perivascular spaces; and (5) seeding of the subarachnoid space during surgical resection of intraparenchymal metastases.

The commonest solid tumours that metastasise to the leptomeninges are breast cancer, lung cancer, melanoma and gastrointestinal cancers. LC occurs in 1–2% of patients with primary brain tumours and approximately 7–15% of patients with lymphomas and 5–15% with leukaemias.

LC has a very poor prognosis, with median survival of 4–6 weeks untreated and 3–6 months following radiotherapy and chemotherapy. Death usually results from progressive neurological dysfunction.

PRESENTATION

LC presents in many ways, but in general, five groups of neurological disturbance occur:

1. Cerebral hemisphere disturbance from either direct infiltration or tumour occlusion of pial blood vessels leading to headache, alteration in mental

status, ataxia, stroke-like syndromes and focal or secondary generalised seizures.

2. Cranial nerve palsies may cause diplopia, facial weakness/numbness/pain, swallowing difficulties, hearing loss and visual disturbance.
3. Spinal cord and nerve root involvement causes weakness, numbness and pain in the affected distribution.
4. Obstruction of CSF flow may cause raised intracranial pressure and hydrocephalus with its associated signs and symptoms.
5. Metabolic interference with normal CNS function leading to encephalopathy.

A high index of suspicion is required to make an early diagnosis and combinations of headache, alteration in mental status, cranial nerve palsies, radiculopathy, incontinence, weakness and sensory abnormalities are common presenting features. LC should always be considered in the cancer patient with multiple neurological symptoms and signs.

DIAGNOSIS

The single most useful test is examination of the CSF, which is abnormal in nearly all patients with LC regardless of CSF cytology. A completely normal CSF is associated with LC in less than 5% of cases. Positive CSF cytology is present in 50% of LC patients, but this increases to 80% following a second CSF examination. The most reliable tumour markers in CSF are HCG, AFP, immunoglobulins from myeloma and CEA. Monoclonal antibody and flow cytometry techniques may be helpful in difficult to diagnose cases.

Contrast-enhanced CT is abnormal in 25–50% of patients with LC. Gadolinium-enhanced MRI is more sensitive than CT and is generally the preferred radiological investigation of choice. Both techniques have a high incidence of false-negatives (CT 58%, MRI 30%). The most common findings are contrast enhancement of the basilar cisterns, cortical convexities and cauda equina, and hydrocephalus without an associated mass lesion. Multifocal subarachnoid lesions are particularly suggestive of LC in a cancer patient.

MANAGEMENT

The main aims are to improve symptoms and quality of life, and prolong survival. Treatment decisions should be made on an individual basis based on the tumour type, likely prognosis, symptoms and performance status. Patients with low volume indolent tumours that are likely to respond to therapy, with no fixed neurological deficits and an excellent performance status, are most likely to benefit from an aggressive treatment approach.

Unfortunately, the majority of patients with LC do not belong to this category and should be managed symptomatically.

Treatment modalities used in LC include radiotherapy, regional chemotherapy, systemic chemotherapy and surgery (limited to insertion of Ommaya reservoirs and ventricular-peritoneal shunts).

For patients fit for an aggressive approach, treatment should encompass the entire neuro-axis. Radiotherapy to the whole craniospinal axis is useful for leukaemic meningitis, but is less effective for solid tumours and is associated with significant myelosuppression. Involved-field radiotherapy to symptomatic and bulk disease is much better tolerated and can be followed by intrathecal (IT) chemotherapy, which is designed to treat subclinical leptomeningeal disease. An Ommaya reservoir can be inserted surgically to make IT administration of chemotherapy much simpler. IT chemotherapy agents include methotrexate (MTX), arabinoside-C and thiotepa and they are typically given twice weekly. Optimal systemic therapy should also be considered for patients with breast cancer and lymphoma.

Treatment complications may be significant and include arachnoiditis infection from IT therapy, mucositis from MTX (can be reduced or prevented with folinic acid), myelosuppression from chemotherapy and radiotherapy, and neurotoxicity. The most significant and feared toxicity is necrotising leucoencephalopathy, which is most commonly seen in patients with a prolonged survival who receive IT MTX following cranial radiotherapy. Its incidence may approach 30% in treated leukaemia and lymphoma patients. White matter changes are seen on neuroimaging in asymptomatic patients and many patients will subsequently develop a progressive dementia and other neurological complications, eventually leading to death.

Poor prognosis patients are best served with supportive care only, although a few may derive symptomatic benefit from involved-field radiotherapy to symptomatic sites, e.g. 20 Gy in five fractions. Multiple brain metastases are often present with LC, and whole brain radiotherapy, e.g. 20 Gy in five fractions or 12 Gy in two fractions, may be offered.

FURTHER READING

Chamberlain M C 2000 Neoplastic meningitis. Current Opinion in Neurology 13:641–648
Grossman S A, Krabak M J 1999 Leptomeningeal carcinomatosis. Cancer Treatment Reviews 25:103–119

Liver metastases

INTRODUCTION

The liver is a major site for metastatic cancer. In one very large autopsy study of over 8000 cancer patients, liver metastases were found in 41% of cases and for tumours found within the portal drainage areas, this figure was up to 75%.

The commonest cancers that metastasise to the liver are colorectal, lung, breast, stomach, pancreas and biliary cancers. Nearly 50% of all patients with colorectal cancer will develop liver metastases, which are the major cause of death. Untreated, prognosis is very poor with median survival of 6 months and 3-year survival less than 3%. With modern chemotherapy (5FU, irinotecan, oxaliplatin), median survival has improved to around 20 months. Surgical resection of colorectal liver metastases may offer 5-year survival rates of 25–30%, but only 10–20% of patients fulfil selection criteria amenable to surgery.

Non-colorectal metastases are considered inoperable in most cases even if technically resectable. This is because the patterns of failure and risks of relapse suggest that liver resection is not useful in this group of patients. However, the possibility of resection should still be assessed on an individual basis. Metastases from functioning neuroendocrine tumours are an exception as they are often slow growing and metastasectomy can relieve symptoms and improve survival. Most reports of surgical cure from other tumour types are anecdotal with success most likely in patients with a long disease-free interval and a solitary metastasis.

As well as surgery, other treatments for liver metastases include chemotherapy, embolisation, alcohol injections, cryoablation, radiofrequency ablation and supportive care measures. The type of treatment is primarily based on the origin of the primary tumour. Inoperable liver metastases are usually incurable, but exceptions include germ cell tumours and lymphomas.

PRESENTATION

Liver metastases may present at the time of the primary diagnosis of the tumour (synchronous) or later in the course of the illness (metachronous).

Most patients are asymptomatic unless the liver disease is advanced, when symptoms such as weight loss, anorexia, nausea, right upper quadrant pain, abdominal distension (ascites or liver mass), ankle swelling, night sweats, pruritus and jaundice may be present. Pain is due to stretching of the liver capsule and is characteristically dull, aching, poorly localised and referred to the right hypochondrium and sometimes the tip of the right shoulder due to diaphragmatic irritation. In addition, sharp knife-like pains are not uncommon.

Clinically, the liver is usually not palpable until there is a large tumour burden, at which point it may have a hard, knobbly tender surface and may be associated with ascites and other stigmata of chronic liver disease.

DIAGNOSIS

Investigations include: liver function tests; clotting; FBC; renal function tests; CEA; CXR; ultrasound of the abdomen; CT scanning with dynamic IV contrast bolus (most metastases are hypovascular and appear as low attenuation lesions within opacified parenchyma). MRI may also provide additional useful information for potentially operable patients.

For patients with an unknown primary, image-guided liver biopsy should be performed unless there are more accessible extrahepatic metastases, e.g. lymph nodes. Tumour markers may also be helpful. For patients with a known primary from the gastrointestinal (GI) tract, breast or lung, it is not usually necessary to obtain histological confirmation unless there has been a long disease-free period.

MANAGEMENT

The management of liver metastases depends on several factors including the type of primary tumour, presence of extrahepatic disease, the location and extent of the liver metastases, co-morbidity (e.g. liver cirrhosis) and the performance status of the patient. The vast majority of patients will have incurable disease with the main aim of treatment being palliation with possible prolongation of survival. Surgery in selected patients offers the only realistic chance of cure. Other therapies such as chemotherapy, embolisation, alcohol injections, cryoablation and radiofrequency ablation are palliative interventions.

SURGERY

Hepatic surgery for non-colorectal liver metastases is rarely indicated. Exceptions include neuroendocrine tumours and hepatocellular carcinoma.

Only 10–20% of patients with colorectal liver metastases are suitable for surgical resection. The goals of potentially curative surgery are:

1. Removal of all metastases with free margins of at least 1 cm
2. Preservation of a functioning liver
3. Preservation of good biliary drainage.

The extent of the resection depends on the size, number, location and relation of the metastases to the vascular and biliary pedicles and on the volume of parenchyma to be left in place after surgery. Up to six of the eight anatomical liver segments or 75% of the volume of the liver can be resected without inducing postoperative liver failure. In general, surgery should at least be considered for patients with no extrahepatic disease with good performance status, when resection margins of at least 10 mm can be obtained safely. The only absolute contraindications are poor general health, clear evidence of extrahepatic disease or inability to resect all disease.

Surgical mortality rates are less than 5% in most centres, and morbidity rates are 20–40% (usually due to transient liver failure, haemorrhage, subphrenic abscess or biliary fistula). Five-year survival rates range from 25 to 40%. Poor prognostic features include resection margins less than 1 cm, more than four metastases, lesions >5 cm, positive lymph nodes, elevated CEA levels (>30 μg/l), advanced primary tumour, synchronous metastases and short disease-free interval.

In patients with operable synchronous liver metastases at diagnosis, the primary tumour is usually resected first followed by liver resection a few months later.

After surgery, two-thirds of patients will develop recurrent disease and 25–50% of these recurrences are confined to the liver. Re-resection is recommended if technically feasible and survival is comparable to primary liver resection.

As only 10–20% of patients with colorectal liver metastases are operable, new modalities have evolved to try and improve the number of patients for resection. These include:

1. Portal embolisation – may be offered in selected cases, when the volume of remnant liver would be too small following an otherwise technically feasible resection. The lobe to be resected is atrophied by embolisation of the relevant portal venous branch, allowing compensatory hypertrophy of the remaining liver (20–50% increase in size over 3 to 6 weeks). Liver resection may then be performed leaving a safe volume of liver remnant.
2. Neoadjuvant chemotherapy with oxaliplatin in combination with 5FU has been shown to increase resection rates in patients with initially inoperable disease confined to the liver. The National Institute of Clinical Excellence (NICE) has therefore recommended this combination for first line use in patients with advanced colorectal cancer confined to the liver, which may become resectable after treatment.

SYSTEMIC CHEMOTHERAPY

Systemic chemotherapy is commonly used in patients with liver metastases but its efficacy depends mainly on the type and extent of the primary tumour. In colorectal cancer 5FU-based therapy has objective response rates of 20–25%, with 40–50% of patients obtaining symptomatic benefit. Overall improvement in median survival is about 6 months. These results have recently improved with new agents such as irinotecan and oxaliplatin. In gastric cancer, similar palliative effects are seen using ECF (epirubicin, cisplatin, 5FU) chemotherapy, but results for other GI cancers are less encouraging. Breast cancer is particularly sensitive to chemotherapy and excellent palliation can be achieved. Dose reductions may be required for some drugs if there is hepatic dysfunction.

REGIONAL CHEMOTHERAPY

Liver metastases obtain most of their blood supply from the hepatic artery, whereas normal liver parenchyma receives most of its supply from the portal vein. Hepatic arterial infusional (HAI) chemotherapy (e.g. with floxuridine (FUDR)) has the potential advantages of producing higher drug levels within the liver with less risk of systemic toxicity. Although encouraging results have been produced, this treatment is still experimental and subject to further clinical studies.

THERMAL ABLATION

Cryosurgery with ultrasound-guided liquid nitrogen probes causes tissue destruction by subzero temperatures. It is safe and effective for the treatment of unresectable primary and metastatic liver tumours.

Radiofrequency ablation (RFA) involves inserting needle electrodes (percutaneously or by laparotomy) into tumours and applying a high frequency alternating current across them. This leads to local temperatures of over 60°C causing thermal injury to tissue. It is suitable for metastases less than 5–6 cm in size, but is not widely available at present.

CHEMOEMBOLISATION

Chemoembolisation combines hepatic artery embolisation with gelatin sponge particles, oil and chemotherapy drugs. This causes tumour ischaemia and high tumour drug concentrations. It has no present role in colorectal cancer, but has shown encouraging results for hepatomas and neuroendocrine tumours.

PERCUTANEOUS ALCOHOL INJECTION

Ultrasound-guided injection of 99.5% alcohol for small tumours less than 3 cm may offer useful palliation for selected patients, but further trials are needed.

GENERAL SUPPORTIVE MEASURES

Patients with advanced liver metastases may experience pain, nausea and vomiting, anorexia, pruritus, peripheral oedema, ascites, confusional states, bleeding/bruising and infections. General supportive measures such as adequate analgesia, steroids, antiemetics, and adequate hydration may improve symptoms significantly. Drainage of ascites and diuretics may also be helpful.

FURTHER READING

Berney T, Mentha G, Roth A D, Morel P 1998 Results of surgical resection of liver metastases from non-colorectal primaries. British Journal of Surgery 85(10):1423–1427
Devita V T, Hellman S, Rosenberg S A 2001 Liver metastases. In: Cancer: Principles and practice of oncology. Lippincott Williams & Wilkins, Philadelphia

Malignant ascites

INTRODUCTION

Malignant ascites is responsible for approximately 10% of all cases of ascites. Intra-abdominal tumours are the commonest cause, with ovarian cancer being the commonest primary tumour accounting for 30–54% of cases, followed by the unknown primary, pancreatic, stomach and uterine cancers. Breast cancer, lung cancer and lymphoma are the commonest extra-abdominal sites.

Malignant ascites is a manifestation of advanced cancer and prognosis is poor for most patients, with median survival of ~20 weeks from diagnosis and less than 10% alive at one year. The outlook is better for patients with ovarian cancer or lymphomas.

In the normal healthy individual, the peritoneal cavity only has a small volume of fluid (~50 ml) because of the homeostatic balance between the hydrostatic pressure, osmotic pressure, and production and resorption of peritoneal fluid. However, disease processes can upset this balance and lead to fluid accumulation and the development of ascites. The main mechanisms in the production of malignant ascites are:

1. Raised hydrostatic pressure due to: (a) lymphatic obstruction by tumour, (b) inferior vena cava obstruction by tumour or thrombosis, (c) hepatic vein obstruction (Budd–Chiari syndrome) by tumour or thrombosis, (d) activation of renin–angiotensin–aldosterone pathway leading to salt and water retention (probably only a factor in patients with massive hepatic metastases).
2. Fluid production exceeding resorptive capacity due to (a) exudative ascites caused by excess protein (albumin) production by tumour, (b) tumour production of vascular endothelial factors (cytokines) leading to 'leaky' vessels with increased permeability to albumin and other proteins.
3. Decreased osmotic pressure due to hypoalbuminaemia.
4. Co-morbid medical conditions such as cardiac failure and cirrhosis of the liver.

CLINICAL FEATURES AND DIAGNOSIS

The commonest symptoms are abdominal distension, discomfort and pain, peripheral oedema and anorexia. Other symptoms include nausea and vomiting (often due to 'squashed stomach syndrome'), shortness of breath, fatigue and decreased mobility. A change in weight is common (weight gain or weight loss).

Clinical signs include abdominal distension, shifting dullness to percussion, and a fluid thrill. Other generalised or localised signs of advanced cancer may also be present.

An ultrasound scan is the easiest and quickest way of confirming the presence of ascites and as little as 100 ml can be detected. A safe site for a diagnostic or therapeutic paracentesis can also be marked on the patient. Aspirated fluid should be sent for cytology, microbiology and biochemistry. Cytology is particularly sensitive for peritoneal carcinomatosis (cytology is positive in >95% of cases). If initial cytology is negative, but clinical suspicion of malignancy is high, then repeat cytology is justified. If the cause of the ascites is still unknown, then further investigations may be appropriate. CT scanning may reveal the primary and is very useful for diagnosing ovarian and pancreatic tumours as well as liver metastases. Other investigations depending on the specific clinical indication include tumour markers (e.g. CEA, CA125, CA19.9), transvaginal ultrasound, barium enema, colonoscopy, gastroscopy, laparoscopy or laparotomy.

MANAGEMENT

There are no evidence-based guidelines in the management of malignant ascites.

As the prognosis is poor in these patients, management is palliative. Treatment should be appropriately tailored to the type of primary tumour causing the ascites. The main interventions are symptomatic paracentesis, diuretic therapy, appropriate systemic therapy, and peritoneovenous shunting. Intraperitoneal therapies remain investigational.

SYMPTOMATIC PARACENTESIS

Symptomatic paracentesis is still the mainstay of treatment, providing relief of symptoms in 90%, but this is usually temporary and may need repeating due to reaccumulation of fluid. The procedure is usually safe to perform 'blind' (without radiological guidance) in symptomatic patients, as the volume of clinically detectable fluid is so large. However, in patients with loculated ascites, large tumour masses or adhesions, drainage of fluid under ultrasound guidance is recommended. Rapid removal of large volumes of ascites should be avoided, as this may lead to hypotension, renal impairment and hyponatraemia. Other complications include peritonitis, hypo-albuminaemia, visceral injury and pulmonary emboli. Up to 10 litres per day may be safely drained, but simultaneous IV fluid replacement with 5% dextrose is a sensible measure when large volumes are removed.

PERMANENT IMPLANTABLE DRAINS

These may prevent the need for repeated paracentesis, which poses the risk of electrolyte disturbance. The drains have been designed to cope with viscous fluids and are less likely to block than peritoneovenous shunts. However, the risk of peritonitis is high (38% in one study) and they are best reserved for patients who develop electrolyte disturbances following repeated paracentesis.

DIURETIC THERAPY

Diuretic therapy is generally less effective in malignant ascites than in cirrhotic ascites. This is because the main mechanism of fluid retention in cirrhosis is activation of the renin–angiotensin–aldosterone pathway (leading to salt and water retention), but this is rarely a major feature in malignant ascites. However, diuretic therapy with spironolactone (100–400 mg daily) and/or furosemide (frusemide) (40–100 mg daily) can be helpful, but may take up to 28 days to achieve full effect. Salt and fluid restriction may also be helpful. Interestingly, patients with massive hepatic metastases and ascites may behave more like cirrhotic patients and respond very well to diuretics.

SYSTEMIC THERAPY

Systemic therapy should be offered to patients with tumours that are likely to be responsive. Very good responses to chemotherapy may be seen in ovarian cancer with complete resolution of ascites and significant prolongation of survival. Ascites due to breast cancer is best treated by chemotherapy if a rapid response is required, otherwise endocrine agents such as tamoxifen or aromatase inhibitors may also be helpful. Therapeutic paracentesis prior to systemic therapy is appropriate if the patient is very symptomatic.

PERITONEOVENOUS SHUNT

Peritoneovenous shunts provide effective palliation in 64–77% of patients with malignant ascites. A Denver shunt (which has a valve and reservoir which can be pumped) is commonly used and is inserted under a short general anaesthetic. The abdominal end is inserted in the hypochondrium and the venous end led subcutaneously into the internal jugular vein and superior vena cava. However, complications are common (25%) and include shunt occlusion, sepsis, fluid overload, DIC and thrombosis. Tumour dissemination may also occur but this is rare. Due to the high complication rate it is generally agreed that shunts are contraindicated in gastrointestinal (GI) malignancy (due to poor prognosis), and should only be used in non-GI malignancies when other options have failed and/or if the patient is of reasonable performance status and likely to survive more than 3 months.

INTRAPERITONEAL THERAPIES

There are currently no large studies on the use of intraperitoneal chemotherapy for malignant ascites and therefore this method is still investigational. The same is true for intraperitoneal radiocolloids such as phosphorus-32 and biological agents such as interferon and tumour necrosis factor (TNF).

FURTHER READING

Parsons S L, Watson S A, Steele R J C 1996 Malignant ascites (review). British Journal of Surgery 1:6–14
Smith E M, Jayson G C 2003 The current and future management of malignant ascites. Clinical Oncology 15:59–72

Malignant bowel obstruction

INTRODUCTION

Malignant bowel obstruction occurs in 3% of all cancers, but is most commonly seen with colon, stomach and ovarian cancers. It is estimated that 25–40% of patients with ovarian cancer and 16% with colon cancer develop malignant bowel obstruction. The cause of the obstruction may be mechanical or a motility disorder (pseudo-obstruction) – see Table 53.1.

PRESENTATION

Malignant bowel obstruction tends to present over weeks or months, with gradually worsening symptoms, although it can present acutely. The obstructive symptoms tend to be intermittent with episodes often resolving

---

TABLE 53.1 Causes of malignant bowel obstruction

Mechanical causes of obstruction	Motility disorders causing obstruction
1. Tumour in the bowel lumen (e.g. polypoid lesions)	1. Tumour infiltration of coeliac or myenteric nerve plexuses
2. Tumour in the bowel wall (e.g. annular lesions or linitis plastica)	2. Hypokalaemia
3. Tumour causing extrinsic compression (e.g. mesenteric and omental masses)	3. Hypercalcaemia
4. Fibrous adhesions (e.g. postoperative small bowel adhesions)	4. Chemotherapy drugs (e.g. vinca alkaloids)
5. Constipation/faecal impaction	5. Opiate drugs
	6. Anticholinergic drugs
	7. Ischaemic bowel (e.g. due to vascular compression or thrombosis)

spontaneously. The problem may be exacerbated by constipation due to immobility or opiate analgesic use.

Symptoms also depend on the level of occlusion. A high obstruction (e.g. duodenum) causes more severe vomiting, but less abdominal distension. Small bowel obstruction causes nausea, vomiting, abdominal distension and severe pain. Large bowel obstruction causes massive abdominal distension and colicky pain, with vomiting late on.

On examination the patient may be cachexic and dehydrated. In upper gastrointestinal (GI) obstruction, there may be epigastric distension, a succession splash and hyperactive bowel sounds. In lower GI obstruction, there may be gross abdominal obstruction, active high-pitched bowel sounds, and resonance to percussion. Perforation should be suspected if there is peritonism and lack of bowel sounds. A rectal examination to exclude faecal impaction should always be performed.

INVESTIGATIONS

These should include electrolytes, renal and liver function tests, FBC, calcium and albumin. Plain abdominal X-ray may show distended bowel loops, fluid levels, evidence of perforation (air under diaphragm) and faecal loading. Further investigations may be appropriate if surgery is being considered. These include small bowel studies, endoscopy and CT scanning.

MANAGEMENT

General measures include fluid resuscitation, electrolyte correction, 'nil by mouth', analgesia and antiemetics. With conservative measures, 12–29% will have resolution of symptoms. Surgery should be considered in patients whose symptoms fail to resolve. The addition of nasogastric intubation is only useful in patients with high obstruction or in patients about to undergo surgery. The main treatment options available are described below.

PHARMACOLOGICAL

Drugs should be given by the parenteral, sublingual or rectal routes. The continuous subcutaneous infusion has now become the preferred route. Colicky pain is often relieved by strong opiates (e.g. diamorphine 10–20 mg s.c. over 24 hours), but the addition of anticholinergics may be of further help (e.g. hyoscine butylbromide 60–300 µg s.c. over 24 hours). Haloperidol (5–10 mg over 24 hours) is a commonly used antiemetic and is often used in combination with cyclizine (100–150 mg s.c. over 24 hours). Methotrimeprazine (levomepromazine) (12.5–75 mg s.c. over 24 hours) is equally as good. Prokinetic agents such as metoclopramide can be helpful in incomplete bowel obstruction, but can exacerbate colicky pain. 5-HT_3 antagonists are reserved for patients with uncontrolled symptoms. Excessive secretions can be controlled with hyoscine or octreotide (e.g. 300–600 μg s.c. over 24 hours). A recent meta-analysis suggests that dexamethasone at a dose of 6–16 mg IV may bring about the resolution of malignant bowel obstruction, but does not improve survival. If no response to steroids is seen within 4–5 days, then they should be stopped.

SURGERY

The role of palliative surgery remains controversial, but it should be considered if conservative measures fail. Time is usually available to make decisions as malignant bowel obstruction rarely presents as an emergency. Surgical options include (1) resection of obstruction with re-anastomosis, (2) bypass procedures, (3) defunctioning colostomy/ileostomy formation and (4) division of adhesions. The mortality rate from surgery is 20%. Survival rates of 43% at 60 days have been reported, but recurrent or continuing symptoms are common. The median survival following surgery ranges from 2 to 11 months. Survival is better after surgery if: (1) the tumour is low grade/stage, (2) the patient is well nourished and of good performance status, (3) there is no evidence of metastatic disease, (4) the obstruction is caused by benign disease (e.g. radiotherapy stricture or surgical adhesions), (5) age less than 65 years.

VENTING GASTROSTOMY/FEEDING TUBES

These are accepted ways of decompressing the stomach and upper GI tract and are often used for patients with intractable nausea, large volume vomiting or severe pain due to gastric distension. Venting gastrostomies are now preferred to nasogastric tubes and they can be introduced by laparotomy, endoscopically or radiologically. The combination of a venting gastrostomy and jejunal feeding tube can successfully ameliorate the symptoms of high outflow upper GI obstruction.

STENTING

Self-expanding metallic stents (inserted under light sedation using radiological or endoscopic techniques) can relieve obstruction in the colon, jejunum, stomach and rectum. Potential problems include stent migration and bowel perforation. They are contraindicated in patients with multiple obstructions and peritoneal carcinomatosis.

Unfortunately, the majority of patients with malignant bowel obstruction remain symptomatic and the need for parenteral hydration should be decided on an individual basis. Subcutaneous fluids can be given in the home setting if necessary.

FURTHER READING

Baines M J 1997 ABC of palliative care: nausea, vomiting and intestinal obstruction. BMJ 315:1148–1150

Ripamonti C, Bruera E 2002 Palliative management of malignant bowel obstruction. International Journal of Gynaecological Cancer 12:135–143

CHAPTER 54

Malignant pericardial effusions

INTRODUCTION

Up to 10% of patients dying from cancer have cardiac or pericardial metastases, but relatively few have symptomatic pericardial effusions. Despite this, pericardial effusion is still the commonest manifestation of metastatic disease to the pericardium. The commonest cancers that cause pericardial effusions are lung, breast, lymphoma and leukaemias. Malignant melanoma has the greatest propensity to spread to the heart, with reports of up to 50% of patients developing cardiac metastases.

Pericardial effusions result from blockage of lymphatic drainage of the heart by cancer cells. Pericardial effusions in the cancer patient may also result from uraemia, previous mediastinal radiation, coexistent cardiac problems, infections or chemotherapy drugs (e.g. busulphan, cytarabine).

Clinical manifestations of pericardial effusions vary greatly depending on the volume, pressure, rate of accumulation and distensibility of the pericardial sac as well as the cardiac status and general health of the patient. The most feared life-threatening complication is cardiac tamponade, which results from impedance of right atrial and ventricular filling by pericardial fluid pressure and results in low output cardiac failure. Urgent treatment may be life-saving, with some patients enjoying excellent quality of life for many months afterwards.

Overall survival in patients with pericardial effusions is less than 6 months, with 85% dying within a year. Patients with breast cancer and lymphomas have a better outlook.

PRESENTATION

Most patients with a malignant pericardial effusion have a previous diagnosis of cancer and are in the late stages of their disease. It is an unusual initial presentation of malignancy. Many patients are asymptomatic and are diagnosed incidentally on CXR or CT scanning. Symptoms are more a function of pressure increase than the actual volume of fluid present. Therefore a patient may remain asymptomatic with up to 1 litre of pericardial fluid if the effusion accumulates slowly, or have severe symptoms with 100 ml of fluid if pericardium is scarred or non-distensible from infiltration.

The commonest symptoms are dyspnoea, cough, chest pain, fever and oedema. If intra-pericardial pressure becomes significantly elevated, cardiac output is compromised, leading to cardiac tamponade with symptoms of dyspnoea, pre-syncope/syncope, chest pain and signs of tachycardia, hypotension, pulsus paradoxus, raised jugular venous pressure, peripheral shutdown, tender hepatomegaly and muffled heart sounds. Shock and inevitably death will ensue without treatment.

DIAGNOSIS

CXR may reveal globular widening of the cardiac silhouette and pleural effusions. ECG may reveal sinus tachycardia, small QRS complexes, or electrical alternans. Two-dimensional echocardiography can assess the volume (as little as 50 ml) and location of the fluid, the presence of cardiac masses and is frequently used for the safe guidance of pericardiocentesis. Fluid sent for cytological analysis will be positive for malignant cells in 65–85% of malignant pericardial effusions.

MANAGEMENT

The two main aims of management after establishing the diagnosis are relief of immediate symptoms and prevention of recurrence. The type of therapy is highly individualised, as it will depend on the cause and severity of the effusion, and the patient's performance status and likely prognosis.

In patients with severe cardiac tamponade, initial measures include high flow oxygen, IV fluids for volume expansion and inotropic support. Pericardiocentesis can be life-saving in this situation and is performed under local anaesthetic with insertion of the needle at 45% dorsally, aiming towards the tip of the scapula. Over 95% will experience improvement in symptoms, with a complication rate of less than 3% if ultrasound guided. However, most patients will experience recurrent effusions and more definitive treatment may be required.

In asymptomatic or mildly symptomatic patients with primary tumours that are likely to respond to systemic therapy, surgical treatment of the effusions may be avoided as many will resolve with the systemic therapy alone. However, in those who fail or are resistant to systemic anti-cancer therapy or who have more significant symptoms, local surgical intervention may be justified.

Since most patients experience reaccumulation of fluid following pericardiocentesis, preventative methods have been developed to address this problem:

1. Subxiphoid pericardiostomy (pericardial window). This is the most widely used technique and is performed under local anaesthesia. A small piece of pericardium is excised and a draining chest tube is placed in the pericardial space and left in situ for 4–5 days to promote local inflammation and fusion of the visceral and parietal pericardium. The recurrence rate is only 3.5% and the complication rate is less than 2%.
2. Percutaneous balloon pericardiostomy. After a successful needle pericardiocentesis a balloon catheter is inserted and inflated to tear open the needle tract and create a window. The success rate is 92%, but the complication rate of 18% (mainly pleural effusions) is less favourable than traditional surgical pericardiostomy (above).
3. Thoracotomy with pericardiectomy. Now obsolete as it has a high mortality rate (13.3%) compared with the less invasive procedures above.
4. Systemic therapy. Chemotherapy is potentially curative for the lymphoma. Malignant pericardial effusions commonly resolve following chemotherapy in breast cancer patients.
5. Sclerosants. Following pericardiocentesis, a catheter can be inserted and sclerosants (e.g. thiotepa, doxycycline, bleomycin) injected into the pericardial space. However, although success has been reported, there have been relatively few studies with small numbers of patients and this is not a widely used method.
6. Radiotherapy. Has been used successfully to treat pericardial effusions due to breast cancer and lymphomas, but is rarely used.

FURTHER READING

Vaitkus P T, Herrman H C, LeWinter M M 1994 Treatment of malignant pericardial effusion. JAMA 272(1):59–64.

Malignant pleural effusions

INTRODUCTION

Malignant pleural effusions (MPEs) are a common problem and account for up to 50% of all pleural effusions. Lung cancer followed by breast cancer are the commonest causes and account for 50–65% of cases. Lymphomas, genitourinary and gastrointestinal cancers account for 25% of cases and in 7–15% there is no identifiable primary.

The presence of an MPE implies advanced disease and the median survival following diagnosis varies from 3 to 12 months depending on the type of underlying malignancy. Although 80% of patients are dead within 6 months, significant palliation can be achieved with appropriate management and therefore virtually all symptomatic patients should be offered treatment.

MPEs result from obstruction and disruption of lymphatic channels anywhere between the pleura and mediastinal nodes by malignant cells. Diseased pleural tissue also produces VEGF (vascular endothelial growth factor), which increases endothelial permeability and also acts as a growth factor for cancerous cells, thus further aggravating the process.

The term 'paramalignant effusions' is used to describe effusions that are not a direct result of neoplastic involvement, but are still indirectly related to underlying malignancy. Examples include post-obstructive pneumonia, pulmonary embolism, obstruction of the thoracic duct, and hypoalbuminaemia due to cachexia. The presence of paramalignant effusions should not deter potentially curative treatment. Radiotherapy and chemotherapy drugs such as methotrexate, procarbazine, bleomycin and cyclophosphamide may also cause effusions in cancer patients.

PRESENTATION

Dyspnoea, which occurs in more than 50% of patients, is the commonest presenting symptom. Generalised symptoms such as fatigue, weight loss, and anorexia are also common because of the advanced nature of the disease. Chest pain is usually localised to the side of the effusion and is dull and aching rather than pleuritic. Most symptomatic patients have a clinically detectable effusion on examination. Cachexia and lymphadenopathy may also be present.

DIAGNOSIS

Investigations should include FBC, liver and renal function, calcium and albumin. CXR will normally show moderate to large effusions ranging from 500 to 2000 ml. Approximately 10% of patients will have massive pleural effusions defined as effusions that occupy the entire hemithorax and 15% will have small effusions (<500 ml) that will be relatively asymptomatic. CT may identify previously undiagnosed small effusions, as well as providing information on lymph node involvement, parenchymal disease, pleural disease and distant metastases. Ultrasound can help in identifying small effusions and directing thoracentesis. The use of MRI is limited, but it may be useful for evaluating chest wall involvement by tumour.

A diagnostic pleural aspiration should be performed and the fluid sent for cytology, biochemistry (glucose, LDH, total protein) and microbiology. Malignant effusions are commonly bloody. Pleural fluid cytology is the simplest way of obtaining the diagnosis and has a diagnostic yield of ~60%. If initial cytology is negative, then it should be repeated as this provides further diagnostic yield. Complications of thoracentesis include pneumothorax, bleeding, infection, and laceration of spleen or liver.

Blind closed pleural biopsies have a similar yield to pleural fluid cytology. If pleural abnormalities are seen on CT, then CT-guided pleural biopsy is the method of choice. If the diagnosis remains elusive, other options include medical thoracoscopy, VATS (video-assisted thoracic surgery) or open biopsy. Medical thoracoscopy is performed under local anaesthesia with a similar technique to chest drain insertion, but with the addition of a thoracoscope or video transmission. Biopsy and visualisation of pleural surfaces allows diagnostic yields in excess of 90% and pleurodesis can also be performed. VATS requires general anaesthesia and single-lung ventilation, but allows more extensive examination and often combines diagnosis with treatment. An open biopsy is preferred if there are pleural space adhesions or the patient cannot tolerate single-lung ventilation. Bronchoscopy should only be considered if there is a history of haemoptysis or clinical features to suggest a bronchial neoplasm.

MANAGEMENT

The approach to the management of MPEs is determined by symptoms, general health and performance status, expected survival, and the likely response of the tumour to systemic treatment. Patients with small cell lung cancer, breast cancer, ovarian cancer and lymphoma often respond to primary chemotherapy, although if the effusion is very symptomatic and affecting performance status, this should be drained prior to starting treatment.

Options for treatment of MPEs are varied and include: observation, therapeutic pleural aspiration, intercostal tube drainage and pleurodesis, thoracoscopic/VATS pleurodesis, pleuroperitoneal shunting and pleurectomy.

OBSERVATION

Indicated for asymptomatic patients with small effusions, although most will need further intervention at some stage.

THERAPEUTIC PLEURAL ASPIRATION

In general, repeated aspiration of 1–1.5 litres of fluid is a reasonable option for patients with a poor performance status and a limited prognosis. Recurrence rates are almost 100% at 1 month and therefore, in patients with a better outlook, attempts should be made to prevent recurrence of the effusion (see below).

INTERCOSTAL TUBE DRAINAGE AND SCLEROSING AGENT INSTILLATION

This is the most widely used method for preventing MPE recurrence. Traditionally, large bore intercostal tubes have been used for drainage and administration of sclerosing agents, but recent evidence suggests that smaller bore tubes (8–14F) are just as effective and better tolerated. Large effusions should be drained in a controlled manner with no more than 1–1.5 litres removed at one time or 500 ml drained per hour, due to the risk of inducing symptoms of cough, chest pain, dyspnoea and vasovagal attacks. Re-expansion pulmonary oedema can also occur following rapid removal of fluid. Even more caution is required in patients who have trapped lung or bronchial obstruction, which should be suspected if there is no contralateral mediastinal shift or if there is ipsilateral mediastinal shift (i.e. toward side of effusion) on CXR. Suction with a pressure of up to $-20\,cmH_2O$ may be used if there is incomplete lung re-expansion or a persistent air leak.

If dyspnoea is not relieved following drainage, then other causes such as lymphangitic carcinomatosis, atelectasis, thromboembolism and tumour embolism should be suspected.

Successful chemical pleurodesis depends on complete lung re-expansion following drainage, but it should still be tried when full re-expansion is not achieved because it may still provide symptomatic relief. Failure of re-expansion is usually due to endobronchial occlusion by tumour or trapped lung due to extensive pleural tumour infiltration. A CXR is required to confirm re-expansion of the lung before administering the sclerosant. Patients selected for pleurodesis should also have significant symptom relief from pleural fluid removal.

Following administration of sclerosing agents, patient rotation is only required when using talc slurry, and the drainage tube should only be clamped for a short period (1 hour). The tube should be removed within 72 hours as long as the lung remains fully expanded and the rate of fluid drainage has decreased (<150 ml/day). The commonly used sclerosing agents are tetracycline, bleomycin and talc. The success rates for tetracycline (e.g. 500 mg) and bleomycin (e.g. 60 units) pleurodesis are approximately 60–65% and these agents are usually diluted in 50–100 cm^3 of sterile saline. Talc is the most effective agent with success rates of 88–100% and may be administered as slurry or poudrage. Talc slurry is made by mixing 2–5 g of talc with 50 ml of normal saline, which is then administered through the chest drain. Common side effects include fever, chills, and chest pain. Fever usually occurs 4–12 hours after instillation and may last for 3 days. A rare but potentially fatal complication is ARDS (adult respiratory distress syndrome) or acute talc pneumonitis, which is associated with doses in excess of 5 g. High dose corticosteroids are the treatment of choice for this complication.

THORACOSCOPY/VATS

Talc poudrage can be performed by medical thoracoscopy or VATS and involves collapsing the lung to give a good view of the pleural cavity followed by insufflation of 2–5 g of talc. The two techniques are equally effective and are also very useful for diagnostic purposes. Complications include empyema and ARDS.

LONG-TERM INDWELLING CATHETERS

Useful for controlling recurrent MPEs in patients with trapped lung in the outpatient setting.

PLEUROPERITONEAL SHUNTING

This is an option for patients within trapped lung and effusions refractory to other treatments. The shunt may be inserted with a limited thoracotomy or VATS. Complications include infection, shunt occlusion and peritoneal tumour seeding.

PLEURECTOMY

Open pleurectomy is effective but has significant morbidity and mortality (10–13% mortality rate). VATS pleurectomy is safer, although both experience and availability of this method are limited.

FAILED PLEURODESIS

Failed pleurodesis may occur due to poor patient selection, suboptimal technique, loculated effusions and trapped lung. Repeat thoracentesis with or without bag drainage is the treatment of choice for patients with a very poor prognosis. Repeat pleurodesis, long-term indwelling catheters, pleuro-peritoneal shunting and VATS pleurectomy are options for fitter patients. Intrapleural fibrinolysis with 250 000 units of streptokinase may be very useful for multiloculated effusions.

FURTHER READING

American Thoracic Society 2000 Official Statement: Management of malignant pleural effusions. American Journal of Respiratory and Critical Care Medicine 162:1987–2001

Antunes G, Neville E 2000 Management of malignant pleural effusions. Thorax 55:981–983

Antunes G et al 2003 BTS Guidelines for the management of malignant pleural effusions. Thorax 58 (suppl II):ii29–ii38

CHAPTER 56

Metabolic problems in cancer

INTRODUCTION

Metabolic disturbances are common in cancer patients and may be as a result of the underlying malignancy and its manifestations, cancer treatment or co-morbid medical conditions.

HYPERCALCAEMIA

This is the commonest life-threatening metabolic disturbance in cancer patients and occurs in 10–20% of all patients at some time during their illness. In hospitalised hypercalcaemic patients, cancer is the most frequent cause. The tumours most commonly associated with hypercalcaemia are breast cancer, non-small cell lung cancer, myeloma, lymphoma, squamous carcinomas of the head and neck, and renal cancers. The presence of hypercalcaemia in malignancy is a poor prognostic factor.

Hypercalcaemia of malignancy occurs when there is increased resorption of calcium from bone and to a lesser degree increased renal tubular reabsorption of calcium. Three main mechanisms occur:

1. Parathyroid related peptide (PTHrP) secreted by cancer cells has a similar homology and mechanism of action to parathyroid hormone (PTH) and causes increased bone resorption, increased renal reabsorption of calcium and phosphaturia. This leads to a humoral hypercalcaemia. Non-metastatic tumours can also cause hypercalcaemia if they secrete PTHrP.
2. Induction of local osteolysis by a variety of tumour-secreted mediators (including PTHrP). This is often a manifestation of late disease.

3. Increased production of calcitriol (vitamin D3) by tumour cells is an important mechanism in patients with lymphoma and myeloma and may respond to steroid therapy.

Clinical manifestations depend on the severity of the hypercalcaemia and initially include non-specific symptoms such as fatigue, anorexia, nausea, vomiting, constipation, confusion and depression. Other symptoms include muscle weakness, polyuria, polydipsia and bone pain. Clinical signs include dehydration, hyporeflexia and bradycardia. Patients with severe hypercalcaemia may experience seizures, stupor, coma and death and it may be mistaken for drug overdose, hypoglycaemia or diabetic ketoacidosis.

Investigations as a minimum should include a full history and examination, renal and liver function tests, free calcium levels and albumin. Further investigations may be appropriate depending on the clinical condition of the patient (e.g. ECG if hypotensive, may reveal bradycardia, prolonged PR interval, wide QRS, short Q-T interval and other conduction defects).

General measures in the management of hypercalcaemia include fluid resuscitation with normal saline and removal of aggravating drugs such as calcium-containing supplements, vitamin D, thiazide diuretics and NSAIDs. Fluid replacement corrects hypovolaemia, hypotension and improves renal function and therefore increases excretion of calcium. Electrolytes including magnesium should be assessed regularly during this period. Bisphosphonates, which work by decreasing calcium release from bone by inhibiting the activity of osteoclasts, are now the drugs of choice for this condition. Pamidronate (60–90 mg IV over 2 hours after rehydration) is the commonest agent used and restores normocalcaemia in 90–100% of patients (usually within 48 hours) for an average period of 2 weeks. Repeated doses can be given every 2–3 weeks. Side effects of flu-like symptoms occur in 20% of patients. Zoledronic acid is a new much more potent bisphosphonate and has already been shown to be more effective and rapid in effect than pamidronate. Other agents that may be of use include:

1. Calcitonin. This peptide hormone inhibits bone resorption and increases renal excretion of calcium. It has a relatively weak hypocalcaemic effect, but has a rapid onset of action (decreases calcium levels within 2–4 hours) and may be useful in conjunction with IV pamidronate in critically ill patients, where a rapid effect is desired.

2. Steroids. Corticosteroids inhibit osteoclast-mediated bone resorption and decrease gastrointestinal (GI) calcium absorption as well as having direct anti-tumour effects in lymphomas, leukaemias and myeloma. However, the hypocalcaemic effect is minimal in most solid tumours and the use of steroids is limited to haematological malignancies and breast cancer patients who have a hypercalcaemic 'flare' following hormonal therapy. Prednisolone 40 mg o.d. is the usual dose.

3. Gallium nitrate. This is a potent inhibitor of bone resorption and restores normocalcaemia in 75–85% of patients. However, it is nephrotoxic and

requires inpatient IV administration over 5 days and is therefore not used in first line management.

4. Oral phosphates. Can be used in patients with mild hypercalcaemia and hypophosphataemia to good effect. However, side effects include nausea and diarrhoea. Usual dose is 250–375 mg q.d.s. p.o.

TUMOUR LYSIS SYNDROME (TLS)

TLS results from the rapid lysis of predominantly malignant cells causing massive release of intracellular contents into the systemic circulation more rapidly than the body can eliminate them. This leads to metabolic complications of hyperkalaemia, hyperphosphataemia, hyperuricaemia and hypocalcaemia, which can lead to acute oliguric renal failure, cardiac arrhythmias, seizures, tetany and sudden death.

It most commonly occurs in haematological malignancies such as the leukaemias and non-Hodgkin's lymphoma. It usually occurs following systemic cytotoxic chemotherapy, but can occur spontaneously and has been occasionally reported following other therapies such as immunotherapy, total body irradiation (TBI) and steroids. It rarely occurs in solid tumours.

TLS is often asymptomatic, but may cause nausea, vomiting, lethargy, weakness, paralysis, renal colic and joint pain. It is important to identify patients at risk in order to instigate prophylactic measures (Table 56.1). The major risk factors are shown in Table 56.2.

TABLE 56.1 Preventive measures for tumour lysis syndrome (should be initiated 24–48 hours prior to therapy)

Daily metabolic screen (renal function, K^+, Na^+, Ca^{2+}, PO_4, urate)
Intravenous fluids for rehydration and to ensure good urine output (100 ml/hour)
Stop drugs that interfere with uric acid excretion (e.g. thiazide diuretics)
Allopurinol 300–900 mg per day
Loop diuretics as required
Sodium bicarbonate can be added to IV fluids for alkalinising of the urine
  (increases solubility of uric acid)

TABLE 56.2 Risk factors for tumour lysis syndrome

Lymphoproliferative malignancy
Bulky chemosensitive disease
High white count
High serum urate
Elevated LDH
Hypovolaemia
Renal impairment
Low urine pH

The management of tumour lysis syndrome is summarised below:

1. Hyperkalaemia (K^+ >6.5 mmol/l) should be urgently managed with calcium gluconate, dextrose and insulin, and calcium resonium.
2. Patients with acute renal failure may require dialysis to avoid fatal complications.
3. Hyperuricaemia (urate >0.5 mmol/l) is managed with allopurinol 300–900 mg daily (p.o. or IV). Acetazolamide may also be helpful.
4. Hypocalcaemia is usually self-correcting if serum phosphorus is corrected and calcium supplementation should be reserved for the symptomatic patient because it may precipitate metastatic calcification. Symptomatic hypocalcaemia (Ca^{2+} usually <2.12 mmol/l) may be corrected with IV calcium (2–3 g calcium gluconate over 1–2 hours) or oral calcium supplements (500–2000 mg in divided doses). If refractory, calcitriol may be used.
5. Hyperphosphataemia (PO_4 >1.4 mmol/l) is treated with the phosphate binder, aluminium hydroxide (500–1800 mg 3–6 times per day). Calcium carbonate is an alternative.

HYPONATRAEMIA

Hyponatraemia is a common problem in malignancy and has many potential causes, which can be categorised into three main groups.

1. Associated with ECF (extracellular fluid) volume depletion: vomiting, diarrhoea, effusions, ascites, ileus, external biliary drainage, diuretic use, renal tubular or cerebral salt wasting.
2. Associated with ECF volume excess: congestive cardiac failure, hypo-albuminaemia, nephrotic syndrome.
3. Associated with normal ECF volume: this is usually due to the syndrome of inappropriate antidiuretic hormone secretion (SIADH). ADH may be released from the posterior pituitary or ectopically from tumours such as small cell lung cancer and head and neck cancer. SIADH is also caused by many other tumours and non-malignant conditions such as pneumonia, meningitis, alcohol withdrawal, and drugs such as vincristine, cyclo-phosphamide, cisplatin, morphine and carbamazepine.

Symptoms are generally non-specific and include anorexia, nausea, fatigue, irritability and confusion. Severe symptoms may occur when the plasma sodium levels drop below 115 mmol/l, becoming life threatening below 105 mmol/l, and include headaches, worsening confusion, seizures and coma (due to acute cerebral oedema).

The aim of management is to restore the normal sodium level and achieve normovolaemia. Treatment for patients with ECF volume excess involves water restriction, and for ECF volume depletion involves replacing sodium and the volume deficit.

In the management of SIADH, the cause should be addressed. Additional options include fluid restriction to 500–1000 ml per day, and demeclocycline (600–1200 mg o.d.). When the syndrome is very severe, hypertonic saline (300 mmol/l slowly IV) can be given and furosemide (frusemide) may also be used, but extreme caution is required due to the risk of inducing central pontine myelinolysis.

HYPOKALAEMIA

This is a very common problem in cancer patients and the main causes are low dietary intake, GI losses (vomiting, diarrhoea, hypersecretion, infections), renal losses (tubular damage by cisplatin, ACTH production by tumours, steroid use, diuretic therapy). It is usually asymptomatic, but when severe may cause weakness and cardiac arrhythmias. Management involves replacement of potassium with oral or IV supplementation and treating the cause.

HYPERURICAEMIA

This most commonly occurs with haematological malignancy, where rapid proliferation of cells is occurring. Uric acid crystal formation in the renal tubules and collecting system leads to renal complications. Arthritis develops due to crystal deposition in the joints. Patients at highest risk are those with leukaemias undergoing treatment, bulky lymphomas, and those with pre-existing renal impairment. Diuretics can also exacerbate the problem.

Initial treatment involves withdrawing exacerbating drugs, and fluid rehydration to dilute uric acid in the urine to increase urate solubility. Alkalisation of the urine to a pH of 7 is also helpful. Allopurinol is the main drug treatment and should be used prophylactically (i.e. given at least 24–28 hours prior to chemotherapy) as well as in the acute setting. It decreases uric acid levels by inhibiting xanthine oxidase (an enzyme that converts hypoxanthine and xanthine to uric acid). A dose of 300–900 mg is usually given. Severe arthritis should be managed with adequate analgesia.

HYPOGLYCAEMIA

The most common causes of hypoglycaemia in malignancy are insulin islet cell tumours, followed by sarcomas and hepatocellular carcinomas.

Mechanisms for hypoglycaemia include the production of insulin and insulin-like factors, excessive glucose consumption by tumours, gross liver disease (decreasing glucose production) and failure of glucose regulatory mechanisms.

Symptoms include dizziness, weakness, sweating, anxiety, nausea and headache, which improve after ingestion of food. Severe hypoglycaemia may cause seizures, focal neurological deficits, stupor and coma.

Treatment of the cause, i.e. the underlying cancer, is the most important way of improving the hypoglycaemia. Mild symptoms can usually be treated with increased food intake. Patients with severe symptoms may benefit from steroids or glucagon. IV glucose may be required for life-threatening hypoglycaemia or to stabilise patients about to undergo specific cancer therapy.

CACHEXIA–ANOREXIA SYNDROME

This is a complex syndrome and is a very common problem in advanced cancer, with up to 80% of patients affected. Cachexia describes the loss and wasting of body tissues. Unlike starvation, where loss of fatty tissue is predominant, there is equal loss of fatty tissue and muscle tissue and so the overall picture of wasting is out of proportion to the degree of anorexia. Increasing oral intake or parenteral feeding does not prevent weight loss. Symptoms of fatigue and weakness are exacerbated. Anorexia is a loss of desire to eat and may result from early satiety, nausea or loss of taste. The precise mechanisms involved in this syndrome are unknown, but cytokines and other tumour products are key factors in the pathogenesis of the metabolic abnormalities.

Survival in these patients is poorer and they tolerate cancer treatment less well. The appearance of the patient 'wasting away' is particularly distressing not only to patients but also to loved ones. Relatives may try too hard to encourage increased food intake and this may lead to relationship problems. The syndrome is worsened by coexisting problems such as dysphagia, nausea, fevers and pain.

Management involves simple measures such as explanation, relieving dysphagia, nausea and vomiting, fevers and providing adequate analgesia. A low dose of steroids, e.g. dexamethasone 2–4 mg, may stimulate appetite and improve well-being, but this is often short-lived (3–6 weeks) and provides little, if any, weight gain. Megestrol acetate (160–800 mg/day) and medroxyprogesterone (500 mg b.d.) stimulate appetite, improve energy levels and may increase weight. Side effects include nausea, fluid retention and increased risk of venous thromboembolism. Metoclopramide helps to reduce nausea and early satiety.

FURTHER READING

Flombaum C D 2000 Metabolic emergencies in the cancer patient. Seminars in Oncology 27(3):322–334

Hussain M H, Cullen K 2002 Metabolic emergencies. In: Johnston P G, Spence R A J (eds) Oncologic emergencies. OUP, Oxford, p 51–73

CHAPTER 57

Paraneoplastic syndromes

INTRODUCTION

Paraneoplastic syndromes are a very broad group of clinical syndromes caused by non-metastatic remote effects of malignant disease. They occur in approximately 10% of cancer patients, although this is likely to be an underestimate. A great variety of paraneoplastic syndromes have been identified and they are clinically important for the following reasons:

1. They may be the first manifestation of an underlying malignancy and hence lead to earlier investigation and treatment.
2. They may cause significant patient morbidity and mortality.
3. They may hinder the treatment of the underlying cancer.
4. Many are treatable and some respond to treatment of the underlying malignancy.
5. Some produce hormones and protein products that are measurable and useful as tumour markers.

The underlying pathophysiology of paraneoplastic syndromes is complex and not fully understood, but the following mechanisms have been implicated:

1. Tumour production of active hormones and/or their precursors, e.g. ADH, ACTH, PTHrP, growth hormone, calcitonin etc.
2. Anti-tumour antibody formation with cross-reactivity with normal tissues.
3. Steroid metabolism by tumours, e.g. leading to increased oestrogen levels, increased vitamin D levels etc.
4. Cytokine production.

MAIN PARANEOPLASTIC SYNDROMES

Table 57.1 lists the main paraneoplastic syndromes.

TABLE 57.1 Paraneoplastic syndromes

Syndrome	Comments
Endocrine/metabolic	Relatively common (see also Ch. 56 on metabolic problems)
SIADH	Most commonly seen with lung cancer
Cushing's	Due to ectopic production of ACTH. Treatment of underlying cancer, ketoconazole and mitotane are helpful
Hypercalcaemia	Most common in squamous carcinomas. PTHrP production
Hypoglycaemia	Due to insulin-like growth factors and somatomedin
Zollinger–Ellison	Due to ectopic gastrin production. Use proton pump inhibitor
Cachexia and anorexia	Complex mechanisms. Cytokines involved
Fever	Due to pyrogens (various cytokines)
Neurological/neuromuscular	Rare. Generally respond poorly to immunosuppressive or anti-tumour treatments
Encephalomyelitis	Inflammatory disorder that can affect the CNS and PNS. The variety of potential clinical effects is large. Most often associated with lung cancer. Presence of anti-Hu antibodies is common
Limbic encephalitis	Associated with SCLC. Confusion, amnesia, psychiatric symptoms. Anti-Hu antibodies found in 50% of cases
Cerebellar degeneration	Mainly seen in SCLC, ovary, and breast cancers. Antibodies commonly detected
Opsoclonus/myoclonus	Rapid uncontrollable eye movements, ataxia and general myoclonus. Steroids and IV immunoglobulin may help
Retinal degeneration	Progressive, painless visual loss, and ring scotoma. Steroids and IV immunoglobulin may help stabilise condition
Neuropathies	Subacute sensory neuropathy is the commonest type and produces sensory loss, areflexia and ataxia. Usually in SCLC
Lambert–Eaton myasthenic syndrome (LEMS)	Autoimmune disorder of neuromuscular junction. Weakness, fatigue and cholinergic symptoms. Associated with SCLC in 60% of cases. Treatment of underlying cancer improves symptoms. Plasmapheresis and immunosuppression helpful
Myasthenia gravis	Fatigability of muscles, especially eye muscles. 85–90% have antibodies to acetylcholine receptor. Thymoma is commonest malignant cause. Tumour removal not usually helpful. Treat with anticholinesterases, steroids and plasmapheresis
Dermatomyositis/polymyositis	Painful inflammatory proximal myopathy. Classic facial heliotrope rash. Elevated creatine kinase, EMG and muscle biopsy are diagnostic. Treat with steroids

(Continued)

TABLE 57.1 (Continued)

Syndrome	Comments
Renal	Relatively uncommon
Glomerulonephritis (GN)	Most common type is membranous GN. Usually associated with Hodgkin's, lung, colon, ovarian, breast and gastric cancers. Treating underlying malignancy and steroids help
Renal tubular disease	Myeloma light chain immunoglobulins cause renal tubular damage and may lead to renal failure. Amyloid has similar effect
Dermatological	Numerous skin disorders have been associated with malignancy, but a direct causal link is rarely demonstrated
Acanthosis nigricans	Hyperpigmented, velvety thickening of skin usually in neck, axillae, palms, soles, perineum and intertriginous regions. Gastric cancer is the commonest underlying malignancy. Others include lung, breast, uterus and ovary
Leser–Trélat sign	Sudden outcropping of itchy seborrhoeic warts. Often associated with acanthosis nigricans. Most common with malignancies of gastrointestinal tract
Paraneoplastic pemphigus	Mucocutaneous ulcers and blistering. Mainly associated with lymphomas and CLL. Poor prognosis
Erythema gyratum repens	Wavy erythematous red bands. Often itchy. Associated with cancers of the breast, lung and gastrointestinal tract
Necrolytic migratory erythema	Associated with malignant pancreatic glucagonomas
Flushing	Usually seen with carcinoids or phaeochromocytomas
Hypertrichosis lanuginosa acquisita	Sudden development of lanugo hair. The commonest underlying cancers are lung, colon, uterus and lymphoma
Sweet's syndrome	Painful erythematous plaques of face and upper limbs, fever, leucocytosis. Associated with leukaemias
Ichthyosis	Development of dry scaly skin. Associated with lymphoma, SCLC, testis and ovarian cancer
Tylosis	Skin thickening of palms and soles. Associated with oesophageal cancer
Inherited dermatological conditions	e.g. Peutz–Jeghers, Gardner's, neurofibromatosis, Cowden's
Haematological	Very common
Anaemias	Normocytic normochromic most common type. Other types include autoimmune haemolytic and microangiopathic haemolytic anaemias
Thrombocytosis	May be due to production of thrombopoietin. Rarely a clinical problem. Treatment is not usually required

(Continued)

TABLE 57.1 *(Continued)*

Syndrome	Comments
Thrombocytopenia	Usually associated with lymphoid malignancies. May respond to steroids or splenectomy
Erythrocytosis	Renal cancer and hepatoma are the main solid tumours that cause this problem. They produce erythropoietin. Treatment is not usually required. Control of the primary tumour often helps
Neutrophilia	Due to tumour production of growth factors such as G-CSF, GM-CSF and other cytokines. No treatment required
Neutropenia	Rare. Probably due to autoantibodies to neutrophils
Eosinophilia	Most commonly seen in Hodgkin's disease
Thrombosis/thrombophlebitis	Very common. Cancer may interfere with the coagulation and fibrinolytic mechanisms. Requires treatment with heparin and warfarin. May need to consider caval filters for recurrent pulmonary emboli. Migratory thrombophlebitis is usually associated with pancreatic cancer
DIC	Rarely severe. Most often occurs with acute promyelocytic leukaemia and adenocarcinomas. Supportive measures and treatment of the underlying cancer are the mainstays of management
Gastrointestinal Protein losing enteropathy	Increased mucosal permeability causes protein loss and hypoproteinaemia. Patients may develop peripheral oedema, weight loss and infections due to low immunoglobulin levels. Most often due to gastrointestinal cancers and lymphomas
Rheumatological Hypertrophic pulmonary osteoarthropathy (HPOA)	Periosteal new bone formation, finger clubbing. Pain and swelling usually around knees, ankles and wrists. Associated with lung cancer. NSAIDs and steroids may help
Arthritis	Arthritis similar to rheumatoid may develop. Usually seen in lung cancer and haematological cancers
Vasculitis	Various vasculitides are associated with haematological cancers, lung, colon and renal cancer

CHAPTER 58

Problems in advanced pelvic malignancy

INTRODUCTION

Uncontrolled pelvic malignancy is a significant cause of morbidity and mortality. Severe treatment-related complications may cause similar problems to the malignancy itself. For example, pelvic surgery and radiation may damage organs, nerves, blood vessels, muscles and the ureters. Advanced cancers of the cervix, ovary, bladder, prostate and rectum are the commonest causes of pelvic problems.

Potential complications of pelvic malignancy and its treatment include the following:

1. Pelvic pain
2. Bowel obstruction
3. Ascites
4. Fistulas
5. Bleeding
6. Diarrhoea and constipation
7. Ureteric and bladder outflow obstruction
8. Lymphoedema and nodal disease
9. Venous thromboembolism (VTE)
10. Anxiety and depression
11. Sexual dysfunction.

GENERAL CONSIDERATIONS

Some patients who present with locally advanced pelvic disease may potentially have curable disease. This will depend on the type of tumour, stage of disease and patient factors such as age, co-morbidity and performance status. In general, these patients require a multi-modality approach with a combination of chemotherapy, radiotherapy and surgery.

Patients with recurrent pelvic disease also present a challenge. Some will be candidates for salvage therapy with curative intent, but for most patients only palliative treatments will be suitable. Salvage therapy is generally reserved for patients with localised central pelvic recurrences with no evidence of distant metastases. A major surgical pelvic exenteration is usually required, which may be preceded by neoadjuvant radiotherapy/chemotherapy.

The aim of treatment for those with incurable disease is control of pelvic symptoms. Local palliative radiotherapy can be very useful in this regard. Several dose schedules may be used, depending on the clinical scenario and the discretion of the radiotherapist. Higher dose palliative radiotherapy schedules are more appropriate for good performance status patients with a better outlook. Shorter schedules are more suitable for less well patients with a poor prognosis. Intracavitary or interstitial brachytherapy can also be of use in selected cases. Systemic chemotherapy may be useful for chemosensitive pelvic cancers such as bladder and ovarian cancers. Hormonal therapy can be very useful for prostate cancer.

SPECIFIC PROBLEMS IN ADVANCED PELVIC MALIGNANCY

PELVIC PAIN

This may be a very disabling symptom. Infiltration of nerves, muscle and bone may cause severe pain. NSAIDs and opiates are usually required. Neuropathic pain is particularly difficult to manage and early referral to the palliative care and pain teams is recommended. Palliative radiotherapy may be very helpful, especially if there is bony involvement. Infections should be actively treated. Antispasmodics should be used as appropriate.

MALIGNANT BOWEL OBSTRUCTION

See Chapter 53 on malignant bowel obstruction.

ASCITES

See Chapter 52 on malignant ascites.

FISTULAS

Fistulas may result from the growth of the cancer itself or as a result of surgical or radiotherapeutic intervention. Fistulation between any of the hollow organs in the pelvis may occur and the commonest types are vesico-vaginal, recto-vaginal, recto-vesical and entero-cutaneous. Symptoms may be very distressing and include pain, offensive discharge, infection and psychosocial problems leading to isolation from family and friends. Diagnostic studies are guided by symptoms and signs and may include cystoscopy, vaginoscopy, proctoscopy, intravenous urogram (IVU), cystogram, barium studies, CT/MRI and EUA.

Management depends on the type of fistula, but general measures include good skin care, treatment of infection to reduce pain and discharge, and psychological support. Palliation of urinary fistulas may be surgically accomplished with uretero-intestinal conduits or bilateral percutaneous nephrostomies. For patients with a life expectancy of less than a few months, nephrostomies are generally preferred because they are simpler to perform. However, there are significant problems with infection, recurrent blockages and dislodgement with nephrostomies and therefore in patients with a longer life expectancy, ureteric-intestinal conduits are the preferred option. More conservative measures involve the use of urethral/suprapubic catheters and incontinence devices. Fistulas involving the bowel are particularly distressing and a diverting colostomy is usually required. An end colostomy is associated with fewer long-term complications than a loop colostomy. Effective palliation for colo-vaginal fistulas can be achieved with self-expanding metal stents.

BLEEDING

General measures to reduce bleeding include stopping drugs such as anticoagulants and NSAIDs and correcting any bleeding diatheses, e.g. platelets, vitamin K and fresh frozen plasma (FFP). Tranexamic acid is sometimes useful. Vaginal bleeding may be controlled with vaginal packing, radiotherapy or arterial ligation if life-threatening. Mild and moderate rectal bleeding often responds to radiotherapy. Bladder washouts may be required for gross haematuria.

Massive terminal haemorrhage requires adequate sedation of the patient with diamorphine (5–10 mg IV or IM) and midazolam (10 mg IV or IM). Green sheets can minimise the distressing appearance of large volumes of blood.

DIARRHOEA AND CONSTIPATION

Potential causes of diarrhoea are numerous and include infection, malabsorption, faecal impaction with leakage, metabolic disturbances, radiotherapy and drugs (e.g. antibiotics, laxatives, cytotoxics and antacids). A severe bout may be life-threatening and requires IV fluid and electrolyte replacement with careful monitoring of pulse, blood pressure and urine output. The cause should be identified and treated accordingly if possible. Drugs commonly used to control diarrhoea include loperamide and opiates.

Constipation also has numerous causes including bowel obstruction by the tumour itself, hypercalcaemia, autonomic disturbance, immobility, depression, dehydration, rectal/anal discomfort, drugs (opiates, loperamide, cyclizine, 5-HT$_3$ inhibitors, vinca alkaloid chemotherapy). The cause should be identified if possible and treated as appropriate. A good fluid intake and mobilisation should be encouraged. An oral laxative (stimulant and softening action) should be started first followed by a rectal laxative if unsuccessful. Faecal impaction can be managed with bisacodyl suppositories, phosphate enemas or manual evacuation.

URETERIC AND BLADDER OUTFLOW OBSTRUCTION

Ureteric obstruction may be unilateral or bilateral and leads to upper tract dilatation, hydronephrosis and progressive renal damage. It may be caused by direct extension of the primary tumour or compression by lymph nodes, or be secondary to retroperitoneal fibrosis (due to RT, surgery or chemotherapy).

Patients usually present with chronic renal impairment, but may present with acute renal failure, urinary tract infections and loin discomfort due to hydronephrosis. Uraemia may cause nausea, fatigue, confusion and seizures. An incidental finding on routine imaging is another common mode of presentation.

Bladder outflow obstruction is usually due to prostate, bladder or penis cancer and leads to bilateral obstruction. The diagnosis can be confirmed with IVU, ultrasound, renography and CT/MRI. Electrolytes and renal function tests should be performed.

The treatment of obstructive uropathy involves correction of fluid and electrolyte disturbances and relief of the obstruction. The obstruction can be relieved by insertion of ureteric stents or by percutaneous nephrostomies. Stents may be difficult or impossible to place in many patients with advanced pelvic disease. Bladder outflow obstruction may be treated with urethral or suprapubic catheterisation.

In poor prognosis patients with advanced cancer, unilateral obstruction that is asymptomatic and not affecting renal function does not require intervention. The decision to intervene when there is bilateral obstruction in a terminally ill cancer patient where no other therapeutic options are available is much more difficult. The patient's own wishes and quality of life must be taken into account.

LYMPHOEDEMA AND NODAL DISEASE

Lymphoedema results from lymphatic and venous obstruction and may be exacerbated by malnutrition and hypoalbuminaemia. Elevation of the legs, elastic compression stockings and massaging can be helpful. Good skin care is essential to help avoid infection (cellulitis). Radiotherapy to bulky nodes is generally not helpful for lymphoedema, but is often used for painful and ulcerating inguinal nodal disease.

VENOUS THROMBOEMBOLISM (VTE)

Pelvic malignancy is a particularly strong risk factor for VTE, as is recent pelvic surgery and older age. There is a reasonable case for full anticoagulation in patients with pelvic malignancy, but the risk of bleeding should be taken into account. For those with proven deep vein thrombosis and/or pulmonary embolism, anticoagulation is needed. However, if the risk of haemorrhage is high, insertion of a vena cava filter to prevent further emboli may be considered.

ANXIETY AND DEPRESSION

This is extremely common and early recognition and intervention is clearly important. Severely depressed patients may be non-compliant with treatment and may have lower pain thresholds.

SEXUAL DYSFUNCTION

Sexual dysfunction results from pain, bleeding, offensive discharge, treatment- or cancer-related pelvic nerve damage, endocrine disturbance, general debilitation, vaginal stenosis, loss of sexual organs (e.g. exenterative surgery) and psychological factors. Specialist referral may be appropriate. Counselling, psychotherapy, good analgesia, relaxation techniques, lubrication, use of vaginal dilators, hormone therapy (e.g. oestrogen replacement), and the use of sildenafil for erectile dysfunction are some examples of the possible treatment options for patients keen to continue their sex life.

FURTHER READING

Booth S, Bruera E (eds) 2004 Palliative care consultations in gynaecology. OUP, Oxford
Segreti E M, Kavanagh B D. Palliative care of the patient with advanced pelvic cancer.
 Available at: http://www.emedicine.com/med/topic3342.htm

Pulmonary metastases

INTRODUCTION

Pulmonary metastases are identified at autopsy in 20–30% of patients who die from cancer and in about 15–25% of these cases, no other evidence of metastatic disease is found. The incidence of pulmonary metastases reflects the prevalence of primary tumours and therefore most are due to breast, lung, colorectal, upper gastrointestinal, prostate and renal cancers. Less common cancers that frequently spread to the lung include sarcomas, choriocarcinoma, melanoma, teratoma, adenoid cystic carcinomas and thyroid cancer.

Most metastatic spread to the lung is via the haematogenous route. Following vascular invasion by the primary tumour, fragments of tumour are dislodged and travel as tumour emboli via the systemic circulation to the lungs, where they may proliferate to form nodules. Pulmonary metastases most commonly affect the outer third of the lungs, especially in the subpleural regions of the lower zones. They are usually multiple and vary in size from 3 mm to 15 cm or more. Less commonly, tumour emboli remain confined to the perivascular interstitium and then invade and spread along lymphatic channels and adjacent interstitial tissue causing lymphangitis carcinomatosa (LC). LC may also result from retrograde lymphangitic spread from hilar nodes and is most commonly seen with adenocarcinomas of the breast, lung, colon, stomach, pancreas and prostate. Endobronchial metastases are rare, but often symptomatic and are usually due to colorectal, breast, kidney and thyroid cancers. Cavitation occurs in 4% of metastases and is usually due to squamous cell carcinomas.

Overall, the prognosis for patients with pulmonary metastases is poor, but subgroups of patients may be cured or enjoy long-term survival. For most cancers, surgery offers the only chance of a permanent cure with up to one-third of patients with resectable disease living over 5 years. Unfortunately, most patients have inoperable disease and for these patients the treatment options are palliative with systemic therapy, localised radiotherapy and supportive care. This is because the vast majority of patients have epithelial malignancies, and synchronous metastases in other sites are very common. However, most patients with pulmonary metastases from sarcomas, teratomas and paediatric malignancy will be candidates for metastasectomy and the overall prognosis is much better. Systemic chemotherapy may achieve complete eradication of disease with teratomas and osteogenic sarcomas.

CLINICAL PRESENTATION

Most pulmonary metastases are detected on routine CXR in otherwise asymptomatic patients. Dyspnoea may result from a large pulmonary tumour burden, airway obstruction or pleural effusions. Sudden dyspnoea can result from pneumothorax, haemorrhage of a lesion or the development of a pleural effusion. Pleural involvement may cause chest pain and apical metastases may result in Pancoast syndrome. Endobronchial disease may present with wheezing and haemoptysis. Patients may also have symptoms related to their primary tumour.

Patients with lymphangitis carcinomatosa usually develop progressive, unrelenting dyspnoea that is often disproportionate to initial radiological findings. A dry cough and chest pain may also be present. Clinical examination may reveal tachypnoea, tachycardia, and occasionally cyanosis and coarse crepitations on auscultation.

IMAGING MODALITIES

For known extrathoracic primary malignancies, the plain CXR remains the standard for screening, surveillance and monitoring for most patients with pulmonary metastases. The typical pattern is of well-circumscribed, multiple, bilateral pulmonary nodules varying in size from a few millimetres to a few centimetres, but occasionally massive (>15 cm) lesions may be present. Lymphangitis carcinomatosa usually appears as reticular or reticulonodular opacification, with associated septal lines (Kerley B lines) and peribronchial cuffing. Pleural effusions and mediastinal lymphadenopathy may also be present. Endobronchial lesions may cause atelectasis and obstructive pneumonia.

CXR often fails to reveal lesions less than 7 mm in size, particularly in the lung apices and bases, and adjacent to the mediastinal structures and the pleura. A patient with a solitary lesion on CXR is likely to have further pulmonary metastatic disease.

CT scanning has a higher resolution than plain CXR and has the advantages of depicting additional and smaller nodules, as well as defining the location of the nodules and the presence of adenopathy. Conventional CT identifies up to 80% of pulmonary nodules >3 mm detected at surgery. Spiral CT scanning has further improved the diagnostic yield, with lesions less than 3 mm now detectable. However, the false-positive rate has also increased with increased sensitivity. Spiral CT of the chest is now the modality of choice for detection of metastatic disease and for surgical planning. It is also preferred for the screening and surveillance of patients with germ cell tumours, osteosarcomas and choriocarcinomas. High resolution CT (HRCT) is the modality of choice for demonstrating lymphangitis carcinomatosis as it can commonly differentiate lymphangitic spread from other diffuse lung diseases.

MRI can better define mediastinal involvement and tissue planes, but adds little information to spiral CT findings.

Positron emission tomography (PET) is not considered superior to CT in the initial detection of pulmonary metastases and is not routinely available. However, its role continues to be evaluated.

DIAGNOSIS

Investigations include: full history and examination; routine bloods including FBC, renal and liver function; CXR; CT of the chest, abdomen and pelvis; appropriate tumour markers, e.g. HCG, AFP, LDH, CEA, CA19.9, CA15.3.

Patients with multiple lung nodules and a known primary cancer will not usually need pathological confirmation. Patients with an unknown primary will need a pathological tissue diagnosis, which should be obtained from the most accessible and safest site. If the pulmonary lesion/s is/are the only site of disease, then tissue can be obtained by percutaneous CT-guided biopsy or bronchoscopy depending on whether the disease is peripherally or centrally located, respectively. Occasionally VATS (video-assisted thoracoscopy surgery) or open biopsy is required. Scintigraphy with radioiodine or radiolabelled octreotide may be useful in diagnosing metastatic disease in patients with thyroid cancer and carcinoid tumours respectively. In lymphangitis carcinomatosa, bronchoalveolar lavage is diagnostic in over 80% of cases.

Solitary pulmonary nodules in patients with a known extrathoracic malignancy should not be presumed as metastatic until confirmed histologically, as solitary pulmonary metastases are uncommon. The primary lesions most likely to produce solitary metastases are cancers of the colon, kidney, testicle, breast and osteosarcomas. A new primary lung cancer or a benign lesion should be high up in the differential diagnosis and every effort should be made to obtain the diagnosis if the patient is fit for any form of treatment.

MANAGEMENT

The management of pulmonary metastases requires a multidisciplinary approach and treatment decisions need to be tailored to the individual patient. The possible treatment modalities are surgery, systemic therapy, radiotherapy and interventional bronchoscopy.

SURGERY

Pulmonary metastasectomy can be used to cure, prolong survival, diagnose and stage cancer. If the aim is to cure or prolong survival then the following criteria should be met before offering pulmonary metastasectomy:

1. Full staging has been completed.
2. The primary tumour site should be free of disease (or completely resectable if still in situ).
3. Metastases should be confined to the lung and be technically resectable with clear margins.
4. The patient must be able to tolerate the procedure and have adequate residual respiratory function.
5. Curative chemotherapy or neoadjuvant therapy is not an option.

The optimum surgical approach remains controversial. Open resection is currently favoured over VATS because it provides access for thorough intraoperative exploration and staging required to identify and resect all lesions not seen on preoperative imaging. However, VATS is sometimes preferred for the patient with limited pulmonary function and a single metastasis with a long disease-free interval. The types of incision for the open surgery approach depend on the site and location of the metastases and include unilateral thoracotomy, median sternotomy and bilateral thoracotomy (clamshell). The aim of resection is to remove all identified or palpated disease with clear margins (at least 0.5–1 cm if possible) and with as much preservation of normal lung parenchyma as possible. This may be achieved by wedge resection, Perelman resection (precision excision with cautery or laser), segmentectomy, lobectomy or pneumonectomy depending on the number and location of metastases and the pulmonary function of the patient. If a metastatic lesion involves the chest wall, pericardium or diaphragm, but is still completely resectable, then an en bloc resection should at least be considered as good results can be achieved.

Surgical morbidity rates are low and mortality rates range between 0 and 2%. Cure can be achieved in approximately 30% of cases. The International Registry of Lung Metastases recently published a data analysis of 5206 patients who underwent pulmonary metastasectomy in multiple centres in Europe, the USA and Canada. Complete surgical resection was achieved in 88% and the actuarial survival of these patients was 36% at 5 years, 26% at

TABLE 59.1 Prognostic groups from the International Registry of Lung Metastases

Group I	Resectable, no risk factors (DFI ≥36 months, single metastasis)	Median survival 61 months
Group II	Resectable, one risk factor (DFI ≤36 months or multiple metastases)	Median survival 34 months
Group III	Resectable, two risk factors (DFI ≤36 months and multiple metastases)	Median survival 24 months
Group IV	Unresectable	Median survival 14 months

DFI, disease-free interval.
NB: Germ cell tumours and Wilms' tumour excluded.

10 years and 22% at 15 years. Median survival was 35 months. The survival rates for incomplete resections were 13% at 5 years and 7% at 10 years. Based on the findings of the Registry, four prognostic groups based on three parameters of prognostic significance (resectability, disease-free interval, number of metastases) were identified (Table 59.1).

In the Registry analysis, 53% relapsed (with a median time to recurrence of 10 months) and of these, 40% underwent a second metastasectomy. The survival of this group of patients was 44% at 5 years and 29% at 10 years. Thus, repeated surgery should be considered if technically feasible. Only 28% of patients eligible for second metastasectomy had epithelial tumours whereas 53% of such patients had sarcomas; this is due to the fact that most sarcoma recurrences are limited and intrathoracic.

SURGERY FOR SELECTED TUMOUR TYPES

Osteosarcoma
The lungs are involved in approximately 85% of metastatic cases. Surgical resection of recurrent disease in the lung has been reported to offer 5-year survival of up to 40%.

Soft tissue sarcoma
Lung metastases are common. Five-year survival following pulmonary resection is 25–38%.

Colorectal cancer
Isolated pulmonary metastases are rare (2–4% of patients). Five-year survival rates of 40–45% are reported following resection. Encouraging results have also been reported in selected patients with synchronous or metachronous liver metastases.

Breast cancer
Isolated pulmonary metastases are very rare (<0.5% of patients). The benefit of pulmonary resection is unclear, but may be an option for selected patients.

Renal cancer
Pulmonary metastases are common. Five-year survival of up to 40% has been reported following resection. Some surgeons advocate radical surgery in patients with limited extrapulmonary disease.

Melanoma
The role of pulmonary resection is unclear, but may be an option for selected patients with isolated disease.

Head and neck cancer
Head and neck cancers commonly metastasise to the lung. Solitary lung lesions are metastatic in 90% of cases and primary lung cancers in 10% of cases. Surgery is thought to improve survival, but further data are needed. Five-year survival of 29–47% is reported.

SYSTEMIC THERAPY OF SELECTED TUMOURS

Germ cell tumours
Combination chemotherapy offers high cure rates even in patients with pulmonary metastases. Macroscopic residual disease following chemotherapy for non-seminomatous germ cell tumours should be resected. Pathological examination reveals differentiated teratoma in ~50%, malignant elements in ~30% and necrosis/fibrosis in ~20%. Fifteen-year survival is ~65%.

Colon cancer
Survival in unresectable disease may be increased with chemotherapy (5FU and folinic acid). New agents such as irinotecan (licensed for second line) and oxaliplatin are improving the outlook of patients with metastatic disease.

Thyroid cancer
Radioiodine may induce complete remission of pulmonary metastases in over 40% of patients, although a clear survival benefit has not been demonstrated. This may be due to the long natural history of this disease. Repeated doses may be given as long as the tumour continues to take up iodine and thyroglobulin levels are elevated. Radiation fibrosis can occur in patients with diffuse pulmonary metastatic disease who have received multiple doses.

Renal cancer
Median survival for unresectable disease is 6–12 months. Immunotherapy with interferon and IL-2 may improve survival, but further studies are needed and are ongoing.

Breast cancer

Chemotherapy is most effective for visceral disease. Anthracycline-based chemotherapy is used first line, with taxanes second line. Hormonal therapy may also be helpful.

Prostate cancer

Pulmonary metastases are usually asymptomatic and invariably associated with bone metastases. They are often refractory to hormonal manipulation.

RADIOTHERAPY

Radiotherapy has a very limited role in the management of pulmonary metastases. It may be useful for treating an identifiable metastasis that is causing haemoptysis, bronchial obstruction or pain due to infiltration of the pleura/chest wall. A single fraction of 8 Gy or 20 Gy in five fractions is appropriate. Brachytherapy may be offered to patients with an endobronchial tumour (single 10–15 Gy fraction).

INTERVENTIONAL BRONCHOSCOPY

Endobronchial stenting, laser therapy, electrocautery or brachytherapy can be offered as palliation for endobronchial tumour. Extrinsic bronchial compression can be managed with stenting.

LYMPHANGITIS CARCINOMATOSA

This distressing condition should be managed as appropriate to the causative malignancy. Supportive therapy with oxygen and high dose steroids (e.g. dexamethasone 8–12 mg o.d.) may be required, especially in the advanced stages. Over 50% of patients with lymphangitis carcinomatosa are dead within 3 months.

FURTHER READING

Davidson R S, Nwogu C E, Brentjens M J, Anderson T M 2001 The surgical management of pulmonary metastasis: current concepts. Surgical Oncology 10:35–42

Dresler C M, Goldberg M 1996 Surgical management of lung metastases: selection factors and results. Oncology 10(5):649–655

International Registry of Lung Metastases 1997 Long-term results of lung metastasectomy: Prognostic analyses based on 5206 cases. Journal of Thoracic and Cardiovascular Surgery 113(1):37–49

Yoneda K Y, Louie S, Shelton D K 2000 Approach to pulmonary metastases. Current Opinion in Pulmonary Medicine 6:356–363

CHAPTER 60

Spinal cord compression

INTRODUCTION

Malignant spinal cord compression (SCC) is one of the most devastating and feared complications of cancer and occurs in approximately 5% of all cancer patients. Breast (29%), lung (17%) and prostate (14%) cancers account for the majority of cases, with lymphoma (5%), renal cancer (4%), myeloma (4%), sarcoma (3%), and others (24%) making up the rest. The thoracic spine (59–78% of cases) is the most frequently involved site, followed by the lumbar spine (16–33%), cervical spine (4–15%) and sacral spine (5–10%).

Anatomically, SCC is classified as epidural, intramedullary or leptomeningeal (within subarachnoid space). Epidural SCC is by far the commonest mechanism and may be caused in three different ways: (1) vertebral body expansion or collapse into the epidural space (~85% of cases), (2) paravertebral tumour invasion through the intervertebral foramina into the epidural space (~10–12%), (3) direct metastasis to the epidural space (~1–3%). As epidural metastases grow, they compress adjacent blood vessels, nerve roots, the thecal sac and spinal cord (or cauda equina), resulting in local and referred pain, radiculopathy and myelopathy. Patients with intramedullary metastases often have synchronous brain metastases and lung cancer is the usual primary lesion. Leptomeningeal disease is discussed in Chapter 50.

Untreated, spinal cord compression leads to progressive painful paralysis, sensory loss and incontinence, often requiring 24-hour nursing care and symptom management. This is devastating not only for the patient, but also for relatives and loved ones. Early diagnosis with recognition of the symptoms and signs and urgent treatment is therefore vitally important to minimise irreversible neurological damage. Better neurological and functional outcomes following treatment are more likely in patients who are ambulatory at diagnosis and who have a gradual onset of weakness rather than a rapid onset. Over 80% of patients who are ambulatory at diagnosis will remain so following treatment. Approximately 7–16% of patients will have a further episode of SCC in the course of their illness.

Unfortunately, although somewhat variable, the prognosis for most patients with SCC is poor, with many surviving only a few months. Median overall survival is reported to be 3 to 6 months. Factors associated with a very poor prognosis include loss of ambulation, bladder and bowel dysfunction, multiple spinal lesions, and lung cancer as the primary diagnosis.

CLINICAL PRESENTATION

In the vast majority of patients there is a prior history of malignancy, but in 8–35% of patients, SCC is the initial manifestation. A recent history of progressive pain, which may be localised, radicular or both, is the most frequent symptom occurring in over 90% of patients. Localised pain is due to vertebral expansion, destruction or fracture and is usually worse at night and on movement, exacerbated in the supine position and relieved in the upright position. Radicular pain is caused by compression of nerve roots or the cauda equina and is often shooting in nature, and depending on the level of compression, may radiate down the arms, legs or in a band-like fashion around the girdle. Pain usually precedes the diagnosis of SCC by days to months.

Weakness is the second commonest symptom (80%), followed by sensory loss (70%) and autonomic dysfunction (50%). The classic pattern of progressive SCC is of pain as the initial symptom, followed by weakness, which may start unilaterally, progressing to bilateral weakness with associated sensory loss below the level of the lesion. Gait difficulties and falls result from weakness and ataxia. Finally, autonomic dysfunction occurs, leading to sphincter incontinence and impotence.

Clinical examination in the early stages may reveal a flaccid paralysis with areflexia, but this progresses to spasticity and hyperreflexia consistent with an upper motor neuron pattern. Lesions involving the upper cervical spine may lead to upper limb weakness or respiratory muscle paralysis causing respiratory failure. Pure cauda equina compression produces lower motor neuron signs.

SCC due to an intramedullary metastasis is rare (1–4% of SCC cases), but causes similar symptoms and signs to epidural SCC. There is often only a single spinal lesion, but it is commonly associated with parenchymal brain metastases.

DIAGNOSIS

Neurological examination and percussion (which exacerbates pain) over the site of the back pain can help localise the lesion. Plain spinal X-ray films reveal bony abnormalities in over 70% of cases. MRI is the imaging modality of choice with a diagnostic accuracy of 95% in SCC. It can also distinguish between a benign and malignant vertebral body collapse with 98% accuracy. MRI advantages over CT include: (1) ability to distinguish cord from other soft tissue masses, (2) ability to assess thecal sac impingement, (3) lower cost. The entire spine should be imaged because multiple sites of compression are present in 26–49% of cases. CT is better than MRI at evaluating vertebral stability and bone destruction and is usually requested prior to spinal surgery. Myelography with or without CT is used if MRI is not possible due to claustrophobia, severe scoliosis, pacemakers, aneurysm clips and ferromagnetic implants.

Further investigations with X-rays, bone scans, CT, MRI and spinal biopsy may be necessary. In patients without a prior history of cancer, a tissue diagnosis should be sought because this may alter the treatment plan. If the spine is the only site of disease, then surgery is usually indicated, as this will usually obtain a histological diagnosis. Spinal biopsy by the percutaneous or open route is an alternative if radiotherapy is to be offered. The percutaneous route gives a positive biopsy in 65% of lytic lesions, but only 25% of blastic lesions. Open biopsy is positive in 85% of cases.

MANAGEMENT

SCC requires emergency treatment. Initial therapy includes the administration of appropriate analgesia, i.e. NSAIDs and strong opiates. Steroids should be given immediately as they have been shown to improve the number of ambulatory patients following radiotherapy. Steroids have a strong anti-inflammatory and analgesic effect, and may also have anti-cancer effects, especially with lymphomas and myeloma. Intravenous bolus dexamethasone is given at a dose of 10–16 mg, followed orally in the same dose for 3–4 days, then tapering off within a few weeks. Early mobilisation should be encouraged for those with no clinical or radiological evidence of spinal instability, as recumbent bed rest can cause muscle wasting, feeding difficulties, dyspepsia and psychological distress. Physiotherapy and occupational therapy should be offered early on.

Radiotherapy and surgery are the main treatment modalities in the management of SCC. Chemotherapy and/or hormonal therapy may be offered in conjunction with these modalities if the tumour is chemo/hormone sensitive and the patient is fit enough to receive treatment.

RADIOTHERAPY (RT)

Palliative RT is the treatment of choice for the majority of patients with SCC because most present with advanced disease and are unsuitable for surgery. Commonly used dose regimens are 20 Gy in five fractions over 5–7 days or

30 Gy in 10 fractions over 2 weeks. For paraplegic patients with a very poor prognosis and severe pain, a single 8 Gy fraction is often more appropriate.

RT reduces pain in 70% and improves power in 45–60%, but only 10–20% of non-ambulatory patients pre-RT become ambulatory following treatment. RT is much less effective in patients with spinal instability and bony compression, and surgery should be considered for these patients (see below).

Radical RT (usually in combination with other treatment modalities) may be indicated for potentially curable tumours such as plasmacytoma, thyroid cancer, seminoma and lymphoma. This highlights the importance of obtaining a histological diagnosis.

See surgery section below for postoperative radiotherapy.

SURGERY

Accepted indications for surgery include:

1. Unknown diagnosis
2. Spinal instability or bony neural compression
3. Good performance status paretic patients with focal cord compression
4. Neurological deterioration despite RT
5. Previous irradiation of the spine (cord) to maximum tolerated dose
6. Intractable pain unrelieved by other measures.

Surgery is usually inappropriate if one or more of the following factors are present:

1. Life expectancy is <3 months
2. There is more than one level of compression
3. Paraplegia has been present for more than 12–24 hours
4. Presence of serious co-morbidity/poor performance status.

Decompression of the spinal cord and mechanical stabilisation are the aims of surgery. The type of surgical procedure depends mainly on the disease site. The vertebral body is the commonest site of metastatic disease, and an anterior approach to surgery offers the most direct and accessible route. The affected vertebral body is resected and replaced with methylmethacrylate cement and instrumentation (e.g. metal cage prostheses or struts) used to attach to adjacent vertebral bodies for maximum stability. Results from surgical series report pain relief in 85–97% of patients, improvement or stabilisation of motor function in 90%, and reduction in incontinence for most patients. However, the procedure has a mortality rate of 3–10%, and a high risk of complications.

Laminectomy (removal of the posterior arch of the vertebral body to decompress the cord) is reserved for posterior vertebral lesions.

Postoperative radiotherapy is normally offered as this will reduce subsequent tumour regrowth and bone destruction that could cause pain and/or loss of surgical fixation devices.

CHEMOTHERAPY, HORMONAL THERAPY AND BISPHOSPHONATES

Specific chemotherapy is not usually used alone as a primary treatment of spinal cord compression, but there are several reports of good neurological recovery in lymphoma, myeloma, germ cell tumours, and neuroblastoma.

There are some reports of good outcomes in breast and prostate cancer patients not suitable for RT or surgery, treated with hormone therapy alone. However, most hormonal responses occur over weeks to months and surgery or RT should always be the initial treatment of choice.

Bisphosphonates should be routinely offered to patients with breast cancer and myeloma following treatment for spinal cord compression, as this has been shown to reduce further skeletal-related events. There is mounting evidence that these drugs should also be routinely used in patients with other types of cancer.

FURTHER READING

Fuller B G, Heiss J D, Oldfield E H 2001 Spinal cord compression. In: DeVita V T, Hellman S, Rosenberg S A (eds) Principles and practice of oncology, 6th edn. Lippincott Williams and Wilkins, Philadelphia

Jacobs W B, Perrin R G 2001 Evaluation and treatment of spinal metastases: An overview. Neurosurgery Focus 11(6)

Loblaw A D, Laerriere N J 1998 Emergency treatment of malignant extradural spinal cord compression: An evidence-based guideline. Journal of Clinical Oncology 16:1613–1624

Mekhail A, Benzel E C, Steinmetz M P 2001 Management of metastatic tumours of the spine: Strategies and operative indications. Neurosurgery Focus 11(6)

CHAPTER 61

Superior vena cava obstruction

INTRODUCTION

Superior vena cava obstruction (SVCO) is a distressing syndrome. The first case of SVCO was due to syphilis (aortitis) and was described by William Hunter in 1757. Until the early part of the 20th century, benign conditions such as syphilitic aortitis and tuberculous mediastinitis accounted for over half of SVCO cases. Malignancy is now the major cause and accounts for approximately 95% of cases. Lung cancer accounts for the vast majority of cases (70–80%), with lymphoma (10%) the next commonest cause. Approximately 5–10% of lung cancer patients will develop SVCO, with small cell being the most frequent histological type. Other primary mediastinal malignancies that cause SVCO include germ cell tumours, thymoma, thyroid and oesophageal cancer. Breast cancer is the commonest metastatic disease to cause SVCO. Benign causes now account for ~10% of cases and the commonest include mediastinal fibrosis and SVC thrombosis (which is often caused by central venous lines).

The superior vena cava is the major drainage vessel for the head, neck, upper extremities and upper thorax. It is located in the middle mediastinum and surrounded by the trachea, right main bronchus, aorta, pulmonary artery and the perihilar and paratracheal lymph nodes. It is 6–8 cm long, 1.5–2 cm wide and is easily compressible. Obstruction leads to collateral circulation mainly via the azygos system, but also via internal mammary veins, lateral thoracic veins, paraspinous veins, and the oesophageal venous network. The subcutaneous veins are also important pathways and their engorgement leads to one of the typical physical signs seen in SVCO.

Traditionally SVCO was thought to be a life-threatening condition and attempts at obtaining a biopsy were regarded as too hazardous. Patients were therefore often given emergency radiotherapy without a histological diagnosis. This practice is now unacceptable as although SVCO is a very distressing condition, it is not life-threatening in itself and diagnostic procedures are now very safe. Treating a potentially very curable lymphoma or germ cell tumour with palliative radiotherapy is not good for the patient or the doctor!

PRESENTATION AND DIAGNOSIS

SVCO is usually diagnosed from its symptoms and signs. Dyspnoea (50–80%), facial swelling and fullness (50%), cough (25%), arm swelling, chest pain and dysphagia are the commonest symptoms. More severe symptoms include dizziness, headache, syncopal episodes, stridor and mental changes. Bending forward, stooping or lying flat may aggravate the symptoms. Physical findings include neck vein and chest wall vein distension (55–65%), facial oedema and chemosis (45%), cyanosis (20%), facial plethora, arm oedema, and papilloedema.

CXR shows mediastinal widening in up to 60% of cases. Other common CXR findings include pleural effusion and a right hilar mass. A completely normal CXR is unusual. The investigations of choice following CXR are venography and contrast-enhanced CT of the chest.

Bilateral arm venography may offer important information to assess whether the vena cava is completely obstructed or is patent and extrinsically compressed. Contrast-enhanced CT of the chest can often demonstrate the level of obstruction and may also identify the cause. To confirm the diagnosis accurately with CT, there must be absent or reduced opacification of the venous system below the level of obstruction and collateral venous channels must be opacified.

The method of obtaining a histological diagnosis will depend on the clinical and radiological findings and may require one or more of the following: sputum cytology (~40% success), CT-guided biopsy of a mass (~80% success), bronchoscopy (~60% success), mediastinoscopy and biopsy (almost 100% success), node biopsy/FNA (~85% success), and thoracocentesis of pleural effusion.

MANAGEMENT

The two main aims in the management of SVCO are symptom relief and treatment of the underlying cause.

General symptomatic measures such as sitting the patient up and administering oxygen may reduce cardiac output and venous pressure. The use of steroids is regarded as standard practice (e.g. dexamethasone 16 mg IV) in spite of the lack of evidence to support this. Diuretics may reduce oedema, but can increase the risk of thrombosis.

In patients with severe symptoms not responding to general measures, the insertion of an endovascular metallic self-expanding stent following percutaneous balloon angioplasty (femoral or arm approach) should be considered. Stenting achieves complete or partial relief of symptoms in 95% of cases and the vast majority will remain free of symptoms until death, with only 10% of patients relapsing with SVCO symptoms. Symptom relief of headache, cyanosis and dyspnoea is often immediate, with facial oedema usually resolving within 24 hours and arm/trunk oedema within 72 hours. Complication rates are low, with bleeding, stent misplacement and migration, occlusion and cardiac arrhythmias being the commonest reported. The role of anticoagulation following stent insertion is controversial.

Radiotherapy has historically been the first line treatment of choice for SVCO as it offers effective symptom relief in 70–95% of patients within 2 weeks, most benefiting within 72 hours. However, since the introduction of metallic endovascular stents, radiotherapy is used much less commonly as a first line measure, especially in severely symptomatic patients when rapid/immediate relief of symptoms is required.

If thrombus is present, thrombolytics may be used alone or prior to stent insertion, e.g. urokinase and rTPA (recombinant tissue plasminogen activator). It is particularly useful in patients with central venous line related SVCO, where line preservation is desirable. Success rates for this group of patients are high, especially if treatment is given within 5 days of the onset of symptoms. Mechanical clot breakers have also been used (e.g. Amplatz thrombectomy device).

Major surgical intervention with a bypass procedure (usually between the innominate or jugular vein of the left side and right atrial appendage) is rarely appropriate in malignant SVCO and should only be considered when symptoms are uncontrolled and all other options have been exhausted.

The treatment of the underlying malignancy will depend on the histological type and the stage of the disease as well as the clinical condition of the patient. Treatment should therefore be individualised. For the vast majority of patients palliation is the most appropriate treatment, but presence of SVCO does not in itself preclude potentially curative radical treatment.

In 1997 Ostler et al suggested a useful treatment algorithm for SVCO (Fig. 61.1).

SMALL CELL LUNG CANCER (SCLC)

The incidence of SVCO is ~10% in SCLC and normally results from massive enlargement of the right paratracheal lymph nodes. Cure is still possible in a few patients (especially those with limited disease). Chemotherapy is the treatment of choice, with 70–90% of patients obtaining symptomatic relief within 7–10 days. Chemotherapy should not be administered into high-pressure arm veins, and the veins of the lower limbs offer alternative safe access.

Consolidation radiotherapy to the chest/mediastinum following chemotherapy adds a small local control and survival benefit in patients with limited disease. Palliative radiotherapy, e.g. 20 Gy in five fractions over 1 week, 17 Gy in two fractions over 1 week or a single 8–10 Gy fraction, can be used for patients unsuitable for chemotherapy.

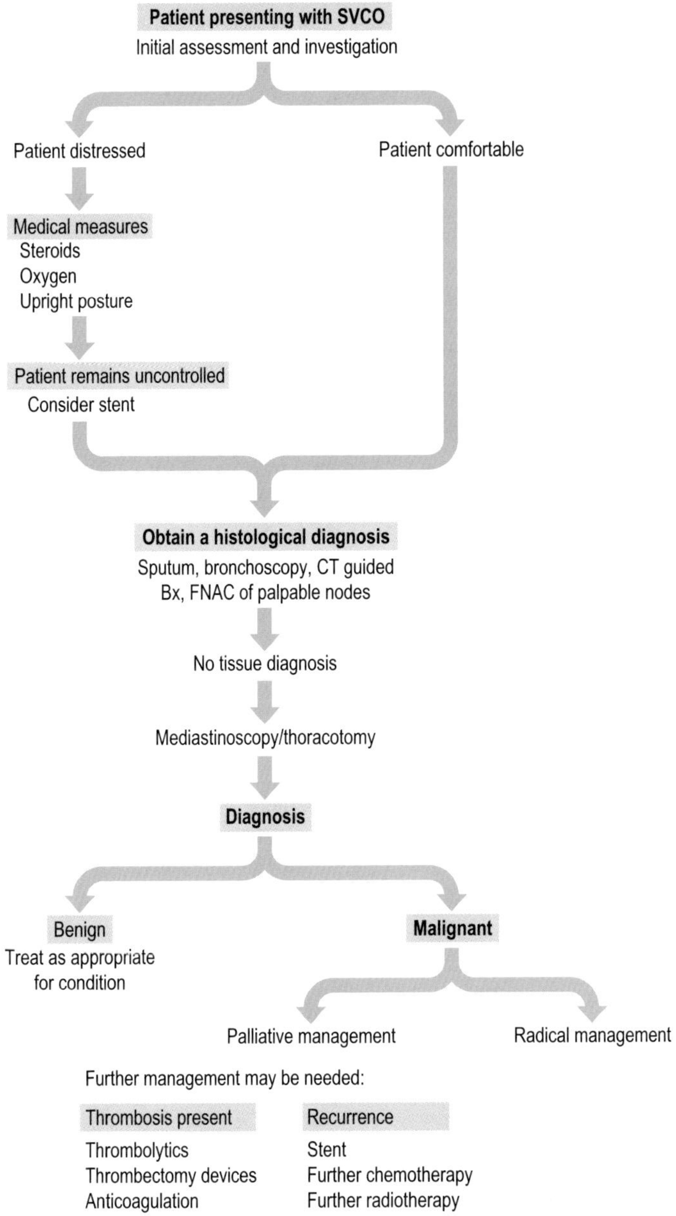

FIGURE 61.1 Management algorithm of SVCO. (Reproduced with permission of Elsevier from Ostler P J, Clarke D P, Watkinson A F, Gaze M N 1997 Superior vena cava obstruction: A modern management strategy. Clinical Oncology 9:83–89.)

NON-SMALL CELL LUNG CANCER (NSCLC)

The incidence of SVCO is ~4% in NSCLC. Radiotherapy is the treatment of choice. If radical radiotherapy is appropriate then a dose of 55–60 Gy in 20–30 fractions or CHART (54 Gy in 32 fractions) should be used. The optimum palliative regimen is unknown, but many centres offer 20 Gy in five fractions. Shorter schedules such as 17 Gy in two fractions over 1 week or a single 8 Gy fraction may be more appropriate for poorer prognosis patients. About 70–90% of patients will experience relief of symptoms within 2 weeks (most within 3 days), which is lifelong for most.

NON-HODGKIN'S LYMPHOMA (NHL) AND HODGKIN'S LYMPHOMA

Chemotherapy is the mainstay of treatment followed by consolidation radiotherapy to bulk disease (>10 cm). Stage I disease may be treated with RT alone.

GERM CELL TUMOURS

Chemotherapy is the mainstay of treatment. Residual masses following teratoma treatment should be surgically resected, but residual seminoma should be treated with salvage chemotherapy or irradiated.

REFERENCES AND FURTHER READING

Nicholson A A, Ettles D F, Arnold A et al 1997 Treatment of malignant superior vena cava obstruction: metal stents or radiation therapy. Journal of Vascular and Interventional Radiology 8(5):781–788

Ostler P J, Clarke D P, Watkinson A F, Gaze M N 1997 Superior vena cava obstruction: A modern management strategy. Clinical Oncology 9:83–89

Rowell N P, Gleeson F V 2002 Cochrane Lung Cancer Group. Steroids, radiotherapy, chemotherapy and stents for superior vena caval obstruction in carcinoma of the bronchus. [Systematic Review] Cochrane Database of Systematic Reviews. Issue 4

Appendices

Normal tissue tolerances to radiotherapy

Normal tissue tolerance is normally defined as the total radiation dose delivered in 2 Gy daily fractions that produces a 5% chance of severe late effects over the next 5 years (TD5/5) (Table A1.1).

Table A1.1 Normal tissue tolerances

Organ	One-third organ volume TD5/5 (Gy)	Whole organ TD5/5 (Gy)	Effect
Brain	60	45	Necrosis/infarction
Brainstem	60	50	Necrosis/infarction
Spinal cord	50–5 cm length	47–20 cm length	Myelitis
Bladder	N/A	65	Contracture/volume loss
Liver	50	30	Liver failure
Kidney	50	23	Clinical nephritis
Lung	45	17.5	Pneumonitis
Heart	60	40	Pericarditis
Skin	$70–10\,cm^2$	$55–100\,cm^2$	Telangiectasia, necrosis, ulceration
Parotid	N/A	32	Xerostomia
Eye lens	N/A	10	Cataract
Retina	N/A	45	Blindness
Optic nerve/chiasm	N/A	50	Blindness
Mandible (temporomandibular joint)	65	60	Limitation of jaw movement
Femoral head	N/A	52	Necrosis
Ribs	50	N/A	Rib fracture
Oesophagus	60	55	Stricture/perforation
Stomach	60	50	Ulceration/perforation
Small intestine	50	40	Obstruction/perforation/fistula
Colon	55	45	Obstruction/perforation/fistula
Rectum	–	60	Severe proctitis/necrosis/fistula formation/stenosis

APPENDIX 2

A–Z of commonly used chemotherapy drugs

(* = Dose-limiting side effect.)

BLEOMYCIN

Classification: Anti-tumour antibiotic.

Mechanism of action: Causes single- and double-stranded DNA breaks leading to inhibition of DNA and RNA synthesis.

Main uses: Squamous carcinomas, germ cell tumours, lymphoma.

Side effects: Rash, skin nodules and hyperpigmentation, mild alopecia, mild nausea and vomiting, hypersensitivity (fever and chills common), *pneumonitis (~10%), *chronic lung fibrosis.

Notes: Risk of pulmonary toxicity increases significantly at doses greater than 500 units. Myelosuppression not a problem.

BUSULPHAN

Classification: Alkylating agent.

Mechanism of action: Causes DNA breaks and crosslinks leading to interference with DNA replication and transcription of RNA.

Main uses: Leukaemias, myeloma.

Side effects: *Myelosuppression, pulmonary toxicity, *hepatic veno-occlusive disease, decreased gonadal function, skin hyperpigmentation. In high dose additional side effects include nausea and vomiting, diarrhoea, mucositis and seizures.

CAPECITABINE

Classification: Cytotoxic antimetabolite.

Mechanism of action: Prodrug that is activated to its active metabolite, fluorouracil, by thymidylate phosphorylase, which is found in higher concentrations in cancer cells than in normal cells. Fluorouracil is metabolised to two active metabolites – fluorodeoxyuridine monophosphate (FdUMP), which inhibits DNA synthesis, and 5-fluorouridine triphosphate (FUTP), which inhibits RNA and protein synthesis.

Main uses: Breast and colorectal cancer.

Side effects: *Hand–foot skin reaction, *stomatitis, *nausea and *vomiting, *diarrhoea, myelosuppression, conjunctivitis, deranged liver function tests (LFTs) (25%), fatigue.

Notes: Dihydropyrimidine dehydrogenase (DPD) is a rate-limiting enzyme in the metabolism of fluorouracil, the active moiety of capecitabine. DPD deficiency is present in about 3% of cancer patients. This population is at a greater risk of severe capecitabine-related toxicities. Capecitabine should be used with caution and may require dose reduction. Currently, screening for DPD deficiency is not readily available. Capecitabine is given by the oral route.

CARBOPLATIN

Classification: Alkylating agent.

Mechanism of action: Platinum complexes form DNA crosslinks, thereby inhibiting DNA synthesis.

Main uses: Ovarian cancer, brain tumours, lung cancer, head and neck cancer, germ cell tumours.

Side effects: *Myelosuppression, nausea and vomiting, metabolic disturbances (low Mg^{2+}, Ca^{2+}, K^+ and deranged LFTs).

Notes: Often used as an alternative to cisplatin in patients with renal dysfunction.

CARMUSTINE (BCNU)

Classification: Alkylating agent.

Mechanism of action: Forms active metabolites that cause DNA crosslinking leading to interference with DNA replication. Also causes interference with DNA repair.

Main uses: Brain tumours, lymphomas.

Side effects: Myelosuppression, nausea and vomiting, renal toxicity, dose-related pulmonary toxicity, vesicant.

CHLORAMBUCIL

Classification: Alkylating agent.

Mechanism of action: Causes DNA breaks and crosslinking, thus interfering with DNA replication and RNA transcription.

Main uses: CLL and NHL.

Side effects: *Myelosuppression, mild nausea and vomiting.
Notes: Generally very well tolerated. Given by the oral route.

CISPLATIN

Classification: Alkylating agent.
Mechanism of action: Platinum complexes form intrastrand, interstrand, and protein DNA crosslinks, thus interfering with DNA synthesis and repair.
Main uses: Germ cell tumours, ovarian cancer, lung cancer, bladder cancer, upper gastrointestinal (GI) cancer, head and neck cancer.
Side effects: *Nausea and vomiting, *nephrotoxicity (tubular necrosis, low Mg, Ca, K), *ototoxicity (most commonly high tone hearing loss and tinnitus, cumulative, dose-related and irreversible), *peripheral neuropathy (usually sensory but may be motor), myelosuppression (moderate), hypersensitivity reactions, vesicant.
Notes: Nausea and vomiting occurs in nearly all patients, so steroids and 5-HT$_3$ inhibitors should be used. Delayed nausea and vomiting is common and continuous antiemetics are required. Renal toxicity can be reduced or prevented with adequate IV hydration (aiming for urine output of at least 100 ml/hour). Cisplatin is a radiation sensitiser and is commonly used in concurrent chemoradiation schedules.

CYCLOPHOSPHAMIDE

Classification: Alkylating agent.
Mechanism of action: Forms active metabolites such as acrolein that cause DNA crosslinks, thus interfering with DNA metabolism.
Main uses: Breast cancer, lung cancer, leukaemia, myeloma, lymphoma.
Side effects: *Myelosuppression, *nausea and vomiting, *haemorrhagic cystitis (10% standard doses, 40% in high dose patients), *acute interstitial pneumonitis, alopecia, infertility, SIADH.
Notes: The risk of haemorrhagic cystitis may be reduced by adequate hydration, frequent voiding of the bladder and the use of mesna.

DACARBAZINE (DTIC)

Classification: Alkylating agent.
Mechanism of action: Alkylation of nucleic acids leads to interference of DNA metabolism.
Main uses: Hodgkin's disease, melanoma.
Side effects: *Myelosuppression, *nausea and vomiting (may be severe), flu-like syndrome (10%).

Notes: Nausea and vomiting is very common and adequate prophylactic and continuing antiemetics are necessary.

DOCETAXEL (TAXOTERE)

Classification: Mitotic inhibitor.

Mechanism of action: Promotes the assembly of tubulin into stable microtubules and inhibits their disassembly, causing inhibition of cell division and eventual cell death.

Main uses: Breast cancer, lung cancer, ovarian cancer.

Side effects: *Myelosuppression, *fatigue, hypersensitivity reactions, fluid retention, alopecia, mild–moderate nausea and vomiting, mucositis, motor/sensory neuropathy, arthralgia/myalgias.

Notes: Premedication with dexamethasone is required to reduce risk of hypersensitivity reaction. Radiation sensitiser.

DOXORUBICIN

Classification: Anti-tumour antibiotic/anthracycline.

Mechanism of action: Damages DNA by intercalation of the anthracycline portion, metal ion chelation, or by generation of free radicals. Can also inhibit topo-isomerase II, which is crucial to the mechanism of DNA replication.

Main uses: Breast cancer, leukaemia, lymphoma, ovarian cancer, sarcomas, lung cancer.

Side effects: *Myelosuppression, acute transient arrhythmias (40%), dose-related cardiac toxicity (*cardiac failure, *cardiomyopathy), nausea and vomiting, diarrhoea, mucositis, infertility, vesicant.

Notes: The risk of drug-induced cardiac failure is 0.1–1.2% at cumulative doses less than $500\,mg/m^2$, but this increases to 30% above this dose level. Cardiac assessment (cardiology referral and echocardiogram) should be offered at the $450\,mg/m^2$ dose level before continuing with treatment.

EPIRUBICIN

Classification: Anti-tumour antibiotic/anthracycline.

Mechanism of action: Damages DNA by intercalation of the anthracycline portion, metal ion chelation, or by generation of free radicals.

Main uses: Breast cancer, upper GI cancer, lymphoma.

Side effects: *Myelosuppression, acute transient arrhythmias (40%), dose-related cardiac toxicity (*cardiac failure, *cardiomyopathy), nausea and vomiting, diarrhoea, mucositis, alopecia, vesicant.

Notes: Cardiac toxicity is rarely a problem if the cumulative dose is kept below 900 mg/m^2.

ETOPOSIDE

Classification: Plant alkaloid mitotic inhibitor (derived from the root of *Podophyllum peltatum* (the May apple or mandrake)).

Mechanism of action: Causes single-strand DNA breaks and inhibits topo-isomerase II, a crucial enzyme in DNA metabolism. It is cell cycle phase specific with most activity in the S- and G2-phases.

Main uses: Germ cell tumours, lung cancer, lymphomas, leukaemias, ovarian cancer.

Side effects: Nausea and vomiting, alopecia, *stomatitis/mucositis (with high dose protocols), *myelosuppression, *deranged LFTs (with high dose protocols), extravasation irritant; risk of secondary AML is ~6% (usually 2–4 years after treatment).

Notes: Can be given orally or intravenously. More nausea and vomiting with the oral route. Cisplatin and etoposide are synergistic. Cisplatin should be administered before etoposide.

FLUDARABINE

Classification: Antimetabolite.

Mechanism of action: It is a fluorinated analogue of adenine and is metabolised to F-ara-ATP, which inhibits DNA synthesis by inhibition of DNA polymerases and prevention of elongation of DNA strands through direct incorporation into the DNA molecule.

Main uses: CLL.

Side effects: *Myelosuppression, CD4 lymphopenia, infectious complications, fever/chills and fatigue (common: 60%), mild nausea and vomiting, diarrhoea, mucositis, *encephalopathy (at high doses).

Notes: Given IV. Antiemetics often not required. High risk of infectious complications and therefore prophylactic co-trimoxazole and aciclovir (if history of shingles) are recommended.

5-FLUOROURACIL (5FU)

Classification: Antimetabolite.

Mechanism of action: It is a fluorinated pyrimidine that is metabolised intracellularly to its active form, fluorodeoxyuridine monophosphate (FdUMP), which inhibits DNA synthesis by inhibiting the normal production of thymidine. It is cell cycle phase specific (S-phase).

Main uses: Colorectal, breast and upper GI cancer.

Side effects: *Plantar–palmar erythema, *mucositis, *diarrhoea, mild nausea and vomiting, conjunctivitis, excessive lacrimation, chemical phlebitis (but not an extravasation hazard), photosensitivity rashes, asymptomatic ECG changes (common), angina (2%), *myelosuppression (but usually mild); acute cerebellar syndrome and encephalopathy are very rare.

Notes: Dihydropyrimidine dehydrogenase (DPD) is a rate-limiting enzyme in the metabolism of fluorouracil. DPD deficiency is present in about 3% of cancer patients. This population is at a greater risk of severe fluorouracil-related toxicities. Fluorouracil should be used with caution and may require dose reduction. Currently, screening for DPD deficiency is not readily available. Myelosuppression is more likely with bolus administration, whereas plantar–palmar erythema, mucositis and severe diarrhoea are more likely with continuous infusional administration.

GEMCITABINE

Classification: Cytotoxic antimetabolite.

Mechanism of action: Gemcitabine, a pyrimidine analogue, is metabolised intracellularly to two active metabolites, gemcitabine diphosphate (dFdCDP) and gemcitabine triphosphate (dFdCTP). The cytotoxic effects are exerted through incorporation of dFdCTP into DNA with the assistance of dFdCDP, causing inhibition of DNA synthesis and induction of apoptosis. It is a radiation-sensitising agent and is cell cycle phase specific (S- and G1/S-phases).

Main uses: Non-small cell lung cancer, pancreatic cancer, bladder cancer.

Side effects: *Myelosuppression (25% severe neutropenia), fever, asthenia, flu-like symptoms, nausea and vomiting (severe in 18%), peripheral oedema, deranged LFTs (common, but usually mild and transient), alopecia (~15%), generalised aches and pains (~10%), skin rashes, peripheral neuropathy (3%), renal dysfunction (uncommon, mild), haemolytic uraemic syndrome (rare).

Notes: For IV administration.

HYDROXYUREA

Classification: Miscellaneous.

Mechanism of action: Inhibitor of ribonucleotide reductase leading to depletion of DNA precursors. May also cause direct damage to DNA. Hydroxyurea is cell cycle phase specific (S-phase).

Main uses: CML.

Side effects: *Myelosuppression, mild nausea and vomiting, mucositis, rashes and hyperpigmentation, drowsiness, elevated creatinine.

Notes: Administered by the oral route.

IFOSFAMIDE

Classification: Alkylating agent.

Mechanism of action: Ifosfamide is a structural analogue of cyclophosphamide and its mechanism of action is presumed to be identical (see above).

Main uses: Cervix, soft tissue sarcoma, germ cell tumours.

Side effects: *Myelosuppression, *haemorrhagic cystitis, alopecia, nausea and vomiting, metabolic acidosis, SIADH, encephalopathy, cardiac arrhythmias (at high dose), sterility, chemical phlebitis (but not an extravasation hazard).

Notes: Mesna reduces incidence of haemorrhagic cystitis from 40% to 3.5%. Adequate hydration is also required to reduce risk. Methylene blue is used to treat encephalopathy.

IRINOTECAN

Classification: Cytotoxic topo-isomerase I inhibitor. Camptothecin.

Mechanism of action: Irinotecan and its active metabolite, SN-38, inhibit the action of topo-isomerase I, an enzyme that produces reversible single-strand breaks in DNA that relieve torsional strain and allow DNA replication to proceed. Irinotecan and SN-38 bind to the topo-isomerase I–DNA complex and prevent re-ligation of the DNA strand, resulting in double-strand DNA breakage and cell death. Irinotecan is cell cycle phase-specific (S-phase).

Main uses: Colorectal cancer, upper GI cancer.

Side effects: *Myelosuppression (severe neutropenia in 25%), *early and late diarrhoea is common (early (<24 hours) is due to the cholinergic syndrome, late (>24 hours) is due to mucosal injury), constitutional symptoms (fever, chills, fatigue, sweating and weight loss are common), nausea and vomiting (moderate/high potential), alopecia (60%), rashes, mucositis, visual disturbance (15%), peripheral oedema, cholinergic syndrome (flushing, rhinitis, hypersalivation, miosis, lacrimation, abdominal cramps), pulmonary syndrome (dyspnoea, fever and reticulonodular pattern on CXR).

Notes: Early onset severe diarrhoea and cholinergic symptoms can be treated with atropine 0.25–1 mg IV or s.c. (monitor pulse and blood pressure). Late diarrhoea can be treated with loperamide.

LOMUSTINE (CCNU)

Classification: Alkylating agent.
Mechanism of action: Reactive metabolites of lomustine cause alkylation and crosslinking of DNA. Other effects include inhibition of DNA synthesis and some cell cycle phase specificity.
Main uses: Brain tumours, lymphomas.
Side effects: *Myelosuppression, nausea and vomiting, transient elevation of LFTs, infertility, pulmonary fibrosis (rare).
Notes: Administered orally. Nausea may be minimised by giving dose at bedtime on an empty stomach.

MELPHALAN

Classification: Alkylating agent.
Mechanism of action: Causes alkylation of DNA resulting in DNA breaks as well as crosslinking of the twin strands, thus interfering with DNA replication and transcription of RNA. Like other alkylators, it is cell cycle phase non-specific.
Main uses: Myeloma.
Side effects: *Myelosuppression, mild nausea and vomiting, diarrhoea, mucositis, skin rashes and pigmentation, amenorrhoea and infertility, pulmonary fibrosis (rare).
Notes: Vesicant. Used in high dose protocols.

METHOTREXATE

Classification: Antimetabolite.
Mechanism of action: Methotrexate and its active metabolites compete for the folate binding site of the enzyme dihydrofolate reductase. Folic acid must be reduced to tetrahydrofolic acid by this enzyme for DNA synthesis and cellular replication to occur. Competitive inhibition of the enzyme leads to blockage of tetrahydrofolate synthesis, depletion of nucleotide precursors, and inhibition of DNA, RNA and protein synthesis. Methotrexate is cell cycle phase specific (S-phase).
Main uses: ALL, breast cancer, bladder cancer, sarcomas, NHL.
Side effects: *Myelosuppression, *mucositis, *haemorrhagic enteritis and intestinal perforation, diarrhoea, nausea and vomiting (especially when used in high dose), skin rashes, photosensitivity, interstitial pneumonitis, transient elevation of LFTs, nephropathy (high doses), chemical meningitis (with intrathecal route, but rare), encephalopathy (high doses).

Notes: Administration by oral, intravenous or intrathecal routes. Folinic acid rescue is required when high doses ($>300\,mg/m^2$) are used. This should be administered 24 hours after starting methotrexate and repeated doses may be required.

MITOMYCIN C

Classification: Antitumour antibiotic.

Mechanism of action: Mitomycin is activated in vivo to an alkylating agent. Binding to DNA leads to crosslinking and inhibition of DNA synthesis and function. Mitomycin is cell cycle phase non-specific.

Main uses: Gastric, bladder, breast and colorectal cancers.

Side effects: *Myelosuppression (late nadir – 24–28 days), nausea and vomiting (may continue for 2–3 days), alopecia, palmar erythema, mild mucositis, interstitial pneumonitis (3–12%) and chronic lung fibrosis (uncommon), *haemolytic uraemic syndrome (cumulative dose dependent – threshold of $50–60\,mg/m^2$), acute encephalopathy (rare).

Notes: Vesicant. Administered intravesically for treatment of superficial bladder cancer. Acute pulmonary toxicity (dry cough, shortness of breath), may be life-threatening and should be managed with steroids.

MITOXANTRONE

Classification: Anti-tumour antibiotic.

Mechanism of action: Exact mechanism of action is unknown but includes intercalation with DNA to cause inter/intrastrand crosslinking. Also causes DNA strand breaks through binding with the phosphate backbone of DNA. Mitoxantrone is cell cycle phase non-specific.

Main uses: Leukaemia, breast cancer, lymphoma.

Side effects: *Myelosuppression, *cardiac failure, *cardiomyopathy, transient arrhythmias, nausea and vomiting, alopecia (15%), mucositis.

Notes: Minimal extravasation hazard. Used in high dose protocols.

OXALIPLATIN

Classification: Cytotoxic alkylating agent.

Mechanism of action: The exact mechanism of action is unknown. It forms reactive platinum complexes, which are believed to inhibit DNA synthesis, by forming interstrand and intrastrand crosslinking of DNA molecules. Oxaliplatin is not generally cross-resistant to cisplatin or carboplatin.

Oxaliplatin is a radiation-sensitising agent. It is cell cycle phase non-specific.

Main uses: Colorectal cancer.

Side effects: *Sensory neuropathy (85–95%), myelosuppression (anaemia and thrombocytopenia are common), nausea and vomiting (may be severe), diarrhoea, transient elevation of LFTs, fever (35%).

Notes: Sensory neuropathy is cumulative, dose related and usually reversible. Sensory symptoms may be exacerbated by the cold (e.g. drinking cold water). Gabapentin is useful for some patients. Pharyngolaryngeal dysaesthesia (sporadic reduced sensitivity of the larynx and pharynx) is seen in 1–2% of patients shortly after drug infusion. GI and haemopoietic side effects are increased when oxaliplatin is used in combination with fluorouracil.

PACLITAXEL (TAXOL)

Classification: Mitotic inhibitor.

Mechanism of action: Extracted from the bark of the Pacific yew (*Taxus brevifolia*). Promotes assembly of microtubules, stabilises them against depolymerisation and inhibits cell replication.

Main uses: Breast, ovarian and lung cancers.

Side effects: *Myelosuppression, *peripheral neuropathy (60%, usually reversible), myalgia/arthralgia (very common), hypersensitivity reactions, nausea and vomiting (usually mild–moderate), alopecia (>80%), diarrhoea, mucositis, cardiotoxictiy (arrhythmias and hypotension during infusion).

Notes: Steroid and antihistamine premedication greatly reduces incidence of hypersensitivity reactions. Irritant extravasation hazard.

PROCARBAZINE

Classification: Miscellaneous.

Mechanism of action: It is a unique antineoplastic agent with multiple sites of action. It inhibits incorporation of small DNA precursors, as well as RNA and protein synthesis, and can also directly damage DNA through an alkylation reaction. Procarbazine is not cross-resistant with other alkylating agents. Cell cycle phase specific (S-phase).

Main uses: Hodgkin's lymphoma, brain tumours.

Side effects: *Myelosuppression, nausea and vomiting (>50%), diarrhoea, mild mucositis, amenorrhoea, azoospermia, infertility, pneumonitis, peripheral neuropathy (10–20%), flu-like symptoms, nightmares, hallucinations and insomnia.

Notes: Administered by the oral route. Procarbazine is a weak monoamine oxidase inhibitor (MAOI) with significant diet and drug interactions. Particularly distressing to the patient are frequent nightmares, depression, insomnia, nervousness and hallucinations, which occur in 10–30% of patients. Nausea may be decreased by taking dose at bedtime or in divided doses.

TEMOZOLOMIDE

Classification: Cytotoxic alkylating agent.
Mechanism of action: Undergoes rapid chemical conversion to the active compound monomethyl triazeno imidazole carboxamide (MTIC), which causes methylation of DNA.
Main uses: Brain tumours.
Side effects: *Myelosuppression (uncommon), nausea and vomiting (moderate to severe), constitutional symptoms (common), male infertility.
Notes: Administered orally.

TOPOTECAN

Classification: Cytotoxic topo-isomerase I inhibitor.
Mechanism of action: Same mechanism of action as irinotecan, but due to different pharmacokinetics it has different antitumour activities and toxicities. It is a radiation-sensitising agent and is cell cycle phase specific (S phase).
Main uses: Ovarian cancer, small cell lung cancer.
Side effects: *Myelosuppression (very common and often severe neutropenia and thrombocytopenia), nausea and vomiting (mild–moderate), constipation, diarrhoea, constitutional symptoms, aches and pains (common), alopecia (50%), cough and dyspnoea (15–20%).
Notes: Neutropenic fever is common (25%).

VINBLASTINE

Classification: Mitotic inhibitor. Vinca alkaloid.
Mechanism of action: Binds to microtubular proteins of the mitotic spindle, leading to crystallisation of the microtubule and mitotic arrest or cell death. Also has some immunosuppressant effect. Cell cycle phase specific.
Main uses: Hodgkin's lymphoma, Kaposi's sarcoma, germ cell tumours.
Side effects: *Myelosuppression, peripheral neuropathy, mucositis (can be severe), mild nausea and vomiting, alopecia, constipation, urinary retention, muscle and tumour pain.

Notes: Vesicant. Neuropathy may also affect cranial nerves (e.g. facial nerve palsies and jaw pain) and autonomic nerves (constipation, paralytic ileus) urinary retention.

VINCRISTINE

Classification: Mitotic inhibitor. Vinca alkaloid.
Mechanism of action: Binds to microtubular proteins of the mitotic spindle, leading to crystallisation of the microtubule and mitotic arrest or cell death. Cell cycle phase specific.
Main uses: ALL, lymphomas, brain tumours, lung cancer, some paediatric malignancies.
Side effects: *Myelosuppression, peripheral neuropathy, optic atrophy, mucositis (can be severe), mild nausea and vomiting, alopecia, constipation, urinary retention. Central neurotoxicities include headache, malaise, dizziness, seizures, mental depression, psychosis and SIADH.
Notes: Vesicant. Intrathecal administration of vincristine is absolutely contraindicated, as it is always fatal. All oncology departments must have a strict intrathecal drug administration policy.

VINORELBINE

Classification: Mitotic inhibitor. Vinca alkaloid.
Mechanism of action: Binds to microtubular proteins of the mitotic spindle, leading to crystallisation of the microtubule and mitotic arrest or cell death. Cell cycle phase specific.
Main uses: Non-small cell lung cancer, breast cancer, lymphoma, ovarian cancer.
Side effects: *Myelosuppression, mild–moderate peripheral neuropathy, mucositis (can be severe), mild nausea and vomiting, alopecia (10%), tumour pain, jaw pain, constipation, urinary retention, pulmonary bronchospasm (5%).
Notes: Vesicant.

Useful oncology related websites

www.asco.org – American Society of Clinical Oncology
www.astro.org – American Society for Therapeutic Radiation Oncology
www.baso.org – Association for Cancer Surgery (formerly known as
    the British Association of Surgical Oncology)
www.bccancer.bc.ca – Canadian site
www.brit-thoracic.org.uk – British Thoracic Society
www.bsg.org.uk – British Society of Gastroenterology
www.btog.org – British Thoracic Oncology Group
www.cancer.gov – National Cancer Institute.
www.cancer.org – American Cancer Society
www.cancerbacup.org.uk – very useful site for cancer patients
www.cancerconsultants.com – general resource centre
www.cancerindex.org – offers multiple oncology links – huge site.
    Use this site to surf almost anywhere in oncology
www.cancerlinks.org – general cancer links
www.cancernetwork.com – multi-source site
www.cancerresearchuk.org – Cancer Research UK
www.cancersourcemd.com – general site
www.cancerworld.com – European site
http://www.dh.gov.uk/Home/fs/en – Department of Health
    homepage website
www.emedicine.com – e-textbook of medicine including oncology
www.esmo.org – European Society for Medical Oncology
http://www.estro.be/estro/Index.html – European Society for
    Therapeutic Radiology and Oncology
http://www.fda.gov/cder/cancer/index.htm – A site containing cancer
    tools, i.e. lists information such as performance status, common toxicity
    criteria and calculators
www.figo.org – International Federation of Gynecology and Obstetrics
www.freebooks4doctors.com – free online medical textbooks
www.freemedicaljournals.com – some free journals online
http://www.gfmer.ch/Medical_journals/Oncology.htm – Geneva
    Foundation for Medical Education and Research. Superb links site with lots
    of free oncology journals, books, atlases, organisations and databases
www.icr.ac.uk – Institute of cancer research
www.mdanderson.org – MD Anderson Cancer Center

www.medscape.com – go to haematology/oncology section for oncology related review articles, conference updates and much more

http://www.moffitt.usf.edu/pubs/ccj/index.html – free online journal of review articles

www.nccn.org – US national comprehensive cancer network. Contains US management guidelines on common cancers

www.ncrn.org.uk – National Cancer Research Network

www.nelh.nhs.uk – National electronic Library for Health

www.nice.org.uk – National Institute for Clinical Excellence. Go to technology appraisals for oncology recommendations

www.oncolink.com – University of Pennsylvania

www.rcr.ac.uk – Royal College of Radiologists website. Contains COIN guidelines for lung, breast, prostate and testicular cancer

www.startoncology.net – European cancer management guidelines

www.statistics.gov.uk – Office for National Statistics. Go to health section to find cancer statistics

www.supportiveoncology.net – free palliative care and supportive oncology journal

www.thedoctorslounge.net – general medicine resource with oncology section

www.theoncologist.com – free online cancer articles

www.raretumours.org – useful resource providing information on rare tumour types

www.ukccsg.org – United Kingdom Children's Cancer Study Group

www.uronet.org – urology site including uro-oncology

www.uroweb.org – European Association of urology

www.worldoncology.net – general cancer resource

Performance status

The concept of performance status is vitally important in oncology and all cancer patients should have their performance status recorded. It is a measuring tool for rating a person's ability to perform usual activities and is very helpful in the following ways:

1. In the assessment of disease progression and how this affects daily living activities of patients.
2. In the evaluation of a patient's response to treatment. Successful treatment may improve performance status, but treatment toxicity may worsen performance status.
3. As a prognostic indicator. Patients with poor performance status often have more advanced disease, medical co-morbidity, nutritional problems and psychological difficulties. They tolerate treatment poorly and have a much poorer quality of life and prognosis.
4. Assessing a patient's suitability for treatment. Poor performance status patients are less likely to be fit for surgery, radiotherapy or chemotherapy. Treatment morbidity and mortality are higher and success rates lower in poor performance status patients and very careful decisions are required in order to avoid causing significant harm.

A particularly difficult area in assessing performance status and suitability for treatment arises when a patient has a poor performance status purely due to a high cancer burden and not because of other problems such as medical co-morbidity. Successful treatment in this situation can dramatically increase the patient's performance status and quality of life. This must be weighed against the potential toxicities of treatment. The patient should be fully informed of the pros and cons of therapy.

Two main scoring systems are in use – the Eastern Co-operative Oncology Group (ECOG)/WHO system and the Karnofsky system.

ECOG/WHO PERFORMANCE STATUS

ECOG/WHO SCORE

0   Fully active, able to carry on all pre-disease performance without restriction
1   Restricted in physically strenuous activity but ambulatory and able to carry out work of a light or sedentary nature, e.g. light housework, office work

2 Ambulatory and capable of all self-care but unable to carry out any work activities. Up and about more than 50% of waking hours

3 Capable of only limited self-care, confined to bed or chair more than 50% of waking hours

4 Completely disabled. Cannot carry on any self-care. Totally confined to bed or chair

5 Dead

KARNOFSKY PERFORMANCE STATUS SCORE

SCORE FUNCTION

100 Normal, no evidence of disease

90 Able to perform normal activity with only minor symptoms or signs of disease

80 Normal activity with effort, some symptoms and signs of disease

70 Able to care for self but unable to do normal activities or work

60 Requires occasional assistance, cares for most needs

50 Requires considerable assistance, frequent medical care

40 Disabled, requires special care and assistance

30 Severely disabled, hospitalisation indicated

20 Very sick, requires active supportive treatment

10 Moribund

0 Dead

Index

Page numbers ending in f refer to figures; page numbers ending in t refer to tables